Recent Results in Cancer Research   171

Managing Editors
P. M. Schlag, Berlin • H.-J. Senn, St. Gallen

Associate Editors
P. Kleihues, Zürich • F. Stiefel, Lausanne
B. Groner, Frankfurt • A. Wallgren, Göteborg

Founding Editor
P. Rentchnik, Geneva

Andreas von Deimling (Ed.)

Gliomas

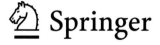 Springer

Editor
Prof. Dr. Andreas von Deimling
Universitätsklinikum Heidelberg
Pathologisches Institut
Abt. Neuropathologie
und
Klinische Kooperationseinheit Neuropathologie
Deutsches Krebsforschungszentrum
Im Neuenheimer Feld 220/221
69120 Heidelberg
Germany
andreas.vondeimling@med.uni-heidelberg.de

ISBN: 978-3-540-31205-5   e-ISBN: 978-3-540-31206-2

DOI: 10.1007/978-3-540-31206-2

Library of Congress Control Number: 2008937134

© 2009 Springer-Verlag Berlin Heidelberg

This work is subject to copyright. All rights are reserved, whether the whole or part of the material is concerned, specifically the rights of translation, reprinting, reuse of illustrations, recitation, broadcasting, reproduction on microfilm or in any other way, and storage in data banks. Duplication of this publication or parts thereof is permitted only under the provisions of the German Copyright Law of September 9, 1965, in its current version, and permission for use must always be obtained from Springer. Violations are liable to prosecution under the German Copyright Law.

The use of general descriptive names, registered names, trademarks, etc. in this publication does not imply, even in the absence of a specific statement, that such names are exempt from the relevant protective laws and regulations and therefore free for general use.

Product liability: The publishers cannot guarantee the accuracy of any information about dosage and application contained in this book. In every individual case the user must check such information by consulting the relevant literature.

Cover design: Frido Steinen-Broo, eStudio Calamar, Spain

Printed on acid-free paper

9 8 7 6 5 4 3 2 1

springer.com

Contents

Part I   Gliomas

1   Astrocytic Tumors 3
Markus J. Riemenschneider and Guido Reifenberger

    1.1   Introduction 3
    1.2   Epidemiological, Neuroradiological, and Clinical Features 4
    1.3   Histopathology 6
    1.4   Immunohistochemistry 9
    1.5   Molecular Genetics 10
    1.6   Molecular Diagnostics 13
    1.7   Pathways to Astrocytoma and Targeted Therapies 15
    1.8   Novel In Vitro and In Vivo Astrocytoma Models 18
    1.9   Conclusion 20
             References 21

2   Molecular Pathology of Oligodendroglial Tumors 25
Christian Hartmann and Andreas von Deimling

    2.1   Epidemiological, Neuroradiological, and Clinical Features 25
    2.2   Pathology 26
    2.2.1   Oligodendrogliomas WHO Grade II 27
    2.2.2   Anaplastic Oligodendrogliomas WHO Grade III 27
    2.2.3   Oligoastrocytomas WHO Grade II 27
    2.2.4   Anaplastic Oligoastrocytomas WHO Grade III 29
    2.2.5   Glioblastomas with Oligodendroglioma Component WHO Grade IV 29
    2.3   Immunohistochemistry 29
    2.4   Molecular Genetics 30
    2.4.1   Combined Losses on Chromosome 1p and 19q
             in Oligodendroglial Tumors 30

2.4.2	Isolated and Combined Losses of 1p and 19q Oligodendroglial and Astrocytic Tumors		31
2.4.3	Mechanism for Combined Losses of 1p and 19q		32
2.4.4	Methods for Detection of Allelic Losses on Chromosome 1p and 19q		32
2.4.5	Tumor Suppressor Gene Identification on 1p and 19q		33
2.4.6	Candidate Genes on 1p		35
2.4.7	Candidate Genes on 19q		36
2.4.8	*IDH1* Mutations in Oligodendroglial Tumors		36
2.4.9	Progression-Associated Genetic Alterations		37
2.5	The Origin of Oligodendrogliomas		38
2.5.1	Phenotype and Genotype of Gliomas		38
2.5.2	Progenitor Cells of Oligodendrocytes and Oligodendroglial Tumors		38
2.6	Prognosis		38
2.6.1	Clinical and Histological/Immunohistological Prognostic Factors		39
2.6.2	Losses on 1p and 19 as a Prognostic Factor		39
2.6.3	MGMT as a Prognostic Factor		40
2.6.4	Other Prognostic Molecular Factors		40
2.7	Conclusions		41
	References		41

3 Ependymal Tumors ... 51
Martin Hasselblatt

3.1	Introduction	51
3.1.1	WHO Classification	51
3.1.2	Synonyms	51
3.1.3	Historical Aspects	52
3.2	Epidemiology and Clinical Features	52
3.2.1	Incidence	52
3.2.2	Age and Sex Distribution	52
3.2.3	Environmental Factors	53
3.2.4	Tumor Localization	53
3.2.5	Typical Clinical Presentation	54
3.2.6	Neuroradiological Imaging	54
3.3	Pathology	54
3.3.1	Macroscopic Features	54
3.3.2	Histological Features	55
3.3.3	Immunohistochemistry	56
3.4	Genetic Susceptibility and Molecular Genetics	57
3.4.1	Genetic Susceptibility	57
3.4.2	Molecular Genetics	57
3.4.3	Tumor Recurrence and Prognosis	59
3.4.4	Potential Molecular Targets for Therapy	60
	References	61

4 Pediatric Gliomas 67
Stefan Pfister and Olaf Witt

4.1	Introduction	67
4.2	Epidemiology and Clinical Features	68
4.3	Histopathology	71
4.4	Molecular Genetics	72
4.5	Molecular Diagnostics	74
4.6	Pathways to Pediatric Astrocytoma	75
4.7	Pathways to Pediatric Ependymoma	76
4.8	Novel Therapies for Pediatric Gliomas	76
4.9	Conclusion	78
	References	78

5 Hereditary Tumor Syndromes and Gliomas 83
David Reuss and Andreas von Deimling

5.1	Neurofibromatosis	83
5.1.1	Historic Aspects	83
5.1.2	Neurofibromatosis Type 1	83
5.1.3	Neurofibromatosis Type 2	87
5.2	Tuberous Sclerosis Complex	90
5.2.1	Molecular Genetics	90
5.2.2	Molecular Pathogenesis	91
5.2.3	Subependymal Giant Cell Astrocytomas	92
5.3	Li-Fraumeni and Li-Fraumeni-Like Syndrome	92
5.4	Melanoma–Astrocytoma Syndrome	93
5.5	Turcot Syndrome	93
5.6	Familial Gliomas	94
	References	94

Part II Management of Gliomas

6 Surgical Management of Intracranial Gliomas 105
Matthias Simon and Johannes Schramm

6.1	Surgical Management: Overview	105
6.2	Surgical Therapy for Gliomas: Indications and Results	106
6.2.1	Low-Grade Gliomas	106
6.2.2	Malignant Gliomas	108
6.2.3	Rare Gliomas	110

	6.2.4	Cytoreductive Surgery for Gliomas in Difficult and Eloquent Locations	111
	6.2.5	Recurrent Gliomas	111
	6.2.6	Pediatric Gliomas	113
	6.2.7	Stereotactic Biopsy and Interstitial Radiosurgery (Brachytherapy)	114
	6.3	Technical Aspects of Glioma Surgery	114
	6.3.1	Electrophysiological Mapping and Monitoring of Eloquent Brain Areas	114
	6.3.2	Imaging of Functional Brain Areas for Glioma Surgery	115
	6.3.3	Image-Guided Surgery: Neuronavigation	116
	6.3.4	Intraoperative Imaging	118
	6.4	Perspectives	119
	6.4.1	Technological Progress and Neurosurgery	119
	6.4.2	Clinical Research and Socioeconomic Issues	119
		References	120

7 Radiation Therapy ... 125
Stephanie E. Combs

	7.1	Low-Grade Gliomas	125
	7.1.1	Dose Prescription: High Versus Low	126
	7.1.2	Timing of Radiation Therapy: Early Versus Delayed	127
	7.2	Anaplastic Gliomas	128
	7.3	Glioblastoma	131
	7.4	Re-irradiation	134
	7.5	Conclusion	135
		References	135

8 Adjuvant Therapy ... 141
Wolfgang Wick and Michael Weller

	8.1	Introduction	141
	8.1.1	General Principles	141
	8.1.2	Current Therapeutic Strategies	143
	8.1.3	Alternative Modes of Application	146
	8.1.4	Alternative Therapies	146
	8.1.5	Gene Therapy	147
	8.2	Astrocytic Tumors	147
	8.3	Oligodendroglial Tumors	149
		References	150

9 Other Experimental Therapies for Glioma ... 155
Manfred Westphal and Katrin Lamszus

	9.1	Introduction	155
	9.2	Surgery	155

9.3	Chemotherapy	156
9.4	Radiation	157
9.5	New Developments	158
9.5.1	Targeted Therapies for Glioma	158
9.5.2	Targeting New Targets by Convection	158
9.6	Immunotherapy	159
9.7	Oncolytic Viruses	160
9.8	Gene Therapy	160
9.9	Stem Cells	161
9.10	Final Remarks	161
	References	161

10 Neurotoxicity of Treatment — 165
Pasquale Calabrese and Uwe Schlegel

10.1	Introduction	165
10.2	Radiation	166
10.3	Radiation-Induced Neurotoxicity	166
10.4	Brain Atrophy	167
10.5	The Effect of Radiation Dosage	168
10.6	Neuropsychological Deficits Associated with Radiotherapy	168
10.7	Quality of Life After Radiotherapy	169
10.8	Other Treatment-Related Parameters Influencing Cognitive Function	170
10.9	Radiotherapy and Chemotherapy	171
10.10	Conclusions	171
10.11	Proposed Neuropsychological and Quality of Life Test Battery	172
	References	173

11 Neuroimaging — 175
R. Klingebiel and G. Bohner

11.1	Introduction	175
11.2	MRI and CT – Technique	176
11.2.1	MRI – General Aspects	176
11.2.2	Imaging Technique	178
11.3	Indications	185
11.3.1	Differential Diagnosis of Cerebral Tumors	185
11.3.2	Peritherapeutic Imaging	187
11.3.3	Posttherapeutic Imaging	188
11.4	Perspectives	189
11.5	Summary	189
	Suggested Reading	190

Part III Concepts

12 Angiogenesis in Gliomas 193
Marcia Machein and Lourdes Sánchez de Miguel

12.1	Introduction	193
12.2	The Angiogenic Factors in Gliomas	196
12.3	Growth Factors and Their Cognate Receptors	196
12.3.1	VEGF	196
12.3.2	Angiopoietins	198
12.3.3	Other Angiogenic Growth Factors	198
12.4	Guidance Molecules	199
12.4.1	Ephrins	199
12.4.2	Delta-Like 4 Ligand-Notch	200
12.4.3	ROBO/Slit	200
12.4.4	Netrins and DCC/UNC Receptors	200
12.4.5	Semaphorins	201
12.5	Endogenous Inhibitors	201
12.5.1	Thrombospondin 1 and 2	202
12.5.2	Angiostatin	202
12.5.3	Endostatin	202
12.5.4	Pigment Epithelial-Derived Factor	202
12.5.5	PEX	203
12.6	Strategies for Therapeutic Angiogenesis Inhibition in Glioma Treatment	203
12.6.1	Inhibition of Endothelial Cell Proliferation and Adhesion Cell Molecules ...	204
12.6.2	Blocking Stimulatory Factors	205
12.6.3	Increase of Endogenous Inhibitors of Angiogenesis	206
12.6.4	Inhibition of Invasive Activity	206
12.7	Perspectives and Unanswered Questions	207
	References	207

13 Gene Regulation by Methylation 217
Wolf C. Mueller and Andreas von Deimling

13.1	Epigenetics	217
13.1.1	Methylation in Normal Cells and Tissues	217
13.1.2	Methylation in Cancer: General Aspects	218
13.2	Strategies of Epigenetic Studies in Gliomas	219
13.3	Methods of Epigenome Analysis	220
13.3.1	General Aspects of Methylation Analysis	220
13.3.2	Bisulfite Sequencing	221
13.3.3	Methylation-Specific PCR	221
13.3.4	Methods of Gene Identification	222
13.3.5	Genome-Wide Methylation Profiling Implementing Methylation: Sensitive Restriction Enzymes	224

	13.3.6	MS-MLPA: A Novel Technique for Methylation Analysis That Does Not Require Bisulfite Modification and Can Be Reliably Applied to FFPE Tissues	224
	13.3.7	Novel Platforms for Genome-Wide, High-Throughput Methylation Analyses in Cancer Samples	225
	13.4	DNA: Methyltransferases and Methylation Pattern Maintenance	225
	13.5	Epigenetically Regulated Genes of Interest in Gliomas	226
	13.6	Diagnostic and Prognostic Value of Epigenetic Analyses: *MGMT* Promoter Methylation in Glioblastomas, Current Concepts, and Possible Future Developments	228
	13.7	Current Therapeutic Strategies to Overcome TSG Silencing	228
	13.7.1	Chromatin Remodeling Agents	228
	13.7.2	Gene Replacement Therapy as a Vision for Restoring Expression of Silenced Genes	230
	13.7.3	Artificial Transcription Factors in Gliomas	230
	13.8	Conclusion and Perspective	231
		References	231

14 Brain Tumor Stem Cells 241
Christian Nern, Daniel Sommerlad, Till Acker and Karl H. Plate

14.1	The Concept of Cancer Stem Cells	241
14.2	Neural Stem Cells in the Adult CNS	243
14.3	Phenotypic and Functional Characterization of Neural Stem Cells	245
14.4	Identification and Enrichment of Brain Tumor Stem Cells	247
14.5	Brain Tumor Histogenesis	249
14.6	Signaling Pathways of Neural Stem Cells and Brain Tumor Cells	251
14.7	The (Cancer) Stem Cell Niche	252
14.8	Therapeutical Aspects	253
14.9	Outlook	254
	References	254

List of Contributors

Till Acker
Neurological Institute (Edinger-Institute)
Neuroscience Center Heinrich-Hoffmann str.7
60528 Frankfurt am Main
Germany
and
Institute of Neuropathology
University Hospital Giessen and Marburg
Amdtstr. 16
35392 Giessen
Germany

Georg Bohner
Department of Neuroradiology
Charité, Universitätsmedizin Berlin
Charitéplatz 1
10117 Berlin
Germany

Pasquale Calabrese
Department of Neurology
Ruhr University Bochum
In der Schornau 23–25
44892 Bochum
Germany

Stephanie E. Combs
Department of Radiation Oncology
University Hospital Heidelberg
Im Neuenheimer Feld 400
69120 Heidelberg
Germany

Andreas von Deimling
Universitätsklinikum Heidelberg
Pathologisches Institut
Abt. Neuropathologie
und
Klinische Kooperationseinheit
Neuropathologie
Deutsches Krebsforschungszentrum
Im Neuenheimer Feld 220/221
69120 Heidelberg
Germany

Christian Hartmann
Universitätsklinikum Heidelberg
Pathologisches Institut
Abt. Neuropathologie
und
Klinische Kooperationseinheit
Neuropathologie
Deutsches Krebsforschungszentrum
Im Neuenheimer Feld 220/221
69120 Heidelberg
Germany

Martin Hasselblatt
Institute of Neuropathology
University of Münster
Domagkstr. 19
48129 Münster
Germany

Randolph Klingebiel
Department of Neuroradiology
Charité – Universitätsmedizin Berlin
Charitéplatz 1
10117 Berlin
Germany

Katrin Lamszus
Department of Neurosurgery
University Hospital Hamburg Eppendorf
Martinistraße 52
20251 Hamburg
Germany

Marcia Ma.chein
Department of Neurosurgery
University of Freiburg Medical School
Breisacher Str. 64
79106 Freiburg
Germany

Wolf C. Müller
Department of Neuropathology
Institute of Pathology
Im Neuenheimer Feld 220/221
69120 Heidelberg
Germany

Christian Nern
Neurological Institute (Edinger-Institute)
Neuroscience Center
Heinrich-Hoffmann-Str. 7
60528 Frankfurt am Main
Germany

Stefan Pfister
Department of Pediatric Hematology
and Oncology
Heidelberg University Hospital
Im Neuenheimer Feld 153
69120 Heidelberg
Germany

and
German Cancer Research Center
Division of Molecular Genetics
Im Neuenheimer Feld 280
69120 Heidelberg
Germany

Karl H. Plate
Neurological Institute (Edinger-Institute)
Neuroscience Center
Heinrich-Hoffmann-Str. 7
60528 Frankfurt am Main
Germany

Guido Reifenberger
Institute of Neuropathology
University of Düsseldorf
Moorenstr. 5
40225 Düsseldorf
Germany

David Reuss
Department of Neuropathology
Institute of Pathology
Im Neuenheimer Feld 220/221
69120 Heidelberg
Germany

Markus J. Riemenschneider
Institute of Neuropathology
University of Düsseldorf
Moorenstr. 5
40225 Düsseldorf
Germany

Lourdes Sánchez de Miguel
Department of Neurosurgery
University of Freiburg Medical School
Breisacher Str. 64
79106 Freiburg
Germany

List of Contributors

Uwe Schlegel
Department of Neurology
Ruhr University Bochum
In der Schornau 23–25
44892 Bochum
Germany

Johannes Schramm
Department of Neurosurgery
University Hospital Bonn
Sigmund-Freud-Straße 25
53105 Bonn
Germany

Matthias Simon
Department of Neurosurgery
University Hospital Bonn
Sigmund-Freud-Straße 25
53105 Bonn
Germany

Daniel Sommerlad
Neurological Institute (Edinger-Institute)
Neuroscience Center
Heinrich-Hoffmann-Str. 7
60528 Frankfurt am Main
Germany

Michael Weller
Department of Neurology
Hertie Institute for Clinical Brain Research
University of Tübingen School of Medicine
Hoppe-Seyler-Str. 3
72076 Tübingen
Germany

Manfred Westphal
Department of Neurosurgery
University Hospital Hamburg Eppendorf
Martinistraße 52
20251 Hamburg
Germany

Wolfgang Wick
Department of Neuro-Oncology
Heidelberg University Hospital
Im Neuenheimer Feld 400
69120 Heidelberg
Germany

Olaf Witt
Department of Pediatric Hematology
and Oncology
Heidelberg University Hospital
Im Neuenheimer Feld 280
69120 Heidelberg
Germany
and
German Cancer Research Center
Clinical Cooperation Unit Pediatric Oncology
Im Neuenheimer Feld 280
69120 Heidelberg
Germany

Part I

Gliomas

Astrocytic Tumors

Markus J. Riemenschneider and Guido Reifenberger

Abstract Astrocytic gliomas are the most common primary brain tumors and account for up to two thirds of all tumors of glial origin. In this review we outline the basic histological and epidemiological aspects of the different astrocytoma subtypes in adults. In addition, we summarize the key genetic alterations that have been attributed to astrocytoma pathogenesis and progression. Recent progress has been made by interpreting genetic alterations in a pathway-related context so that they can be directly targeted by the application of specific inhibitors. Also, the first steps have been taken in refining classical histopathological diagnosis by use of molecular predictive markers, for example, *MGMT* promoter hypermethylation in glioblastomas. Progress in this direction will be additionally accelerated by the employment of high-throughput profiling techniques, such as array-CGH and gene expression profiling. Finally, the tumor stem cell hypothesis has challenged our way of understanding astrocytoma biology by emphasizing intratumoral heterogeneity. Novel animal models will provide us with the opportunity to comprehensively study this multilayered disease and explore novel therapeutic approaches in vivo.

Markus J. Riemenschneider (✉)
Department of Neuropathology
Heinrich-Heine-University, Moorenstr. 5
40225 Duesseldorf,
Germany
E-mail: m.j.riemenschneider@gmx.de

1.1 Introduction

Astrocytic gliomas are the most common group of primary central nervous system (CNS) tumors and account for up to two thirds of all tumors of glial origin. The World Health Organization (WHO) classification of CNS tumors (Louis et al. 2007) recognizes a total of seven distinct histological entities of astrocytic neoplasms (Table 1.1). These may be roughly separated into two major groups: (1) the more common group of diffusely infiltrating astrocytic tumors, comprising diffuse astrocytoma, anaplastic astrocytoma, and glioblastoma multiforme, as well as (2) the less common group of astrocytic tumors exhibiting a more circumscribed growth, namely, pilocytic astrocytoma, pleomorphic xanthoastrocytoma (PXA), and subependymal giant cell astrocytoma. In the new WHO classification of 2007 (Louis et al. 2007), gliomatosis cerebri was added to the astrocytic tumor group because it is no longer considered as a distinct entity but as a variant of diffusely growing astrocytic glioma with unusually extensive infiltration of large parts of the brain and occasionally even the spinal cord. In addition, the pilomyxoid astrocytoma has been newly recognized as a histologically and clinically distinct variant of pilocytic astrocytoma with less favorable prognosis (Tihan et al. 1999). However, because pilocytic astrocytomas constitute the most common primary brain tumors in children,

Table 1.1 Classification and grading of astrocytic tumors according to the WHO classification of tumors of the central nervous system

Tumor type	WHO grade
Diffusely infiltrating astrocytic gliomas	
Diffuse astrocytoma	II
Fibrillary astrocytoma	II
Protoplasmic astrocytoma	II
Gemistocytic astrocytoma	II
Anaplastic astrocytoma	III
Glioblastoma	IV
Giant cell glioblastoma	IV
Gliosarcoma	IV
Glioblastoma with oligodendroglial component	IV
Gliomatosis cerebri	(III)[a]
Astrocytic gliomas with more circumscribed growth	
Pilocytic astrocytoma	I
Pilomyxoid astrocytoma	II
Pleomorphic xanthoastrocytoma	II
Pleomorphic xanthoastrocytoma with anaplastic features	Not determined
Subependymal giant cell astrocytoma	I

[a]Gliomatosis cerebri usually corresponds to WHO grade III. However, in most instances, grading has to be performed on small biopsy samples, which in the classic (type 1) lesions without any solid focus may underestimate grade due to the sometimes rather low density of diffusely infiltrating tumor cells. In contrast, biopsies from the solid area of a type 2 lesion often corresponds to anaplastic astrocytoma (WHO grade III) or glioblastoma (WHO grade IV)

they will not be covered here but are described in detail in Chap. 4 on "Pediatric Gliomas."

Historically, the German pathologist Rudolf Virchow (1821–1902) was the first to separate the gliomas from other primary brain tumors, such as the meningiomas, the melanomas and so-called sarcomatous tumors of the CNS. The first systematic classification of gliomas according to defined histological criteria and their putative histogenetic origin dates back to the seminal publication of Bailey and Cushing in 1926 (Bailey and Cushing 1926). These authors also systematically related histological features to patients' outcome, thereby providing the first basis for brain tumor grading. Today, the astrocytic tumors, like all other CNS tumors, are worldwide uniformly diagnosed and graded according to the criteria of the WHO classification of CNS tumors, which were published in an updated form in 2007 (Louis et al. 2007).

1.2
Epidemiological, Neuroradiological, and Clinical Features

The incidence of astrocytic tumors tends to be highest in western countries. Caucasians are more frequently affected than people from African or Asian descent (Ohgaki and Kleihues 2005). The Central Brain Tumor Registry of the United States (CBTRUS 2005) indicates incidence rates of astrocytic gliomas being twice as high in whites as in blacks. In Japan, however, gliomas are only about half as frequent as in the United States (Kuratsu et al. 2001). Males are slightly more commonly affected, with a male to female ratio of about 1.3:1. A potential increase in brain tumor incidence of about 1–2% per year has been reported, which primarily seems to affect the elderly population (Greig et al. 1990). However, it cannot be excluded that this increase may be mainly due to the refinement and widespread availability of modern neuroradiological imaging techniques, which have greatly facilitated tumor detection (Legler et al. 1999).

According to CBTRUS data, diffuse astrocytoma of WHO grade II has an annual incidence rate of 1.3/1 million population. The mean age of diagnosis is 46 years and the 5-year survival rate is about 45%. Anaplastic astrocytoma has a slightly later median age of onset of about 50 years. The annual incidence is about 4.9/1 million population and prognosis is significantly worse with a 5-year survival rate of only 28%. Glioblastoma manifests at a median age of 64 years with an annual incidence of about 3/100,000 population. Thus, glioblastoma is the most frequent primary brain tumor. It accounts for approximately 12–15% of all intracranial neoplasms and 50–60% of all astrocytic tumors. Despite aggressive multimodal treatment, the prognosis of glioblastoma is very poor, with nearly all patients succumbing to their disease within the first 2 years (2-year survival rate is 8.2%, 5-year survival rate 2.9%).

So-called long-term glioblastoma survivors are patients who survive for longer than 36 months after diagnosis. Although a number of studies have reported on such patients, it cannot be excluded that at least in some of the reports, long-term survival may be related to the inclusion of patients with malignant oligodendroglial tumors or pleomorphic xanthoastrocytoma (Kraus et al. 2000). A recent study of the German Glioma Network reported on the thus far largest series of 55 glioblastoma long-term survivors (Krex et al. 2007). While no specific clinical, socioeconomic, or molecular parameters could be directly linked to long-term survival, this study clearly indicated that young age at diagnosis, good initial clinical performance score, and the presence of *MGMT* promoter methylation in the tumor cells are favorable factors overrepresented in glioblastoma long-term survivors.

Diffusely infiltrating astrocytomas may arise in all parts of the brain. However, they are mostly observed in the cerebral hemispheres and most frequently affect the frontal and temporal lobes. Tumor infiltration can extend into the adjacent cortex, the basal ganglia, or even the contralateral hemisphere. A diffuse astrocytic glioma or, less commonly, a diffuse oligodendroglial or mixed glioma, that infiltrates the brain extensively, involving three or more lobes (frequently bilaterally), often extending to infratentorial structures and to the spinal cord is referred to as "gliomatosis cerebri."

On computed tomography (CT) scans, diffuse astrocytomas of WHO grade II present as ill-defined, homogeneous masses of low density. On magnetic resonance imaging (MRI), they are typically hypointense on T1-weighted and hyperintense on T2-weighted images. While gadolinium enhancement is not common in low-grade diffuse astrocytomas and generally suggestive of malignant transformation, at least partial contrast enhancement is commonly seen in WHO grade III lesions. However, a subset of anaplastic astrocytomas lack contrast enhancement on MRI, thus underlining the crucial importance of histology for the correct grading of these neoplasms. Glioblastoma typically presents with ring enhancement on neuroimaging, with the contrast enhancement corresponding to the vital and highly vascularized peripheral area of the neoplasm surrounding a central area of tumor necrosis that lacks enhancement.

Glioblastoma (WHO grade IV) may arise from diffuse astrocytoma (WHO grade II) and anaplastic astrocytoma (WHO grade III) through malignant progression. These tumors usually develop in younger patients (< 45 years of age) and are referred to as secondary glioblastoma.

Time of progression may range from less than 1 year to more than 10 years with a median time interval of about 4–5 years. Primary glioblastoma, which develops de novo without a history of a lower-grade lesion, accounts for the vast majority of cases. Patient age in these cases is significantly higher, with a median age of diagnosis around 55–60 years and a clinical history usually shorter than 3 months. In the past few years there has been increasing evidence that the terms "primary" and "secondary" glioblastoma do not only describe subgroups of patients with different clinical history but may even account for distinct disease entities that are associated with distinct patterns of genetic aberrations (Kleihues and Ohgaki 1999). However, prognosis seems to be equally poor in both cases and histological features do not differ between primary and secondary glioblastomas.

Clinically, patients with astrocytic gliomas often initially present with epileptic seizures. Focal clinical symptoms are variable and depend on tumor location. While for low-grade lesions neurological deficits may be subtle, higher-grade tumors may present with symptoms that appear more severe. Clinical history in these cases is often short and rapid tumor growth may coincide with perifocal edema causing mass shift and symptoms of increased intracranial pressure.

Pleomorphic xanthoastrocytoma (PXA) belongs to the group of astrocytic gliomas exhibiting a more circumscribed growth pattern and accounts for less than 1% of all astrocytic neoplasms. Histologically, the vast majority of PXA cases correspond to WHO grade II and patients demonstrate a relatively favorable prognosis (Giannini et al. 1999). However, rare cases show histological features of anaplasia, in particular increased mitotic activity and/or necrosis. Such tumors are referred to as "PXA with anaplastic features" and are more likely to demonstrate a less favorable outcome. On recurrence, some PXA may progress to high-grade gliomas, including glioblastoma multiforme, as demonstrated in several case reports (Giannini et al. 2007). While the tumor usually initially manifests within the first 2 decades of life, occasionally older patients are affected. PXAs are typically located superficially in the cerebral hemispheres, most often the temporal lobe, with frequent involvement of the leptomeninges. This is also the reason why patients often present with a long-standing history of seizures. In contrast to diffuse astrocytoma of WHO grade II, PXA radiologically presents as a contrast-enhancing, often cystic mass lesion.

Subependymal giant cell astrocytoma (SEGA) is closely associated with tuberous sclerosis, with an estimated 6–16% of tuberosis sclerosis patients developing one or more of these tumors. Neuroimaging typically demonstrates a contrast-enhancing intraventricular tumor, most often located in the region of the foramen of Monro. Obstructive hydrocephalus is a common feature. The most common clinical symptoms are either worsening of a preexisting epilepsy or symptoms of increased intracranial pressure. Patients diagnosed with a SEGA should be clinically checked for the presence of other manifestations of tuberous sclerosis, if not already known to have the syndrome.

1.3
Histopathology

Diffuse Astrocytoma. Histologically, diffuse astrocytomas are well-differentiated tumors lacking signs of anaplasia. They consist of neoplastic astrocytic cells embedded in a loosely structured, often microcystic fibrillary tumor matrix (Fig. 1.1d). According to the prevailing cell type, three major variants of diffuse astrocytoma are distinguished. The most common subtype is *fibrillary astrocytoma*, which is composed of multipolar tumor cells with scant cytoplasm and fine cell processes. Nuclear atypia may be present, distinguishing tumor cells from reactive astrocytes, but mitoses are generally rare or completely absent. Occasional or regional gemistocytic

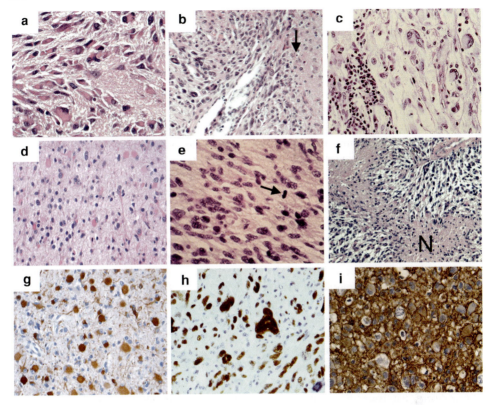

Fig. 1.1 Histological and immunohistochemical features of astrocytic tumors. (**a-c**) Astrocytomas with circumscribed growth. (**a**) Subependymal giant cell astrocytoma is composed of mainly large and plump, polygonal cells with abundant, glassy cytoplasm within a variably fibrillated matrix. (**b, c**) Cells in pleomorphic xanthoastrocytoma show nuclear and cytoplasmatic pleomorphism and xanthomatous change. Note the relatively sharp border between the tumor and the surrounding brain tissue (*arrow* in **b**) and reactive lymphocytic infiltration (**c**). (**d–f**) Diffusely infiltrating astrocytomas. (**d**) Diffuse astrocytoma of WHO grade II is a moderately cellular tumor composed of uniform fibrillary or gemistocytic astrocytic tumor cells with no signs of anaplasia. (**e**) Anaplastic astrocytoma shows increased cellularity, nuclear atypia, and mitotic activity (*arrow*). (**f**) Glioblastoma with the histological hallmarks of prominent microvascular proliferation and pseudopalisading necrosis (*N*). (**g–i**) Typical immunohistochemical features in diffusely infiltrating astrocytomas: Staining of gemistocytic astrocytoma cells for the glial fibrillary acid protein (GFAP, **g**), strong nuclear positivity for the p53 tumor suppressor protein in a giant cell glioblastoma (**h**) and overexpression of the epidermal growth factor receptor (EGFR) in a case of glioblastoma (**i**)

astrocytes can be observed in fibrillary astrocytoma. These cells exhibit a characteristically large eosinophilic cytoplasm with eccentric nuclei and strong immunohistochemical expression of glial fibrillary acid protein (GFAP; Fig. 1.1g). Tumors consisting of more than 20% gemistocytic astrocytes are classified as *gemistocytic astrocytoma*. Several reports indicate that gemistocytic tumor cell differentiation is a prognostically unfavorable feature as these tumors tend to undergo malignant progression more rapidly (Schiffer et al. 1988; Peraud et al.

1998). A rare astrocytoma variant is *protoplasmatic astrocytoma*. In these cases, neoplastic astrocytes exhibit a small cell body with few, flaccid cell processes and only weak GFAP expression. Mucoid degeneration or formation of microcysts is commonly observed.

Due to their high degree of cellular differentiation, diffuse astrocytomas are referred to as low-grade lesions and correspond to WHO grade II. However, they have an inevitable tendency for recurrence and malignant progression to anaplastic astrocytoma and, finally, secondary glioblastoma.

Anaplastic Astrocytoma. Basic histological features and tumor cell types are similar to those described for diffuse astrocytomas. However, anaplastic astrocytoma is characterized by a higher degree of nuclear pleomorphism, increased cellularity, and an elevated mitotic activity (Fig. 1.1e). Hypercellularity may be regional. Occasional multinucleated tumor cells and atypical mitoses may be observed. Necrosis is generally absent and, if present, demands for the diagnosis of glioblastoma. Small tumor vessels are still lined with a single, flat layer of endothelial cells. However, the beginning of microvascular proliferation may be observed, but is still limited to occasional tumor vessels and not glomerulum- or garland-like, as observed in glioblastoma. Anaplastic astrocytomas correspond to WHO grade III and tend to recur and progress to secondary glioblastoma.

Glioblastoma. Key histological features that distinguish glioblastomas from lower-grade astrocytic lesions are the presence of prominent microvascular proliferation and necroses (Fig. 1.1f). Pathological vessels are most commonly found around necrotic areas and exhibit a typical glomerulum- or garland-like appearance. In addition, vascular thrombosis is frequently observed and may contribute to the formation of ischemic tumor necrosis. Necroses can either appear as large areas of destroyed tumor tissue or can manifest in small, band-like foci surrounded by radially orientated, densely packed tumor cells in a "pseudopalisading" pattern.

The tumor cells in glioblastoma are highly pleomorphic, including relatively well-differentiated fibrillary or gemistocytic astrocytes, spindle cells, small cells with pathologic nuclear/cytoplasmic ratio, as well as multinucleated giant cells. Mitotic activity is high and atypical mitoses may be numerous. Metaplastic changes are occasionally present leading to epithelial differentiation (so-called glioblastoma with epithelial differentiation or adenoid glioblastoma) or formation of bone or cartilage. Further uncommon differentiation patterns include the presence of numerous PAS-positive granular tumor cells ("granular cell glioblastoma") or prominent tumor cells with lipidization ("heavily lipidized glioblastoma"). Occasional glioblastomas are composed of a monomorphic population of small anaplastic cells with sparse cytoplasm and round or carrot-shaped hyperchromatic nuclei (Miller and Perry 2007). These *small cell glioblastomas* should be distinguished from highly anaplastic oligodendrogliomas and cerebral primitive neuroectodermal tumors.

Gliosarcoma comprises up to 2% of all glioblastomas and displays a biphasic pattern with both glial and mesenchymal (sarcomatous) differentiation. Interestingly, molecular genetic studies clearly demonstrated that both tumor components are of monoclonal origin (Actor et al. 2002).

Another variant is *giant cell glioblastoma*, which accounts for less than 5% of all glioblastomas. While multinucleated giant cells may appear in a high fraction of classic glioblastomas, they dominate the histological picture in the giant cell variant. The giant cells are extremely bizarre and the number of nuclei may reach up to more than 20. In some cases, the cells are embedded in a reticulin fiber-rich matrix. Giant cell glioblastomas frequently show a more circumscribed growth, which may contribute to their somewhat better prognosis. Interestingly, giant cell glioblastoma, though clinically manifesting as a primary glioblastoma, shares a high incidence of *TP53* mutations with secondary glioblastoma and frequent *PTEN* mutation with primary glioblastoma (Meyer-Puttlitz et al. 1997; Peraud et al. 1999; Fig. 1.1h).

A fraction of glioblastomas present histological features associated with oligodendroglial differentiation. These cases are referred to as *glioblastoma with oligodendroglial component*. There is evidence that these tumors clinically behave better than classic glioblastoma but worse than anaplastic oligodendroglioma and anaplastic oligoastrocytoma without necrosis (Miller et al. 2006).

Gliomatosis Cerebri. Gliomatosis cerebri is rare and preferentially develops in adults with an age peak between 40 and 50 years. The diagnosis of gliomatosis cerebri is established by a tissue biopsy combined with neuroimaging findings, which demonstrate extensive tumor growth involving three or more cerebral lobes, frequently bilateral tumor spread, and infiltration of the basal ganglia, brain stem structures, cerebellum, and sometimes even spinal cord. The biopsy specimens show an infiltrating glioma typically composed of monomorphic, often elongated tumor cells that grow diffusely in the brain parenchyma. The vast majority of cases exhibit astrocytic features, while cases of oligodendroglial or mixed oligoastrocytic gliomatosis have also been reported. The formation of so-called secondary structures, such as perineuronal satellitoses as well as perivascular and subpial aggregates, is often seen in cortical infiltration areas. The classic form of gliomatosis cerebri (type I) presents without any solid mass lesion and does not show marked microvascular proliferation and necrosis. In contrast, type II lesions are characterized by the presence of a focal mass lesion, most frequently corresponding to anaplastic astrocytoma or glioblastoma, in addition to the diffusely infiltrating areas of gliomatosis.

Pleomorphic Xanthoastrocytoma. Histologically, pleomorphic xanthoastrocytomas are relatively compact and well-circumscribed tumors growing in the cerebral cortex and invading the meninges. The adjacent cortex often shows dysplastic features. The tumors are composed of pleomorphic astrocytic tumor cells, including bipolar spindle cells growing in fascicles, epithelioid cells, as well as multinucleated giant cells, with variable subsets of the neoplastic cells displaying cytoplasmatic lipidization (Fig. 1.1b, c). A pericellular or perilobular reticulin network, eosinophilic protein droplets, and prominent lymphocytic infiltrates are further characteristic features. Rare histologic variants include tumors with angiomatous, epithelioid, or gangliocytic components. While the vast majority of pleomorphic xanthoastrocytomas correspond to WHO grade II, a few cases exhibit five or more mitoses per ten HPF (microscopic high-power fields) and/or necrosis. These tumors are designated *pleomorphic xanthoastrocytoma with anaplastic features* (Giannini et al. 1999). No definite WHO grade has been assigned to these rare cases, but compared to classic cases their prognosis appears less favorable.

Subependymal Giant Cell Astrocytoma. Histology reveals a circumscribed, moderately cellular tumor composed of pleomorphic large astrocytic cells with abundant glassy eosinophilic cytoplasm, round ganglioid nuclei, and distinct nucleoli (Fig. 1.1a). Smaller spindle cells growing in streams as well as calcifications are also commonly encountered. Mitoses are usually absent or rare. Subependymal giant cell astrocytoma corresponds to WHO grade I. Occasionally, increased mitotic activity and/or necrosis can be noted, but are not necessarily linked to malignant behavior.

1.4
Immunohistochemistry

Astrocytic tumors stain generally positive for a couple of more or less lineage-specific markers, with glial fibrillary acid protein

(GFAP) being the diagnostically most relevant marker. Expression of vimentin, S-100 protein, microtubule-associated protein 2 (MAP2), and alpha B-crystallin is also commonly observed in astrocytic tumors; however, these antigens are also expressed in most other glial tumors and many non-glial neoplasms. The fraction of GFAP-positive tumor cells varies considerably from case to case. As mentioned before, protoplasmatic astrocytomas are only weakly GFAP-positive, while the fibrillary and gemistocytic astrocytoma variants show more consistent and stronger GFAP staining (Fig. 1.1g). In gemistocytic astrocytes, GFAP immunoreactivity is often accentuated in the subplasmalemmal region due to the intracytoplasmatic distribution of intermediate filaments. With increasing malignancy, GFAP immunoreactivity may become weaker or even get completely lost, as in small anaplastic glioma cells. In gliomatosis cerebri, the infiltrating tumor cells may also be GFAP-negative. Thus, differential diagnosis may become challenging in such cases or in gliomas displaying metaplastic changes. For example, adenoid glioblastomas occasionally exhibit expression of epithelial markers, such as cytokeratins, and thus have to be distinguished from intracerebral metastases. Also, rare cases of gliosarcomas primarily may appear as spindle-cell sarcomas, with glial differentiation difficult to detect even by means of immunohistochemistry.

Apart from the expression of glial lineage markers, several transformation-associated proteins are expressed in astrocytomas. For example, nuclear positivity for the p53 tumor suppressor protein is present in about 60% of WHO grade II and III astrocytomas, but absent in pilocytic astrocytomas, subependymal giant cell astrocytomas, and the vast majority of pleomorphic xanthoastrocytomas. In glioblastomas, p53 immunoreactivity is also commonly observed in secondary glioblastomas and giant cell glioblastomas (up to 80%; Fig. 1.1h), while primary glioblastomas only stain positive in about 30% of cases. In contrast, immunoreactivity for the epidermal growth factor receptor (EGFR) is a common feature in primary glioblastomas (about 60% of the cases; Fig. 1.1i) and rare in secondary glioblastomas as well as other astrocytic neoplasms (Kordek et al. 1995). In pleomorphic xanthoastrocytomas, expression of the CD34 antigen is often found not only in vascular endothelial cells but also in tumor cells (Reifenberger et al. 2003). Subependymal giant cell astrocytomas show variable expression of GFAP and S-100. In addition, immunoreactivity for neuronal markers such as synaptophysin or neurofilaments may be detectable.

Labeling indices for the proliferation-associated antigen Ki-67 (MIB-1) differ considerably from tumor to tumor, and mean values determined for the individual WHO grades have large overlap. However, in diffuse astrocytic gliomas a threshold value of more than 5% is often used as an additional criterion to distinguish between WHO grade II and III lesions. The Ki-67 index in pleomorphic xanthoastrocytomas and subependymal giant cell astrocytomas usually does not exceed the 5% level.

1.5 Molecular Genetics

Diffuse Astrocytoma. The *TP53* tumor suppressor gene at 17q13.1 is mutated in about 60% of diffuse astrocytomas (Ichimura et al. 2000). Even higher frequencies of up to 80% of *TP53* mutations are detectable in the gemistocytic variant (Watanabe et al. 1998). Interestingly, *TP53* mutations in most cases are already present in the first biopsy and their frequency does not increase in recurrences, suggesting that *TP53* mutations are among the earliest events in astrocytoma development (Fig. 1.2). This hypothesis is supported by the fact that brain tumors in patients harboring a *TP53* germline mutation predominantly correspond to astro-

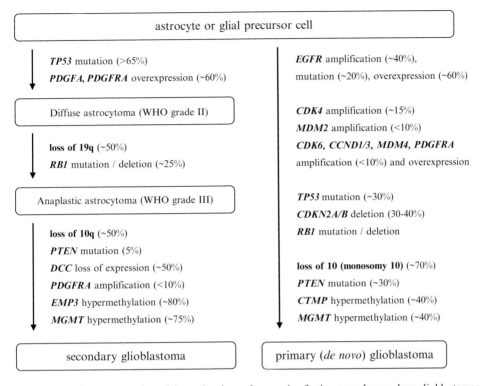

Fig. 1.2 Schematic representation of the molecular pathogenesis of primary and secondary glioblastomas (According to Ohgaki and Kleihues 2007 with modifications)

cytic tumors, usually anaplastic astrocytoma or glioblastoma. In line with Knudson's double-hit hypothesis, *TP53* mutations in diffuse astrocytomas are commonly associated with loss of heterozygosity (LOH) at polymorphic loci on 17p resulting in complete loss of wild-type p53 in the tumor cells. Diffuse astrocytomas without *TP53* alterations frequently exhibit promoter methylation and loss of expression of the $p14^{ARF}$ gene at 9p21, the gene product of which regulates MDM2-mediated degradation of p53 (Watanabe et al. 2007). Other genes that have been reported to be epigenetically silenced in more than 50% of diffuse astrocytomas include the *MGMT* gene at 10q26 (Watanabe et al. 2007), the protocadherin-gamma subfamily A11 (*PCDH-gamma-A11*) gene at 5q31 (Waha et al. 2005), and the *EMP3* gene at 19q13 (Kunitz et al. 2007).

Interestingly, *MGMT* hypermethylation was found to be associated with *TP53* mutation but is mutually exclusive to $p14^{ARF}$ hypermethylation (Watanabe et al. 2007).

Another common alteration in diffuse astrocytomas is overexpression of the platelet-derived growth factor receptor alpha (PDGFRA) and its ligand PDGFalpha, thereby enabling an autocrine growth stimulation of the tumor cells (Hermanson et al. 1992). *PDGFRA* amplification, however, is restricted to a small subset of high-grade gliomas, in particular glioblastomas (Fleming et al. 1992).

Karyotyping and comparative genomic hybridization analyses revealed trisomy 7 or gains of chromosome 7q as a common genomic imbalance, which is detectable in up to 50% of diffuse astrocytomas. Further chromosomal aberrations comprise losses on 22q, 19q, 13q, 10p, 6, and the sex chromosomes as well as gains on 5p, 9, and 19p (for review, see Reifenberger and Collins 2004). In contrast to oligodendrogliomas, combined losses on 1p and 19q are rare in diffuse astrocytomas.

Anaplastic Astrocytoma. Anaplastic astrocytomas share a similarly high frequency of gains on chromosome 7, allelic losses on 17p, and *TP53* mutations with diffuse astrocytomas. In addition, anaplastic astrocytomas often carry deletions on chromosomes 6, 9p, 11p, 19q, and 22q. The deletions on 9p preferentially target the cell-cycle regulatory genes *CDKN2A, p14^{ARF}*, and *CDKN2B* at 9p21. Inactivation of *p14^{ARF}* serves as an alternative means to impair the p53 pathway in cases without *TP53* mutations (Ichimura et al. 2000). Deletions or mutations of *CDKN2A* (coding for p16^{INK4a}) and *CDKN2B* (coding for p15^{INK4b}), the gene products of which function as inhibitors of complexes between D-type cyclins and the cyclin-dependent kinases CDK4 and CDK6, alter cell cycle regulation at the G_1/S-phase transition by aberrantly activating the retinoblastoma (pRB) pathway. Up to 20% of anaplastic astrocytomas carry homozygous deletions involving *CDKN2A* and *CDKN2B*, while amplification and overexpression of the *CDK4* gene at 12q13-q14 is present in up to 10% of cases (Reifenberger et al. 1994). Furthermore, about 25% of anaplastic astrocytomas have mutations in the retinoblastoma gene (Ichimura et al. 1996). In contrast to glioblastomas, *EGFR* amplification is only rarely observed in anaplastic astrocytomas (< 10% of cases). Similarly, mutations in the *PTEN* tumor suppressor gene at 10q23 are rare. If present, however, *PTEN* mutations are associated with poor prognosis (Smith et al. 2001).

Glioblastoma. Glioblastomas are characterized by complex chromosomal, genetic, and epigenetic changes affecting a variety of tumor suppressor genes and proto-oncogenes. The most common chromosomal aberrations detected by conventional karyotyping are monosomy 10, trisomy 7 and, in about 50% of the cases, "double minute chromosomes" or "homogenously staining regions," which are cytogenetic correlates of gene amplification (Bigner and Vogelstein 1990).

The concept of *primary glioblastoma* (glioblastoma arising de novo) and *secondary glioblastoma* (glioblastoma arising from a lower-grade precursor lesion) has shed light on different genetic pathways in glioblastoma formation (Ohgaki and Kleihues 2007; Fig. 1.2). The more common primary glioblastomas bear frequent *EGFR* amplification as well as *PTEN* tumor suppressor gene mutations. *TP53* mutations are found in only 30% of the cases; however, *p14^{ARF}* alterations as well as *MDM2* or *MDM4* amplification can serve as alternative means to bypass p53-regulated growth control in primary glioblastoma. Secondary glioblastomas carry *TP53* mutations in more than 60% of cases, while *EGFR* and *MDM2* or *MDM4* amplification as well as *PTEN* mutations are rare. Allelic losses on 19q and 13q, promoter hypermethylation of the *RB1* gene, and overexpression of *PDGFRA* are more common in secondary than in primary glioblastoma (Ohgaki and Kleihues 2007). In addition, epigenetic silencing of various genes, including *MGMT* and *EMP3*, is more common in secondary than in primary glioblastomas. Collectively, these data suggest that primary and secondary glioblastomas constitute genetically different disease entities (Fig. 1.2). However, as indicated before, both entities share comparable histological features and an equally poor prognosis. The fact that the different alterations eventually target the same cellular pathways, namely, the p53, pRb1, PTEN/PI3K/AKT, and mitogen-activated protein kinase pathways, and thereby lead to the similar functional aberrations, may explain this phenomenon (Reifenberger and Collins 2004).

Giant cell glioblastomas clinically manifest as primary glioblastomas but share features of both primary and secondary glioblastoma. While they carry *PTEN* mutations in the same frequency as primary glioblastomas (about 30–40%), *TP53* mutations are detectable in up to 90% cases and *EGFR* amplification and/or overexpression is usually absent (Meyer-Puttlitz et al. 1997; Peraud et al. 1999; Fig. 1.1h).

The molecular genetics of *gliosarcoma* is fairly similar to that of primary glioblastomas, except for *EGFR* amplification, which seems to be less frequent (Reis et al. 2000). Microdissection of the gliomatous and sarcomatous tumor components followed by CGH analysis revealed common genetic aberrations in both components, thus arguing for a monoclonal origin of both components (Actor et al. 2002).

Combined deletions of 1p and 19q, i.e., the characteristic genomic aberration in oligodendroglial tumors, are rare in glioblastomas (less than 10% of the cases), and not overrepresented in glioblastomas from long-term survivors (Krex et al. 2007). However, some studies reported that 1p/19q deletion may be more common in glioblastomas with an oligodendroglial component, which in part may account for the better survival associated with this particular glioblastoma subgroup (Miller et al. 2006).

Gliomatosis Cerebri. Molecular studies on gliomatosis cerebri have identified *TP53* mutations in 11–44% of the cases (Herrlinger et al. 2002; Mawrin 2005). Individual tumors demonstrated a *PTEN* mutation and/or *EGFR* amplification, while *CDK4* or *MDM2* amplifications as well as homozygous *CDKN2A* deletions were not detected. In line with a monoclonal tumor origin, molecular analysis of tissue samples from multiple spatially distinct regions in gliomatosis cerebri revealed identical *TP53* mutations (Kros et al. 2002). However, specific molecular changes driving the widespread tumor infiltration in gliomatosis cerebri remain to be uncovered.

Pleomorphic Xanthoastrocytoma. Loss on chromosome 9 is the most common genomic imbalance in pleomorphic xanthoastrocytoma, which is detectable by CGH analysis in 50% of cases. Other losses affect chromosomes 17 (10%), 8, 18, and 22 (4% each). Chromosomal gains could be identified on chromosomes X (16%), 7, 9q, 20 (8% each), 4, 5, and 19 (4% each) (Weber et al. 2006). *TP53* mutations are seen in a small fraction of tumors (< 10% of cases; Giannini et al. 2001; Kaulich et al. 2002). A recent study reports on frequent homozygous deletions of the tumor suppressor genes *CDKN2A, p14^{ARF}*, and *CDKN2B* on 9p21.3. Interestingly, transcript levels of the *TSC1* gene on 9q were also found to be consistently low in PXAs; however, the causative mechanism still remains unclear, as there was no evidence for *TSC1* mutations or promoter methylation (Weber et al. 2006).

Subependymal Giant Cell Astrocytoma. Biallelic inactivation of either the *TSC1* or the *TSC2* tumor suppressor gene is typical for these tumors (Chan et al. 2004). Since the corresponding gene products have an inhibitory function on the mTOR pathway, their mutational inactivation leads to aberrant activation of mTOR signaling, which in turn represents an interesting novel target for specific pharmacologic inhibition. A comparative genomic hybridization study on subependymal giant cell astrocytomas indicated that chromosomal imbalances are rare or absent (Rickert and Paulus 2002).

1.6
Molecular Diagnostics

Correct histopathological diagnosis is of utmost importance for evaluating prognosis and providing patients with an adequate therapeutic regimen. However, when merely employing conventional histology and immunohistochemistry many astrocytoma cases are diagnostically challenging. In addition, it is well known that survival of individual glioma patients may vary considerably within each histological group, even after adjustment for relevant prognostic factors such as age, performance score, and extent of resection. This points to a role of tumor-inherent molecular factors in the response to therapy and eventually survival. However, despite the identification of numerous chromosomal and genetic aberrations in the different types of astrocytic gliomas, the molecular diagnostics of these tumors is just beginning to become of clinical relevance. Particularly in regard to the prediction of chemosensitivity to alkylating drugs commonly used to treat malignant gliomas, such as the nitrosoureas and temozolomide, considerable progress has been made in the last few years. The *MGMT* (O^6-methylguanine–DNA methyltransferase) gene on chromosome 10q26 encodes a DNA repair protein that removes alkyl groups from the O^6 position of guanine, an important site of DNA alkylation (Gerson 2004). Chemotherapy-induced alkylation in this location triggers cytotoxicity and apoptosis. High levels of the MGMT repair protein thus may counteract the therapeutic effect of alkylating agents and thereby lead to treatment failure. Epigenetic silencing of *MGMT* by means of promoter hypermethylation has been identified as the main mechanism reducing MGMT expression and thereby diminishing its DNA repair activity. Importantly, *MGMT* promoter methylation has been associated with the response of glioblastomas to alkylating chemotherapy using nitrosourea compounds (Esteller et al. 2000), temozolomide (Hegi et al. 2005), or a combination of both (Herrlinger et al. 2006). Based on *MGMT* promoter methylation analysis in glioblastomas from patients treated in a large prospective clinical trial, patients whose tumors had a methylated *MGMT* promoter survived significantly longer than patients whose tumors lacked *MGMT* promoter methylation when treated with combined radio-/chemotherapy (Hegi et al. 2005). In patients treated with radiotherapy alone, *MGMT* promoter methylation did not influence survival, thus indicating that the *MGMT* promoter status is a predictive factor for response to chemotherapy but not radiotherapy. As *MGMT* promoter methylation can be easily assessed by methylation-specific polymerase chain reaction (MSP) analysis, it is now a frequently requested molecular assay at neuropathological centers.

High-Throughput Approaches. Advances in high-throughput profiling techniques nowadays allow for the simultaneous screening of thousands of genes within a single tumor. Thereby, characteristic molecular signatures can be assessed at the genomic level by means of array-based comparative genomic hybridization (array-CGH), as well as at the transcript level by mRNA expression profiling. After employing bioinformatic approaches, these signatures may be used to assign tumors to defined molecular subgroups providing refined diagnostic and prognostic information. In this regard, it was shown that gene expression-based classification of morphologically ambiguous high-grade gliomas correlates better with prognosis than the histological classification (Nutt et al. 2003). Furthermore, molecular classification of gliomas on the basis of genomic profiles obtained by array-CGH closely parallels histological classification and was able to distinguish, with few exceptions, between different astrocytoma grades as well as between primary and secondary glioblastomas (Roerig et al. 2005). Another array-CGH study suggested that glioblastomas can be subdivided into clinically relevant subsets on the basis of genomic profiles (Korshunov et al. 2006). Along these lines, comprehensive molecular profiling at the gene and transcript levels identified distinct prognostic subclasses of high-grade astrocytomas, which could be assigned to different stages in neurogenesis (Phillips et al. 2006). Interestingly, tumors displaying neuronal lineage markers presented with longer survival, while patients whose tumors expressed neural stem cell markers had shorter survival times. Markers of proliferation, angiogenesis, and mesenchyme contributed to the definition of the prognostically poor astrocytoma subgroup. Moreover, the authors could derive a two-gene (*PTEN* and *DLL3*) expression signature from their profiles suggesting that markers within the Akt and Notch signaling pathways can be employed as meaningful prognostic markers (Phillips et al. 2006). Expression profiling of pediatric glioblastomas similarly identified at least two tumor subsets, one being associated with poor prognosis and Ras and Akt pathway activation as well as increased expression of genes related to proliferation and to a neural stem-cell phenotype. The other subset showed a better prognosis, lacked Akt and Ras pathway activation, and is speculated to originate from astroglial progenitors (Faury et al. 2007).

The main drawback of large-scale profiling techniques, however, is that their use in routine neuropathological diagnostics is limited as these methods are quite expensive and not generally available. Thus, it seems desirable to identify single diagnostically or prognostically relevant genes or defined genetic signatures, merely comprising a small number of genes or proteins, respectively.

1.7
Pathways to Astrocytoma and Targeted Therapies

The Cell-Cycle Regulatory Pathways pRB and p53. The pRB pathway plays a central role in regulating G_1/S transition and is commonly affected in anaplastic astrocytomas and glioblastomas. Under mitogenic stimuli, CyclinD expression is upregulated and the CyclinDs bind to Cdk4 or Cdk6, thereby phosphorylating the Rb1 protein and releasing E2F transcription factors, resulting in the activation of S-phase genes like CyclinE. The formation of the CDK4/CyclinD complex can be negatively regulated by *CDKN2A* (encoding p16^{INK4a}) and *CDKN2B* (encoding p15^{INK4B}), which are two of the INK4 family of CDK inhibitors that specifically bind to Cdk4 and Cdk6, competing with and thereby blocking their binding to the CyclinDs. Specific pRB pathway alterations in astrocytomas comprise *RB1* mutations and loss of expression as well as amplifications of *CDK4* found in the same frequency in both primary and secondary glioblastomas (Schmidt et al. 1994; He et al. 1995; Ichimura et al. 1996; Table 1.2). Deletions of *CDKN2A* and *CDKN2B* are more frequently detected in primary glioblastomas (Jen et al.

Table 1.2 Synopsis of the most relevant tumor suppressor genes and proto-oncogenes involved in astrocytoma pathogenesis

Gene	Location	Typical alteration	Function of the protein
Tumor suppressor genes			
TP53	17p13	Mutation	Regulation of apoptosis, cell cycle progression and DNA repair
RB1	13q14	Mutation, hypermethylation	Cell cycle regulation
CDKN2A	9p21	Homozygous deletion, hypermethylation	Cell cycle regulation by inhibition of CDK4 and 6
p14^{ARF}	9p21	Homozygous deletion, hypermethylation	Cell cycle regulation by inhibition of Mdm2
PTEN	10q23	Mutation	Negative regulation of PI3K
TSC1/TSC2	9q34/16p13	Mutation, phosphorylation	Negative regulation of mTOR
Proto-oncogenes			
EGFR	7p11	Amplification and overexpression	Growth factor receptor
PDGFRA	4q12	Amplification and overexpression	Growth factor receptor
MET	7q31	Amplification and overexpression	Growth factor receptor
CDK4	12q13	Amplification and overexpression	Promotion of G_1/S-phase progression
CDK6	7q21–22	Amplification and overexpression	Promotion of G_1/S-phase progression
CCND1	11q13	Amplification and overexpression	Cyclin D_1, G_1/S-phase progression
CCND2	6p21	Amplification and overexpression	Cyclin D_3, G_1/S-phase progression
MDM2	12q15	Amplification and overexpression	Inhibition of p53
MDM4	1q32	Amplification and overexpression	Inhibition of p53
MYCC	8q24	Amplification and overexpression	Transcription factor

1994), and promoter hypermethylation may also account for the inactivation of these two genes (Schmidt et al. 1997).

The p53 pathway regulates a plethora of cell functions, including responses to DNA damage, hypoxia, apoptosis, inappropriate oncogene activation, and defects in DNA methylation (Prives and Hall 1999). Alterations in the p53 signaling pathway are a common finding in diffuse astrocytomas of all WHO grades. While mutation or loss of the p53 tumor suppressor gene is frequent already in diffuse astrocytomas of WHO grade II and recurrences arising from these tumors, including secondary glioblastomas (Watanabe et al. 1997), alterations of other pathway components more often substitute for *TP53* mutations in primary glioblastomas. A subset of glioblastomas and anaplastic astrocytomas exhibits amplification of the *MDM2* and *MDM4* genes (Reifenberger et al. 1996; Riemenschneider et al. 1999, 2003), which can inhibit p53 function through inhibitory binding to p53. Thus, *MDM2* and *MDM4* amplification/overexpression constitutes an alternative mechanism to escape from p53-regulated cell cycle control. Another way to impair p53 function is deletion or methylation of the tumor suppressor gene *p14^{ARF}* on chromosome 9q21 (Nakamura et al. 2001). *p14^{ARF}* (the human homologue of *p19^{ARF}*) is encoded through an alternative reading frame from the same chromosomal locus as exon 1 of the *CDKN2A* (*p16^{INK4A}*) tumor suppressor gene and has the ability to inhibit MDM2-mediated degradation of p53 (Quelle et al. 1995; Pomerantz et al. 1998; Table 1.2).

Growth Factor Receptor Signaling and the PI3K/AKT Pathway. Activated EGFR and PDGFRA signaling pathways are a common finding in diffuse astrocytomas and affect multiple cell functions such as cell proliferation, growth, differentiation, migration, and survival. Many diffuse astrocytomas of WHO grade II exhibit overexpression of *PDGFRA* (Hermanson et al. 1992), while amplification and overexpression of *EGFR* and *PDGFRA* are a finding characteristic of high-grade lesions, in particular glioblastoma (Table 1.2; Figs. 1.1i and 1.2). Ligands of both EGFR and PDGFRA are secreted by the tumor cells themselves and can stimulate their receptors in an autocrine fashion (Ekstrand et al. 1991). In about half of the cases, *EGFR* amplification is associated with a structural rearrangement of the *EGFR* gene resulting in the formation of a deletion-mutant receptor, which is referred to as EGFRvIII. The *EGFRvIII* gene has an in-frame deletion of 801 base pairs, corresponding to exons 2–7 in the mRNA, resulting in the deletion of amino acids 6–273 in the extracellular ligand-binding domain and the generation of a glycine at the fusion point (Wikstrand et al. 1998). Functionally, the mutated vIII receptor is constitutively active, thus mimicking the effects of ligand-stimulated EGFR in increasing cell proliferation. Clinically, recent data indicate that EGFRvIII mutant glioblastomas constitute a distinct subset of tumors with more aggressive behavior, in which established prognostic factors in glioblastoma were not predictive of outcome (Pelloski et al. 2007).

One of the major pathways involved in signal transduction downstream of growth factor receptors is the PI3-kinase/AKT pathway, which has attracted considerable attention within recent years. Activated growth factor receptors can bind and activate the PI3-kinase, which then phosphorylates phosphatidylinositol-4,5-diphosphate (PIP2) to phosphatidylinositol-3,4,5-triphosphate (PIP3) leading to activation of protein kinaseB/AKT. This process is controlled by the tumor suppressor PTEN (phosphatase and tensin homolog deleted on chromosome 10), which has the ability to dephosphorylate PIP3 to PIP2 and thereby inhibits AKT (Knobbe et al. 2002). Another recently identified negative regulator of AKT is the carboxyl-terminal modulator protein (CTMP), which was reported to demonstrate hypermethylation and transcriptional downregulation in up to 40% of glioblastomas (Knobbe et al. 2004). In conveying the downstream signaling effects of AKT, the serine/threonine protein kinase mammalian target of rapamycin (mTOR) has been proposed to play a central role. AKT can either directly or indirectly (via the TSC-complex) phosphorylate mTOR, leading to subsequent activation of S6K and STAT3, as well as suppression (i.e., phosphorylation) of 4E-BP1 with the effects of cell cycle progression and inhibition of apoptosis (Bjornsti and Houghton 2004; Riemenschneider et al. 2006).

Growth factor receptor signaling pathways have gained attention recently in regard to targeted molecular therapies. In non-small cell lung cancers it could be demonstrated that the presence of certain activating mutations of *EGFR* conveyed responsiveness to the tyrosine kinase inhibitor Gefitinib (Bell et al. 2005). In contrast to the frequent vIII mutations in the extracellular ligand-binding domain of *EGFR* in glioblastomas, those activating mutations affect the ATP-binding pocket of the tyrosine kinase domain, leaving the receptor ligand-dependent (Lynch et al. 2004). Also among patients with glioblastoma, about 10–20% appear to benefit from the EGFR inhibitors erlotinib and gefitinib (Table 1.3). However, the infrequency of mutations in the *EGFR* kinase domain of glioblastomas suggests that such mutations do not account for responsiveness to EGFR kinase inhibitors. A recent study reported that coexpression of EGFRvIII and PTEN, as detected by immunohistochemistry, may serve as a predictor of responsiveness to EGFR kinase inhibitors in glioblastomas (Mellinghoff et al. 2005).

Another example on why careful pathway dissection is necessary for advancing molecular targeted therapies is the use of mTOR inhibitors in patients whose tumors have loss of *PTEN*. Rapamycin, a complex macrolide and potent fungicide, immunosuppressant, and anticancer

Table 1.3 Selected molecular targets and specific inhibitors under evaluation in glioma therapy (Modified from Rich and Bigner 2004)

Target	Function	Specific inhibitor	Drug type
EGFR	Tyrosine kinase growth factor receptor	Gefitinib (ZD1839)	Tyrosine kinase inh.
		Erlotinib (OSI774)	Tyrosine kinase inh.
		AEE788	Tyrosine kinase inh.
PDGFRA	Tyrosine kinase growth factor receptor	Imatinib mesylate (STI571)	Tyrosine kinase inh.
		SU6668	Tyrosine kinase inh.
		MLN518/608	Tyrosine kinase inh.
VEGFR	Tyrosine kinase growth factor receptor	SU5416	Tyrosine kinase inh.
		PTK787/ZK222584	Tyrosine kinase inh.
PKC	Protein kinase	Tamoxifen	Anti-estrogen
		LY317615	Small molecule
RAS	Proto-oncogene	Tipifarnib (R115777)	Farnesyl transferase inh.
		Lonafarnib (SCH66366)	Farnesyl transferase inh.
PI3K	Lipid kinase	Wortmannin	Antibiotic
		LY294002	Antibiotic
MTOR	Serine/threonine protein kinase downstream of AKT	Rapamycin	Antibiotic
		CCI-779	Antibiotic
		RAD001	Antibiotic
		AP23573	Antibiotic
Integrins avß3 and avß5	Cell adhesion molecule	Cilengitide (EMD121974)	Cyclic RGD peptide

agent, is a highly specific inhibitor of mTOR (Singh et al. 1979). A phase II study of CCI-779, an ester of rapamycin, in patients with recurrent glioblastoma led to radiographic improvement in 36% of patients, and was associated with a significantly longer median time to progression (Table 1.3). Interestingly, high levels of phosphorylated p70S6 kinase in baseline tumor samples appeared to predict a patient population more likely to benefit from treatment (Galanis et al. 2005). While these results may represent a further promising step in the treatment of glioblastoma patients, they also show quite plainly that no single agent is likely to produce striking results in these aggressive tumors and that better therapeutic results may only be achieved by identification of novel therapeutic targets and the combination of different agents.

Invasion- and Adhesion-Associated Pathways. Another reason why the efficacy of treating malignant gliomas remains largely unsatisfying is that astrocytoma cells have the ability to invade deeply into the surrounding brain tissue, thus making local therapeutic approaches ineffective. Many extracellular factors regulating glioma cell invasion have been well established. Astrocytoma cells have been shown to modulate their microenvironment by secreting proteolytic enzymes, like matrix-metalloproteinases (Rao 2003), as well as extracellular matrix components, like fibronectin, laminin, vitronectin, and collagen type IV (Friedlander et al. 1996; Mahesparan et al. 1999). Complex signaling pathways are also involved in the regulation of astrocytoma cell migration and invasion. Activation of EGFR and/or PTEN/PI3K/AKT signaling can enhance tumor cell invasion (Guha and Mukherjee 2004; Rao and James 2004). Similar effects can be achieved by binding of various different integrin subtypes to autocrinely secreted extracellular matrix components (Friedlander et al. 1996; Goldbrunner et al. 1996). Of note, integrin and growth factor receptor signaling pathways have been shown to overlap in their activating effects on the focal adhesion kinase (FAK), which serves as central relays in integrating different upstream pathways in their effects on migratory and invasive cell properties making FAK an ideal candidate molecule for novel targeted molecular therapies (Riemenschneider et al. 2005). Small molecule inhibitors against FAK have recently demonstrated potent antimigratory effects in various cancer cell lines (Huang et al. 2005; Choi et al. 2006a, b). In addition, the blockade of integrins may lead to indirect targeting of FAK. EMD121974, for example, is a potent antagonist to αvß3 and αvß5 integrins and is currently being evaluated in phase I and II studies in adults with recurrent anaplastic gliomas or newly diagnosed GBMs (Eskens et al. 2003).

Except for FAK, the proline-rich tyrosine kinase (Pyk2) interacts with many of the same proteins, although the consequences of these interactions remain to be elucidated (Lipinski et al. 2003). Other important molecules involved in astrocytoma cell migration and invasion are members of the Rho family of small GTPases (RhoA and Rac1), including signaling by lysophosphatidic acid (LPA) and sphingosine-1-phosphate (S1P), as well as the nuclear factor (NF)-κB family of transcriptions factors (for review, see Salhia et al. 2006).

1.8
Novel In Vitro and In Vivo Astrocytoma Models

The Tumor Stem Cell Hypothesis. Modeling of astrocytic gliomas has made tremendous advances in the past few years and has accelerated our insight into the molecular and cellular mechanisms of astrocytoma growth. A recent milestone in the field is the identification of a potential tumor stem cell (TSC) fraction (Vescovi et al. 2006), which is characterized by expression of the CD133 antigen and other stem cell-associated markers. Dirks and colleagues isolated the CD133-positive cell subpopulation from human brain tumors and could demonstrate that these cells exhibited stem cell properties, i.e., self-renewal, in vitro. Moreover, when transplanted into NOD-SCID (non-obese diabetic, severe combined immunodeficient) mouse brains, only CD133-positive cells produced tumors, which were exact phenocopies of the patients' original lesions, while CD133-negative cells – even when injected in higher concentrations – were not able to produce tumors (Singh et al. 2004).

However, it has to be mentioned that there is some controversy in the field regarding the exceptional tumor initiating capabilities of CD133-positive glioma cells. In a recent study, tumor cells from 22 primary and secondary glioblastomas were cultured under medium conditions favoring the growth of neural and cancer stem cells (Beier et al. 2007). Remarkably, only a subset of primary glioblastomas contained a significant CD133-positive subpopulation and both CD133-positive and -negative tumor cells were similarly tumorigenic in nude mice, suggesting that CD133-negative tumor cells may also exhibit stem cell properties. Nevertheless, CD133-positive cells were characterized by higher proliferation indices, thus suggesting a possible prognostic significance of this cell fraction.

Recent evidence suggests that TSCs may also be accountable for the radioresistance of glioblastomas through preferential activation of the DNA damage checkpoint response and an increase in DNA repair capacity (Bao et al. 2006). In comparison to their negative counterparts, CD133-positive TSCs were enriched after radiation in both cell culture and the brains of immunocompromised mice. Radioresistance of CD133-positive glioma stem cells could be reversed with a specific inhibitor of the Chk1 and Chk2 checkpoint kinases. Thus, the CD133-positive tumor cell fraction may represent the cellular population that confers glioma radioresistance and could be the source of tumor recurrence after radiation. Consequently, targeting DNA damage checkpoint response in cancer stem cells may provide a novel therapeutic glioblastoma model.

Further studies indicate that primary human tumor-derived TSCs and their matched glioma cell lines showed marked phenotypic and genotypic differences (Lee et al. 2006). In contrast to the traditionally serum-cultured cell lines, tumor stem cells derived from glioblastomas and cultured in bFGF and EGF more closely recapitulated the genotype, gene expression patterns, and in vivo biology of human glioblastomas. Thus, TSC cultures may serve as a more reliable model than many commonly utilized glioma cell lines for understanding the biology of primary human tumors.

Novel Animal Models. Recent progress has also been made in regard to genetically engineered mouse models. Their detailed description is beyond the scope of this review and the reader is referred to a number of excellent review articles specifically addressing this issue (Holland 2001; Reilly and Jacks 2001; Begemann et al. 2002; Gutmann et al. 2003; Hesselager and Holland 2003). Mutant mice can be generated either by genetic germ-line modifications or somatic gene transfer and provide a powerful tool for investigating the importance of single molecular alterations or pathways in astrocytoma pathogenesis. By such experiments it could be shown that Ras- and AKT-dependent pathways, but also inactivation of pRB- and p53-signaling, are of essential importance for astrocytoma formation in vivo (Holland et al. 2000; Uhrbom et al. 2002; Xiao et al. 2002). The histology of CNS tumors generated in such models has been reviewed by an international consortium and guidelines for the classification of these tumors have been defined (Weiss et al. 2002). Most interestingly, those engineered tumors appear to more and more realistically mimic their human counterparts. In this regard, a novel animal model was generated by the double knockout of the *TP53* tumor suppressor gene and the neurofibromatosis type 1 (*NF1*) gene, which leads to the activation of Ras signaling

(Zhu et al. 2005). The resultant mice developed astrocytomas with 100% penetrance. The murine tumors exhibited key features of human astrocytomas with diffuse infiltration of the surrounding brain tissue and malignant progression over time. Of note, early presymptomatic lesions resided within the subventricular zone (SVZ) of the lateral ventricle, one region of the CNS that is supposed to contain neurogenic stem cells.

Taken together, these findings clearly indicate that these novel animal astrocytoma models may be exploited as powerful tools in the preclinical evaluation of novel therapies. Moreover, they may also help to provide further insight into the pathways and molecular alterations underlying astrocytoma pathogenesis and may even help to address the yet unresolved issue of identifying the astrocytoma cell of origin.

1.9
Conclusion

This review outlines the tremendous advances that have been made over the last 2 decades regarding our understanding of the molecular alterations underlying astrocytoma oncogenesis and progression. Classification of astrocytic tumors according to WHO criteria is still primarily based on the recognition of key histological features. In terms of molecular diagnostics, however, *MGMT* promoter hypermethylation has been established as a first predictive molecular marker in glioblastomas, which is more and more commonly implemented in the diagnostic procedure in neuropathological centers and provides important predictive information on chemosensitivity. No doubt, the facilitated accessibility of high-throughput profiling techniques will further accelerate the progress of molecular diagnostics and may also refine our knowledge about the key pathogenic pathways involved in astrocytomas. These pathways can then be targeted by the use of novel specific inhibitors, enabling us to provide patients with more individualized therapeutic approaches in addition to surgery, radiotherapy, and conventional chemotherapy. Several of these drugs are already in clinical phase I and II trials. The development of novel animal models will allow us to test new agents in a preclinical setting and most realistically access their therapeutic potential for subsequent clinical trials. Finally, another future challenge will be to address the issue of tumor heterogeneity by, for example, specifically targeting the infiltrating cells in the invasive rims of the tumors or a potential tumor stem cell fraction with high pathogenic ability.

Note added in proof

During the production of this review two novel large-scale multi-dimensional studies were released reporting on the integrative genomic analysis of human glioblastoma:

The Cancer Genome Atlas Research Network investigated 91 human glioblastomas for mutations in 601 selected genes (Cancer Genome Atlas Research Network 2008). Major novel findings were the detection of NF1 mutations in 14% and ERBB2 mutations in 8% of tumors. Parsons and colleagues sequenced 20,661 genes in 22 human glioblastomas and thereby identified recurrent mutations in the active site of isocitrate dehydrogenase 1 (IDH1) in a large fraction of young patients and in most patients with secondary glioblastomas (Parsons DW et al. 2008). Direct sequencing in a series of 685 brain tumors revealed highest frequencies of somatic IDH1 mutations in diffuse astrocytomas (68%), oligodendrogliomas (69%), oligoastrocytomas (78%) and secondary glioblastomas (88%). Primary glioblastomas and other entities were characterized by a low frequency or absence of mutations in amino acid position 132 of IDH1 (Balss et al. 2008). The very high frequency of IDH1 mutations in WHO grade II astrocytic and oligodendroglial gliomas suggests a role in early tumor development and may be exploited for differential diagnostic purposes.

References

Actor B, Cobbers JM, Buschges R et al. (2002) Comprehensive analysis of genomic alterations in gliosarcoma and its two tissue components. Genes Chromosomes Cancer 34:416–427

Bailey P, Cushing H (1926) A classification of tumors of the glioma group on a histogenetic basis with a correlated study of prognosis. Lippincott, Philadelphia

Balss J, Meyer J, Mueller W et al. (2008) Analysis of the IDH1 codon 132 mutation in brain tumors. Acta Neuropathol 116:597–602.

Bao S, Wu Q, McLendon RE et al. (2006) Glioma stem cells promote radioresistance by preferential activation of the DNA damage response. Nature 444:756–760

Begemann M, Fuller GN, Holland EC (2002) Genetic modeling of glioma formation in mice. Brain Pathol 12:117–32

Beier D, Hau P, Proescholdt M et al. (2007) CD133(+) and CD133(-) glioblastoma-derived cancer stem cells show differential growth characteristics and molecular profiles. Cancer Res 67:4010–4015

Bell DW, Lynch TJ, Haserlat SM et al. (2005) Epidermal growth factor receptor mutations and gene amplification in non-small-cell lung cancer: molecular analysis of the IDEAL/INTACT gefitinib trials. J Clin Oncol 23:8081–8092

Bigner SH, Vogelstein B (1990) Cytogenetics and molecular genetics of malignant gliomas and medulloblastoma. Brain Pathol 1:12–18

Bjornsti MA, Houghton PJ (2004) The TOR pathway: a target for cancer therapy. Nat Rev Cancer 4:335–348

Cancer Genome Atlas Research Network (2008) Comprehensive genomic characterization defines human glioblastoma genes and core pathways. Nature 455:1061–1068.

CBTRUS (2005) Statistical Report: Primary Brain Tumors in the United States, 1998–2002. Published by the Central Brain Tumor Registry of the United States

Chan JA, Zhang H, Roberts PS et al. (2004) Pathogenesis of tuberous sclerosis subependymal giant cell astrocytomas: biallelic inactivation of TSC1 or TSC2 leads to mTOR activation. J Neuropathol Exp Neurol 63:1236–1242

Choi HS, Wang Z, Richmond W et al. (2006a) Design and synthesis of 7H-pyrrolo[2,3-d]pyrimidines as focal adhesion kinase inhibitors. Part 2. Bioorg Med Chem Lett 16:2689–2692

Choi HS, Wang Z, Richmond W et al. (2006b) Design and synthesis of 7H-pyrrolo[2,3-d]pyrimidines as focal adhesion kinase inhibitors. Part 1. Bioorg Med Chem Lett 16:2173–2176

Ekstrand AJ, James CD, Cavenee WK et al. (1991) Genes for epidermal growth factor receptor, transforming growth factor alpha, and epidermal growth factor and their expression in human gliomas in vivo. Cancer Res 51:2164–2172

Eskens FA, Dumez H, Hoekstra R et al. (2003) Phase I and pharmacokinetic study of continuous twice weekly intravenous administration of Cilengitide (EMD 121974), a novel inhibitor of the integrins alphavbeta3 and alphavbeta5 in patients with advanced solid tumours. Eur J Cancer 39:917–926

Esteller M, Garcia-Foncillas J, Andion E et al. (2000) Inactivation of the DNA-repair gene MGMT and the clinical response of gliomas to alkylating agents. N Engl J Med 343:1350–1354

Faury D, Nantel A, Dunn SE et al. (2007) Molecular profiling identifies prognostic subgroups of pediatric glioblastoma and shows increased YB-1 expression in tumors. J Clin Oncol 25:1196–1208

Fleming TP, Saxena A, Clark WC et al. (1992) Amplification and/or overexpression of platelet-derived growth factor receptors and epidermal growth factor receptor in human glial tumors. Cancer Res 52:4550–4553

Friedlander DR, Zagzag D, Shiff B et al. (1996) Migration of brain tumor cells on extracellular matrix proteins in vitro correlates with tumor type and grade and involves alphaV and beta1 integrins. Cancer Res 56:1939–1947

Galanis E, Buckner JC, Maurer MJ et al. (2005) Phase II trial of temsirolimus (CCI-779) in recurrent glioblastoma multiforme: a North Central Cancer Treatment Group Study. J Clin Oncol 23:5294–5304

Gerson SL (2004) MGMT: its role in cancer aetiology and cancer therapeutics. Nat Rev Cancer 4:296–307

Giannini C, Scheithauer BW, Burger PC et al. (1999) Pleomorphic xanthoastrocytoma: what do we really know about it? Cancer 85:2033–2045

Giannini C, Hebrink D, Scheithauer BW, Dei Tos AP and James CD (2001) Analysis of p53 mutation and expression in pleomorphic xanthoastrocytoma. Neurogenetics 3:159–162

Giannini C, Paulus W, Louis DN, Liberski P (2007) Pleomorphic xanthoastrocytoma. p.22ff. In: Louis DN, Ohgaki H, Wiestler OD, and Cavenee WK (2007) WHO Classification of Tumours of the Central Nervous System, 3rd edition. IARC Press, Lyon, France

Goldbrunner RH, Haugland HK, Klein CE et al. (1996) ECM dependent and integrin mediated tumor cell migration of human glioma and melanoma cell lines under serum-free conditions. Anticancer Res 16:3679–3687

Greig NH, Ries LG, Yancik R, Rapoport SI (1990) Increasing annual incidence of primary malignant brain tumors in the elderly. J Natl Cancer Inst 82:1621–1624

Guha A, Mukherjee J (2004) Advances in the biology of astrocytomas. Curr Opin Neurol 17:655–662

Gutmann DH, Baker SJ, Giovannini M, Garbow J, Weiss W (2003) Mouse models of human cancer consortium symposium on nervous system tumors. Cancer Res 63:3001–3004

He J, Olson JJ, James CD (1995) Lack of p16INK4 or retinoblastoma protein (pRb), or amplification-associated overexpression of cdk4 is observed in distinct subsets of malignant glial tumors and cell lines. Cancer Res 55:4833–4836

Hegi ME, Diserens AC, Gorlia T et al. (2005) MGMT gene silencing and benefit from temozolomide in glioblastoma. N Engl J Med 352:997–1003

Hermanson M, Funa K, Hartman M et al. (1992) Platelet-derived growth factor and its receptors in human glioma tissue: expression of messenger RNA and protein suggests the presence of autocrine and paracrine loops. Cancer Res 52:3213–3219

Herrlinger U, Felsberg J, Kuker W et al. (2002) Gliomatosis cerebri: molecular pathology and clinical course. Ann Neurol 52:390–399

Herrlinger U, Rieger J, Koch D et al. (2006) Phase II trial of lomustine plus temozolomide chemotherapy in addition to radiotherapy in newly diagnosed glioblastoma: UKT-03. J Clin Oncol 24:4412–4417

Hesselager G, Holland EC (2003) Using mice to decipher the molecular genetics of brain tumors. Neurosurgery 53:685–694; discussion p 695

Holland EC, Celestino J, Dai C et al. (2000) Combined activation of Ras and Akt in neural progenitors induces glioblastoma formation in mice. Nat Genet 25:55–57

Holland EC (2001) Gliomagenesis: genetic alterations and mouse models. Nat Rev Genet 2:120–129

Huang YT, Lee LT, Lee PP, Lin YS, Lee MT (2005) Targeting of focal adhesion kinase by flavonoids and small-interfering RNAs reduces tumor cell migration ability. Anticancer Res 25:2017–2025

Ichimura K, Schmidt EE, Goike HM, Collins VP (1996) Human glioblastomas with no alterations of the CDKN2A (p16INK4A, MTS1) and CDK4 genes have frequent mutations of the retinoblastoma gene. Oncogene 13:1065–1072

Ichimura K, Bolin MB, Goike HM et al. (2000) Deregulation of the p14ARF/MDM2/p53 pathway is a prerequisite for human astrocytic gliomas with G1-S transition control gene abnormalities. Cancer Res 60:417–424

Jen J, Harper JW, Bigner SH et al. (1994) Deletion of p16 and p15 genes in brain tumors. Cancer Res 54:6353–6358

Kaulich K, Blaschke B, Numann A et al. (2002) Genetic alterations commonly found in diffusely infiltrating cerebral gliomas are rare or absent in pleomorphic xanthoastrocytomas. J Neuropathol Exp Neurol 61:1092–1099

Kleihues P, Ohgaki H (1999) Primary and secondary glioblastomas: from concept to clinical diagnosis. Neurooncol 1:44–51

Knobbe CB, Merlo A, Reifenberger G (2002) Pten signaling in gliomas. Neurooncol 4:196–211

Knobbe CB, Reifenberger J, Blaschke B, Reifenberger G (2004) Hypermethylation and transcriptional downregulation of the carboxyl-terminal modulator protein gene in glioblastomas. J Natl Cancer Inst 96:483–486

Kordek R, Biernat W, Alwasiak J et al. (1995) p53 protein and epidermal growth factor receptor expression in human astrocytomas. J Neurooncol 26:11–16

Korshunov A, Sycheva R, Golanov A (2006) Genetically distinct and clinically relevant subtypes of glioblastoma defined by array-based comparative genomic hybridization (array-CGH). Acta Neuropathol (Berl) 111:465–474

Kraus JA, Wenghoefer M, Schmidt MC et al. (2000) Long-term survival of glioblastoma multiforme: importance of histopathological reevaluation. J Neurol 247:455–460

Krex D, Klink B, Hartmann C et al. (2007) Long-term survival with glioblastoma multiforme. Brain 130:2596–2606

Kros JM, Zheng P, Dinjens WN, Alers JC (2002) Genetic aberrations in gliomatosis cerebri support monoclonal tumorigenesis. J Neuropathol Exp Neurol 61:806–814

Kunitz A, Wolter M, van den Boom J et al. (2007) DNA hypermethylation and Aberrant Expression of the EMP3 Gene at 19q13.3 in Human Gliomas. Brain Pathol 17:363–370

Kuratsu J, Takeshima H, Ushio Y (2001) Trends in the incidence of primary intracranial tumors in Kumamoto, Japan. Int J Clin Oncol 6:183–191

Lee J, Kotliarova S, Kotliarov Y et al. (2006) Tumor stem cells derived from glioblastomas cultured in bFGF and EGF more closely mirror the phenotype and genotype of primary tumors than do serum-cultured cell lines. Cancer Cell 9:391–403

Legler JM, Ries LA, Smith MA et al. (1999) Cancer surveillance series [corrected]: brain and other central nervous system cancers: recent trends in incidence and mortality. J Natl Cancer Inst 91:1382–1390

Lipinski CA, Tran NL, Bay C et al. (2003) Differential role of proline-rich tyrosine kinase 2 and focal adhesion kinase in determining glioblastoma migration and proliferation. Mol Cancer Res 1:323–332

Louis DN, Ohgaki H, Wiestler OD, Cavenee WK (2007) WHO Classification of Tumours of the Central Nervous System, 3rd edition. IARC Press, Lyon, France

Lynch TJ, Bell DW, Sordella R et al. (2004) Activating mutations in the epidermal growth factor receptor underlying responsiveness of non-small-cell lung cancer to gefitinib. N Engl J Med 350:2129–2139

Mahesparan R, Tysnes BB, Read TA et al. (1999) Extracellular matrix-induced cell migration from glioblastoma biopsy specimens in vitro. Acta Neuropathol (Berl) 97:231–239

Mawrin C (2005) Molecular genetic alterations in gliomatosis cerebri: what can we learn about the origin and course of the disease? Acta Neuropathol (Berl) 110:527–536

Mellinghoff IK, Wang MY, Vivanco I et al. (2005) Molecular determinants of the response of glioblastomas to EGFR kinase inhibitors. N Engl J Med 353:2012–2024

Meyer-Puttlitz B, Hayashi Y, Waha A et al. (1997) Molecular genetic analysis of giant cell glioblastomas. Am J Pathol 151:853–857

Miller CR, Dunham CP, Scheithauer BW, Perry A (2006) Significance of necrosis in grading of oligodendroglial neoplasms: a clinicopathologic and genetic study of newly diagnosed high-grade gliomas. J Clin Oncol 24:5419–5426

Miller CR, Perry A (2007) Glioblastoma. Arch Pathol Lab Med 131:397–406

Nakamura M, Watanabe T, Klangby U et al. (2001) p14ARF deletion and methylation in genetic pathways to glioblastomas. Brain Pathol 11:159–168

Nutt CL, Mani DR, Betensky RA et al. (2003) Gene expression-based classification of malignant gliomas correlates better with survival than histological classification. Cancer Res 63:1602–1607

Ohgaki H, Kleihues P (2005) Epidemiology and etiology of gliomas. Acta Neuropathol (Berl) 109:93–108

Ohgaki H, Kleihues P (2007) Genetic pathways to primary and secondary glioblastoma. Am J Pathol 170:1445–1453

Parsons DW, Jones S, Zhang X et al. (2008) An integrated genomic analysis of human glioblastoma multiforme. Science 321:1807–1812.

Pelloski CE, Ballman KV, Furth AF et al. (2007) Epidermal growth factor receptor variant III status defines clinically distinct subtypes of glioblastoma. J Clin Oncol 25:2288–2294

Peraud A, Ansari H, Bise K, Reulen HJ (1998) Clinical outcome of supratentorial astrocytoma WHO grade II. Acta Neurochir (Wien) 140:1213–1222

Peraud A, Watanabe K, Schwechheimer K et al. (1999) Genetic profile of the giant cell glioblastoma. Lab Invest 79:123–129

Phillips HS, Kharbanda S, Chen R et al. (2006) Molecular subclasses of high-grade glioma predict prognosis, delineate a pattern of disease progression, and resemble stages in neurogenesis. Cancer Cell 9:157–173

Pomerantz J, Schreiber-Agus N, Liegeois NJ et al. (1998) The Ink4a tumor suppressor gene product, p19Arf, interacts with MDM2 and neutralizes MDM2's inhibition of p53. Cell 92:713–723

Prives C, Hall PA (1999) The p53 pathway. J Pathol 187:112–126

Quelle DE, Zindy F, Ashmun RA, Sherr CJ (1995) Alternative reading frames of the INK4a tumor suppressor gene encode two unrelated proteins capable of inducing cell cycle arrest. Cell 83:993–1000

Rao JS (2003) Molecular mechanisms of glioma invasiveness: the role of proteases. Nat Rev Cancer 3:489–501

Rao RD, James CD (2004) Altered molecular pathways in gliomas: an overview of clinically relevant issues. Semin Oncol 31:595–604

Reifenberger G, Collins VP (2004) Pathology and molecular genetics of astrocytic gliomas. J Mol Med 82:656–670

Reifenberger G, Reifenberger J, Ichimura K, Meltzer PS, Collins VP (1994) Amplification of multiple genes from chromosomal region 12q13–14 in human malignant gliomas: preliminary mapping of the amplicons shows preferential involvement of CDK4, SAS, and MDM2. Cancer Res 54:4299–4303

Reifenberger G, Ichimura K, Reifenberger J et al. (1996) Refined mapping of 12q13-q15 amplicons in human malignant gliomas suggests CDK4/SAS and MDM2 as independent amplification targets. Cancer Res 56:5141–5145

Reifenberger G, Kaulich K, Wiestler OD, Blumcke I (2003) Expression of the CD34 antigen in pleomorphic xanthoastrocytomas. Acta Neuropathol (Berl) 105:358–364

Reilly KM, Jacks T (2001) Genetically engineered mouse models of astrocytoma: GEMs in the rough? Semin Cancer Biol 11:177–191

Reis RM, Konu-Lebleblicioglu D, Lopes JM, Kleihues P, Ohgaki H (2000) Genetic profile of gliosarcomas. Am J Pathol 156:425–432

Rich JN, Bigner DD (2004) Development of novel targeted therapies in the treatment of malignant glioma. Nat Rev Drug Discov 3:430–446

Rickert CH, Paulus W (2002) No chromosomal imbalances detected by comparative genomic hybridisation in subependymal giant cell astrocytomas. Acta Neuropathol (Berl) 104:206–208

Riemenschneider MJ, Buschges R, Wolter M et al. (1999) Amplification and overexpression of the MDM4 (MDMX) gene from 1q32 in a subset of malignant gliomas without TP53 mutation or MDM2 amplification. Cancer Res 59:6091–6096

Riemenschneider MJ, Knobbe CB, Reifenberger G (2003) Refined mapping of 1q32 amplicons in malignant gliomas confirms MDM4 as the main amplification target. Int J Cancer 104:752–757

Riemenschneider MJ, Mueller W, Betensky RA, Mohapatra G, Louis DN (2005) In situ analysis of integrin and growth factor receptor signaling pathways in human glioblastomas suggests overlapping relationships with focal adhesion kinase activation. Am J Pathol 167:1379–1387

Riemenschneider MJ, Betensky RA, Pasedag SM, Louis DN (2006) AKT activation in human glioblastomas enhances proliferation via TSC2 and S6 kinase signaling. Cancer Res 66:5618–5623

Roerig P, Nessling M, Radlwimmer B et al. (2005) Molecular classification of human gliomas using matrix-based comparative genomic hybridization. Int J Cancer 117:95–103

Salhia B, Tran NL, Symons M et al. (2006) Molecular pathways triggering glioma cell invasion. Expert Rev Mol Diagn 6:613–626

Schiffer D, Chio A, Giordana MT, Leone M, Soffietti R (1988) Prognostic value of histologic factors in adult cerebral astrocytoma. Cancer 61:1386–1393

Schmidt EE, Ichimura K, Reifenberger G, Collins VP (1994) CDKN2 (p16/MTS1) gene deletion or CDK4 amplification occurs in the majority of glioblastomas. Cancer Res 54:6321–6324

Schmidt EE, Ichimura K, Messerle KR, Goike HM, Collins VP (1997) Infrequent methylation of CDKN2A(MTS1/p16) and rare mutation of both CDKN2A and CDKN2B(MTS2/p15) in primary astrocytic tumours. Br J Cancer 75:2–8

Singh K, Sun S, Vezina C (1979) Rapamycin (AY-22,989), a new antifungal antibiotic. IV. Mechanism of action. J Antibiot (Tokyo) 32:630–645

Singh SK, Hawkins C, Clarke ID et al. (2004) Identification of human brain tumour initiating cells. Nature 432:396–401

Smith JS, Tachibana I, Passe SM et al. (2001) PTEN mutation, EGFR amplification, and outcome in patients with anaplastic astrocytoma and glioblastoma multiforme. J Natl Cancer Inst 93:1246–1256

Tihan T, Fisher PG, Kepner JL et al. (1999) Pediatric astrocytomas with monomorphous pilomyxoid features and a less favorable outcome. J Neuropathol Exp Neurol 58:1061–1068

Uhrbom L, Dai C, Celestino JC et al. (2002) Ink4a-Arf loss cooperates with KRas activation in astrocytes and neural progenitors to generate glioblastomas of various morphologies depending on activated Akt. Cancer Res 62:5551–5558

Vescovi AL, Galli R, Reynolds BA (2006) Brain tumour stem cells. Nat Rev Cancer 6:425–436

Waha A, Guntner S, Huang TH et al. (2005) Epigenetic silencing of the protocadherin family member PCDH-gamma-A11 in astrocytomas. Neoplasia 7:193–199

Watanabe K, Sato K, Biernat W et al. (1997) Incidence and timing of p53 mutations during astrocytoma progression in patients with multiple biopsies. Clin Cancer Res 3:523–530

Watanabe K, Peraud A, Gratas C et al. (1998) p53 and PTEN gene mutations in gemistocytic astrocytomas. Acta Neuropathol (Berl) 95:559–564

Watanabe T, Katayama Y, Yoshino A et al. (2007) Aberrant hypermethylation of p14ARF and O6-methylguanine-DNA methyltransferase genes in astrocytoma progression. Brain Pathol 17:5–10

Weber RG, Hoischen A, Ehrler M et al. (2006) Frequent loss of chromosome 9, homozygous CDKN2A/p14(ARF)/CDKN2B deletion and low TSC1 mRNA expression in pleomorphic xanthoastrocytomas. Oncogene

Weiss WA, Israel M, Cobbs C et al. (2002) Neuropathology of genetically engineered mice: consensus report and recommendations from an international forum. Oncogene 21:7453–7463

Wikstrand CJ, Reist CJ, Archer GE, Zalutsky MR, Bigner DD (1998) The class III variant of the epidermal growth factor receptor (EGFRvIII): characterization and utilization as an immunotherapeutic target. J Neurovirol 4:148–158

Xiao A, Wu H, Pandolfi PP, Louis DN, Van Dyke T (2002) Astrocyte inactivation of the pRb pathway predisposes mice to malignant astrocytoma development that is accelerated by PTEN mutation. Cancer Cell 1:157–168

Zhu Y, Guignard F, Zhao D et al. (2005) Early inactivation of p53 tumor suppressor gene cooperating with NF1 loss induces malignant astrocytoma. Cancer Cell 8:119–130

Molecular Pathology of Oligodendroglial Tumors

2

Christian Hartmann and Andreas von Deimling

Abstract The term oligodendroglioma was created by Bailey, Cushing, and Bucy based on the observation that these tumors share morphological similarities with oligodendrocytes (Bailey and Cushing 1926; Bailey and Bucy 1929). However, a convincing link between oligodendrocytes and oligodendrogliomas still needs to be shown. Oligoastrocytomas or mixed gliomas are histologically defined by the presence of oligodendroglial and astrocytic components. According to the WHO classification of brain tumors, oligodendroglial tumors are separated into oligodendrogliomas WHO grade II (OII), anaplastic oligodendrogliomas WHO grade III (OIII), oligoastrocytomas WHO grade II (OAII), anaplastic oligoastrocytomas WHO grade III (OAIII), and glioblastomas with oligodendroglioma component WHO grade IV (GBMo) (Louis et al. 2007). The perception of oligodendroglial tumors has changed in recent years. The diagnosis of oligodendroglioma or oligoastrocytomas is made much more frequently than 10 years ago. Treatment modalities have been advanced and novel concepts regarding the origin of oligodendroglial tumors have been developed. This review focuses on recent developments with impact on the diagnosis and understanding of molecular mechanisms in oligodendroglial tumors.

Christian Hartmann (✉)
Universitätsklinikum Heidelberg
Pathologisches Institut
Abt. Neuropathologie
und
Klinische Kooperationseinheit
Neuropathologie
Deutsches Krebsforschungszentrum
Im Neuenheimer Feld 220/221
69120 Heidelberg
Germany
E-mail: Christian.hartmann@med.uni-heidelberg.de

2.1 Epidemiological, Neuroradiological, and Clinical Features

Oligodendrogliomas occur 1.5–2.1 times more frequently in men than in women (Mork et al. 1986; Zulch 1986). The average age of onset of oligodendrogliomas is between 35 and 55 years with a peak incidence around 45 years (Mork et al. 1986; Zulch 1986). Often OII occur in patients under 40 years of age and OIII arise in patients over 40 years of age (Ludwig et al. 1986). The incidence of oligodendrogliomas has risen over the last few years, reaching levels of 25% of primary brain tumors. This rise is most likely due to the improvement in the therapy of oligodendroglial tumors and the feeling of the diagnostician not to withhold potentially effective treatment for patients with glioma containing any feature reminiscent of oligodendroglial tumors (Coons et al. 1997; Ironside et al. 2002). The frequency of anaplastic tumors among the oligodendroglial gliomas varies strongly between 3.5% and 50% (Winger et al. 1989; Shaw et al. 1992). The incidence of oligoastrocytomas also ranges from 2% to 19%, which is most likely a consequence of the lack of stringent diagnostic criteria (Jaskolsky et al. 1987; Louis et al. 2007).

The etiology of oligodendrogliomas remains unclear with only few studies and some case reports pointing to tumor-initiating factors. None of the hereditary tumor syndromes is associated with oligodendrogliomas. However, familiar oligodendrogliomas were reported in single cases (Ferraresi et al. 1989; Kros et al. 1994). In rabbits, application of N-methyl-N-nitrosourea induced tumors with histological features of oligodendrogliomas (Kleihues et al. 1970). The involvement of SV40 and JS viruses in the induction of oligodendrogliomas is uncertain and conflicting data have been reported (Herbarth et al. 1998; Huang et al. 1999). In one patient an oligodendrogliomas might have been induced by radiation therapy (Huang et al. 1987). In two patients that sustained head injuries, oligodendrogliomas arose at the site of brain damage due to contusion (Perez-Diaz et al. 1985). Furthermore, a few case reports proposed an association between multiple sclerosis and oligodendrogliomas (Giordana et al. 1981; Sega et al. 2006).

Within the group of gliomas, epileptic seizures are most frequently encountered in oligodendrogliomas. Often an epileptic seizure is the first symptom of an oligodendroglioma. Other typical clinical symptoms of oligodendrogliomas are headaches in combination with signs of increased intracranial pressure. Depending on the location of the tumor, varying focal neurological symptoms occur. OII are slowly growing tumors. Cases with seizures as a first symptom usually present a clinical history of about 1 year. Intervals of more than 5 years are not uncommon and in children more than 10 years between onset of seizures and diagnosis of oligodendroglioma has been reported (Greenfield et al. 2002).

Compared to white matter, oligodendrogliomas usually appear on computed tomography (CT) images as a well-demarcated hypo- or isodense lesion. Frequently calcifications can be found, mostly around the periphery of the tumor in a so-called gyriform or ribbon-like pattern. On magnetic resonance imaging (MRI) oligodendrogliomas typically appear as hypointense lesions on T1 and hyperintense on T2 images. The margins are sharply demarcated and perifocal edema is rather small. Varying signal intensities are found in rare cases due to hemorrhages or cystic degeneration. Gadolinium contrast enhancement shows low accuracy in predicting OIII. Enhancement was also found in OII, and on the other hand lack of enhancement was seen in OIII (Ginsberg et al. 1998; Lebrun et al. 2004; White et al. 2005). However, noninvasive grading of oligodendrogliomas appears to be more promising with techniques such as proton magnetic resonance spectroscopic imaging (MRSI) (Rijpkema et al. 2003; Xu et al. 2005). In a small series FDG-PET showed raised glucose utilization within the tumor in six of eight WHO Grade II gliomas with 1p/19q LOH and in none of the WHO Grade II gliomas without this genetic alteration (Stockhammer et al. 2007).

2.2 Pathology

Usually oligodendrogliomas arise in the white matter of the cerebral hemispheres. They occur with a distribution frequency of 3:2:2:1 in the frontal, parietal, temporal, and occipital lobes (Chin et al. 1980; Lee and Van Tassel 1989; Tice et al. 1993). Only in rare cases oligodendrogliomas can be observed in the cerebellum, brainstem, or spinal cord (Greenfield et al. 2002).

Macroscopically, oligodendrogliomas appear as soft, gelatinous grayish-pink masses with relatively well-delineated borders compared with astrocytic gliomas. A gritty texture in unfixed tissue indicates calcification, characteristically in the periphery of the tumor and in adjacent cortical structures. Regions of cystic degeneration can be found in large tumor masses, necrosis only in OIII (see below). Hemorrhages can be found even in OII. Oligodendrogliomas exhibit a tendency to infiltrate adjacent leptomeningeal structures. More rarely, infiltration of the dura might occur, thereby leading to an initial impression of a meningioma.

2.2.1
Oligodendrogliomas WHO Grade II

OII are monomorphous gliomas with moderate cellularity, isomorphic round to oval nuclei and, on paraffin section, a clear perinuclear halo, a so-called honeycomb or fried egg appearance. The typical perinuclear halo is based on an artifact due to tissue fixation (Ironside et al. 2002). These perinuclear halos cannot be observed in unfixed tissue sections such as smear preparations or frozen sections. Furthermore, numerous delicate, branching vessels with a 'chicken wire' or 'retiform' appearance are characteristic of oligodendrogliomas (Fig. 2.1a). Frequently calcification is seen in OII (Fig. 4.1b). Some mitoses are allowed according to the definition of OII (Louis et al. 2007).

2.2.2
Anaplastic Oligodendrogliomas WHO Grade III

OIII are defined by increased cellularity, cytological atypia with pleomorphic cells or multinucleated giant cells, brisk mitotic activity, vascular proliferation ranging from increased cellularity of branching vessels, microvascular proliferation (Fig. 4.1d) to glioblastoma-like garlands or glomeruloid vessels, and necrosis that may show geographic aspects or exhibit perinecrotic palisading of tumor cells (Louis et al. 2007).

2.2.3
Oligoastrocytomas WHO Grade II

OAII are defined as tumors composed of components resembling both oligodendroglioma and astrocytoma. Different authors suggested various cut-off values for the astrocytic component to separate oligodendrogliomas from oligoastrocytomas. Values between 1% (Kim et al. 1996), 25% (Mork et al. 1986), and 50% (Hart et al. 1974) have been proposed. For good reasons, WHO did not define a cut-off value to separate oligoastrocytomas from oligodendrogliomas and astrocytomas. The evaluation of slides is based on the assumption that the plane visualized is representative of the entire tumor. However, the proportion of astrocytic and oligodendroglial components may vary considerably in different planes. Further, due to surgical procedures not all tumor material is evaluated by histological examination. Two groups of oligoastrocytomas defined by different morphology have been described: The "biphasic" tumors with two clearly distinct components and the "diffuse" neoplasm with astrocytic tumor cells scattered in between oligodendroglial cells (Hart et al. 1974). However, it needs to be shown that these scattered astrocytic tumor cells are indeed neoplastic cells and not reactive and hypertrophic astrocytes. Another problem in the diagnosis of OAIII is the presence of an increased mitotic rate in absence of other clearly anaplastic features. The WHO allows a higher rate of mitoses in OII than in astrocytoma WHO grade II. It is not yet been resolved whether a moderately increased mitotic activity in oligoastrocytomas requires different grading depending on whether the mitoses are predominantly seen in the oligodendroglial or in the astrocytic component, i.e., WHO grade II or WHO grade III. Several reports indicated that the presence of some mitoses in oligoastrocytomas are WHO grade III and require more aggressive treatment (Miller et al. 2006; van den Bent et al. 2006).

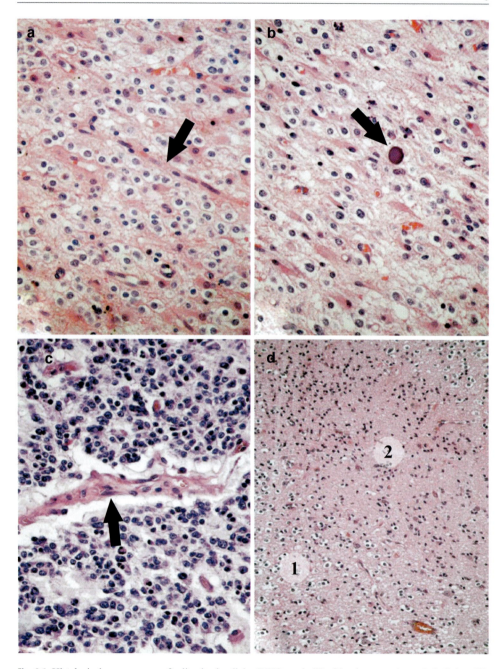

Fig. 2.1 Histological appearance of oligodendroglial tumors. (**a**) Oligodendroglioma WHO grade II with delicate branching capillaries. (**b**) The same tumor with small calcifications. (**c**) Anaplastic oligodendroglioma WHO grade III with microvascular endothelial proliferation. (**d**) "Biphasic" oligoastrocytoma WHO grade II with an oligodendroglial component (1) and an astrocytic component (2)

2.2.4
Anaplastic Oligoastrocytomas WHO Grade III

OAIII show histological features of anaplasia including nuclear and cellular atypia, high cellularity, and high mitotic activity. Microvascular proliferation may be present; however, the issue of necrosis is not sufficiently addressed by the WHO. Recent studies showed that patients with OAIII containing necrosis had a shorter overall survival than patients with OAIII not containing necrosis (Miller et al. 2006; van den Bent et al. 2006). Therefore, the current WHO classification suggests classifying and grading anaplastic tumors with oligodendrocytic and astrocytic differentiation and with necrosis as glioblastoma (GBMo) with oligodendroglial component WHO grade IV (Louis et al. 2007). On the other hand, a recent study demonstrated that in such tumors necroses were not of prognostic significance if the oligodendroglial component showed the classical features of oligodendroglioma. In that study, the classic features of oligodendroglioma were highly associated with combined 1p and 19q deletions (Giannini et al. 2008).

2.2.5
Glioblastomas with Oligodendroglioma Component WHO Grade IV

Anaplastic oligoastrocytomas with necrosis may be termed glioblastomas with oligodendroglial component WHO grade IV (GBMo). This diagnosis was introduced in the WHO 2007 brain tumor classification based on the observation that such tumors have a poorer clinical performance than anaplastic oligoastrocytomas without necrosis. GBMo seem to have a better prognosis than ordinary GBM (He et al. 2001; Kraus et al. 2001; Homma et al. 2006). However, according to the WHO GBMo is not yet an established GBM variant but is seen as a pattern of differentiation (Louis et al. 2007).

2.3
Immunohistochemistry

Multiple immunohistochemical markers have been proposed to distinguish oligodendrogliomas from astrocytomas. However, due to inconsistent results none of these markers has been established for routine diagnostics. Specific immunohistochemical markers would be very helpful for reducing the high interobserver variation in the diagnosis of OIII (Giannini et al. 2001). Based on the concept of a link between oligodendrocytes and oligodendrogliomas, multiple immunohistochemical markers were evaluated that are expressed in oligodendrocytes. For example, expression of the myelin basic protein (MBP) (Tanaka et al. 1988; Kashima et al. 1993), galactocerebroside (Kennedy et al. 1987; de la Monte 1989), and myelin-associated glycoprotein (MAG) (Perentes and Rubinstein 1987) was found only in some oligodendrogliomas or in portions of the tumors. Furthermore, no oligodendroglioma-specific expression of the oligodendrocytic lineage markers platelet-derived growth factor receptor alpha (PDGFRA), proteolipid protein (PLP), and chondroitin sulfate proteoglycan (NG2) was found (Landry et al. 1997; Shoshan et al. 1999). Recently, the transcriptional activity of the oligodendrocytic linage genes 1 and 2 (OLIG1, OLIG2) raised new hope for separating oligodendrogliomas from astrocytomas (Lu et al. 2001; Marie et al. 2001; Hoang-Xuan et al. 2002). However, multiple follow-up studies found Olig-1 and Olig-2 expression in astrocytic tumors as well (Ohnishi et al. 2003; Aguirre-Cruz et al. 2004; Ligon et al. 2004). Nevertheless, it was shown that Olig-expressing tumor cells do not express GFAP (Azzarelli et al. 2004; Mokhtari et al. 2005). Nuclear expression of endothelin beta receptors (EDNRB) was described in oligodendroglial tumors and only rarely in glioblastomas (Anguelova et al. 2005). However, an independent study confirming these data has not been reported yet. Due to these frustrating efforts to establish oligodendroglioma-specific immunohistochemical markers, glial fibrillary acid protein (GFAP) which binds to cells of astrocytic differentiation but not to typical oligodendroglial cells is used as a "negative" marker. However, strong expression of GFAP is also seen in so-called mini-gemistocytes, well compatible with the diagnosis of oligodendroglioma (Louis et al. 2007). Recently, strong expression of cartilage glycoprotein-39/YKL-40 (CHI3L1) has been described in glioblastomas and no or weak binding only in anaplastic oligodendrogliomas WHO grade III. The distinction of both glioma entities by YKL-40 was better than that achieved with GFAP (Nutt et al. 2005). However, further studies are required to demonstrate the value of YKL-40 in routine diagnostics (Louis et al. 2007).

2.4
Molecular Genetics

2.4.1
Combined Losses on Chromosome 1p and 19q in Oligodendroglial Tumors

The genetic hallmarks of oligodendroglial tumors are combined chromosomal deletions on the short arm of chromosome 1 (1p) and the long arm of chromosome 19 (19q). Up to 90% of all OII carry this alteration (von Deimling et al. 1992; Bello et al. 1994, 1995a, b; Reifenberger et al. 1994; Kraus et al. 1995). The rate of combined losses on 1p and 19q is lower in OIII with approximately 50–70% of tumors carrying this alteration (Cairncross et al. 1998; Smith et al. 2000; Mueller et al. 2002). It has been pointed out that oligodendrogliomas with combined losses on 1p and 19q demonstrate a more "classical" histological phenotype. In contrast, oligodendrogliomas without losses on 1p and 19q exhibited more frequently astrocytic features (Burger et al. 2001; Sasaki et al. 2002; Ueki et al. 2002; McDonald et al. 2005). These findings reflect the high interobserver variation in the diagnosis of oligodendroglial tumors and indicates that molecular analysis for 1p and 19q deletions is a helpful diagnostic parameter.

Oligodendroglial tumors with combined losses on 1p and 19q typically occur at an extratemporal location. In contrast, oligodendroglial tumors with an intact 1p/19q status accumulated in the temporal lobe (Zlatescu et al. 2001; Mueller et al. 2002).

A higher apoptotic index was observed in oligodendrogliomas with combined losses on 1p and 19q than in oligodendrogliomas without losses. This variation in apoptotic activity might explain the differences in clinical behavior in both oligodendroglioma variants (Wharton et al. 2007). Because of the frequency of combined 1p and 19q deletions in low-grade oligodendroglial tumors, it is assumed that these alterations have an initiating role in tumorigenesis. The high rate of combined 1p and 19q losses prompted speculations on defining OII by molecular rather than by histological criteria (Reifenberger and Louis 2003). The lower frequency of 1p and 19q deletions in OIII may point to a higher degree of genetic heterogeneity possibly due to the difficult distinction of OIII from other malignant gliomas such as GBMo.

Combined losses of 1p/19q are found in approximately 50% of oligoastrocytomas (von Deimling et al. 2000; Mueller et al. 2002). These losses are mutually exclusive to LOH 17p and *TP53* mutations (Maintz et al. 1997; von Deimling et al. 2000; Mueller et al. 2002; Ueki et al. 2002), indicating either an oligodendroglioma genotype characterized by losses on 1p/19q or an astrocytoma genotype characterized by *TP53* mutations (Fig. 2.2). In oligoastrocytomas 1p/19q losses occur in the oligodendroglial and astrocytic component, thereby indicating a clonal origin of oligoastrocytomas and supporting the concept of at least two genetic variants of oligoastrocytomas (Kraus et al. 1995). However, in a few cases differing genetic alterations were observed in the oligodendroglial and astrocytic tumor component (Dong et al. 2002; Qu et al. 2007). This implies that oligoastrocytomas are predominantly of monoclonal origin. Furthermore, *TP53* mutations were seen mostly in temporal oligoastrocytomas but not in extratemporal tumors (Mueller et al. 2002). At least two models might explain these findings. The environment of the temporal and extratemporal location might vary and, thereby, provide different growth advantages for oligodendroglial tumors with and without 1p/19q losses. On the other hand, different cells of origin with a varying susceptibility for 1p/19q losses might be the source for temporal and extratemporal oligodendroglial tumors.

Combined losses of 1p/19q are found in approximately 5% of GBM, suggesting an oligodendroglioma rather than an astrocytoma genotype and, therefore, a better prognosis than GBM without this alteration. There is an overlap between GBM with combined losses of 1p/19q and GBM with an oligodendroglial component (He et al. 2001). However, two studies imply that patients with GBM with combined losses of 1p/19q do not have a better prognosis than patients with normal GBM. In a series of 220 GBM, combined losses of 1p/19q were identified in 9% of cases. However, there was no difference in survival between patients with and without combined 1p/19q losses (Houillier et al. 2006). In a different study GBM long-time survivors were tested for 1p/19q losses. Only 2 of 32 tumors carried combined 1p/19q losses, thereby indicating that this genetic lesion is not a marker for longer survival (Krex et al. 2007).

Combined 1p/19q losses were also observed in gliosarcomas. A recent study identified this lesion in five of seven recurrent gliosarcomas which were diagnosed as oligodendrogliomas at first resection. Interestingly, the lesions were present in both the glial and sarcomatous component. The authors suggested the name "oligosarcoma" for this gliosarcoma variant (Rodriguez et al. 2007).

2.4.2 Isolated and Combined Losses of 1p and 19q Oligodendroglial and Astrocytic Tumors

While the combination of 1p/19q losses is typical for oligodendroglial tumors, a deletion of either chromosomal region is also seen in astrocytic tumors. In fact, 19q losses have been demonstrated to frequently occur in the progression of astrocytoma toward malignancy (von Deimling et al. 1994; Hartmann et al. 2002). Likewise, 1p deletions have been described in malignant astrocytic tumors. Therefore, coincidence of 1p and 19q deletions is also expected in some astrocytic tumors. However, the extent of deletions on the chromosomal arms 1p and 19q differ between oligodendroglial and astrocytic tumors. While the entire 1p and 19q arms are lost in oligodendroglial tumors, these deletions are much smaller in astrocytic tumors. Interestingly and in line with classical clinicopathological correlations, small 1p deletions in astrocytic tumors are associated with a poor prognosis contrasting the finding of favorable prognosis indicated by losses of the entire 1p and 19q arms in oligodendroglial tumors (Idbaih et al. 2005; Ichimura et al. 2008).

Due to the clinically important differences between the losses of the entire 1p and 19q arms versus losses involving only parts of chromosomal arms 1p and 19q, it has been suggested to analyze not only telomeric but also centromeric locations on 1p (Boulay et al. 2007).

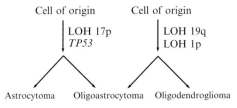

Fig. 2.2 Model for oligoastrocytomas. The major fraction of oligoastrocytomas exhibits either genetic alterations typical for astrocytoma or for oligodendroglioma

2.4.3
Mechanism for Combined Losses of 1p and 19q

Recently, a centromeric or pericentromeric t(1;19)(q10,p10) translocation was identified as the mechanism leading to the combined loss of the two chromosomal arms (Griffin et al. 2006; Jenkins et al. 2006). In fact, chromosome 1 and 19 translocation was already observed earlier in a single cell line, but has not been recognized as a general feature of these tumors (Magnani et al. 2005).

Optical fusion of signals from a chromosome 1 probe and a 19p12 probe using fluorescence in situ hybridization (FISH) was observed in 90% of the cases that showed combined losses of 1p and 19q. In total 55% of oligodendrogliomas, 47% of oligoastrocytomas, and 0% of astrocytomas demonstrated this t(1;19)(q10,p10) translocation. Overall survival time was nearly similar for patients that were evaluated for 1p/19q losses or t(1;19)(q10,p10) translocation (Jenkins et al. 2006).

The centromeric regions of chromosomes 1 and 19 (and interestingly chromosome 5 as well) show a high sequence homology. Presumably, the specific chromosomal karyo-architecture of the oligodendroglioma precursor cell results in centromeric co-localization of chromosome 1 and 19 that might promote centromeric instability in this cell type, thus promoting translocation events (Jenkins et al. 2006). Interestingly, in two cases a t(1;19)(q10,p10) translocation but no 1p/19q losses were observed (Jenkins et al. 2006). This finding might indicate that there is a small portion of oligodendrogliomas with a reciprocal whole-arm exchange at the centromere. Further, it may suggest that the rate of oligodendrogliomas with chromosome 1 and 19 alterations is even higher than that detected by methods focusing on 1p/19q deletions only (Fig. 2.3). On the other hand, t(1;19)(q10,p10) translocations were described in only 90% of the cases that demonstrated 1p/19q losses (Jenkins et al. 2006). This might be due to insufficient translocation detection but could also be caused by losses without translocation.

Further confirmatory studies have not been reported yet. Recently, 1p/19q deletions without evidence of a t(1;19)(q10,p10) translocation have been reported in short-term culture of oligodendroglioma (Gadji et al. 2008).

2.4.4
Methods for Detection of Allelic Losses on Chromosome 1p and 19q

Different methods for detection of 1p/19q losses are employed in routine diagnostics. PCR-based microsatellite analysis with several markers is still considered the most robust needing only a small amount of tumor DNA (Hartmann et al. 2005). However, this method is quite labor-intensive and also requires constitutional DNA, usually extracted from peripheral blood leukocytes. A novel technique, multiplex ligation-dependent probe amplification (MLPA), has the advantage of not requiring constitutional DNA (van Dijk et al. 2005). Furthermore, processing of MLPA PCR is faster and allows a higher resolution due to the simultaneous assessment of more than 40 markers (Fig. 2.4). Both methods cannot detect the t(1;19)(q10,p10) translocation. The method most familiar to pathologists is FISH, which is rapid and is suitable for routine laboratories specialized in histology. A big advantage is that FISH is performed on paraffin-embedded material used for standard diagnostic protocols. In addition, FISH does not require control tissues such as peripheral leukocytes required for microsatellite analysis or MLPA. However, FISH usually covers only a single position on the chromosome thus not giving conclusive information on the extent of the potential deletion. This could be circumvented by demonstrating the translocation with FISH using centromeric probes (Griffin et al. 2006; Jenkins et al. 2006). However, the kits commercially available are not suitable for detecting the translocation. In addition FISH is at danger of being misinter-

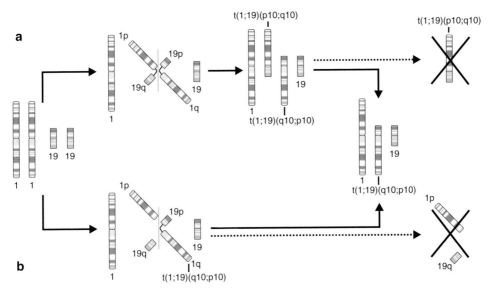

Fig. 2.3 Models for t(1;19)(q10,p10) translocation mechanisms in oligodendroglial tumors based on data from Griffin et al. 2006 and Jenkins et al. 2006. (**a**) The centromeric or pericentromeric regions of one chromosome 1 and one chromosome 19 come close to each other, the repetitive DNA strains break and 19p recombines with 1q arm to t(1;19)(q10;p10) and 1p recombines with 19q to t(1;19)(p10;q10). In this intermediate phase, no losses of 1p/19 can be detected. In a second step the t(1;19)(p10;q10) fusion chromosome is eliminated from the tumor cell and, therefore, a loss of 1p/19q occurs. This translocation model would imply that there are oligodendrogliomas that do not show losses on 1p/19q but demonstrate a translocation. Interestingly, such tumors were identified in small numbers (Jenkins et al. 2006). (**b**) An alternative mechanism. After centromeric or pericentromeric fracture of one chromosome 1 and one chromosome 19, only the 19p and 1q arm fuse leading to a t(1;19)(q10;p10). The remaining 1p/19q arms will be eliminated directly. In this model, the number of tumors that show losses of 1p/19q and a t(1;19)(q10;p10) translocation should be nearly identical

preted because artifacts and signals tend to fade after long-term storage.

The most attractive method to separate oligodendroglial tumor with losses on 1p/19q from those without would be based on immunohistochemistry. However, no reliable immunohistochemical marker has been identified so far. Different microarray expression studies already have been performed on oligodendroglial tumors but no suitable markers were identified (Watson et al. 2001; Fuller et al. 2002; Kim et al. 2002; Mukasa et al. 2002; Nutt et al. 2003; Mukasa et al. 2004; Tews et al. 2006). Proteome analysis by two-dimensional protein gel electrophoresis might be a more successful approach. Indeed, differently expressed proteins were identified between oligodendrogliomas with and without losses on 1p by this strategy (Okamoto et al. 2007), but it remains to be shown whether some of these proteins are useful immunohistochemical markers for 1p/19 loss.

2.4.5
Tumor Suppressor Gene Identification on 1p and 19q

The observation of a centromeric or pericentromeric t(1;19)(q10,p10) translocation with a complete loss of 1p and 19q challenges the concept of the presence of at least one tumor suppressor gene (TSG) on 1p and 19q each with relevance

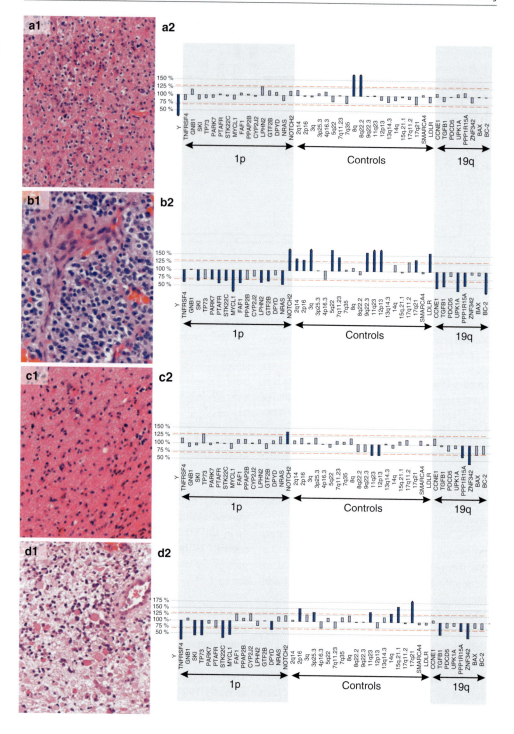

for oligodendroglial tumors (Griffin et al. 2006; Jenkins et al. 2006). In many tumors, reproducible chromosomal translocations join two genes to a fusion gene which acquires tumor-promoting properties. The t(1;19)(q10,p10) translocation might lead to such activation and all attempts to identify an altered TSG on the remaining copies of 1p and 19q may be fruitless. Nevertheless, to date no genes have been observed in the centromeric or pericentromeric regions of chromosomes 1 and 19 which may be candidates for a tumor-promoting fusion protein (Jenkins et al. 2006). The highly repetitive nature of centromeric DNA complicates sequencing but there is evidence that genes map within centromeric regions (Cooke 2004). The observation of oligodendrogliomas that show a t(1;19)(q10,p10) translocation but no losses of 1p/19q (Jenkins et al. 2006) may indicate an intermediate phase with the presence of a temporary t(1;19)(p10;q10) fusion chromosome (Fig. 2.3, model a). If the t(1;19)(q10,p10) translocation results in an oncogenic fusion gene, the tumor cells should have no additional benefit by removing the t(1;19)(p10;q10) fusion chromosome in a second step. However, if the primary benefit of the t(1;19)(q10,p10) translocation for tumor cells is the loss of 1p/19q, the elimination of the temporary t(1;19)(p10;q10) fusion chromosome in a second step may indicate that candidate TSGs on 1p/19q are important for induction of oligodendrogliomas.

2.4.6
Candidate Genes on 1p

Many candidate TSGs have been suggested but have not been confirmed in consecutive studies. One of the interesting genes is *CDKN2C*, which carried point mutations (Husemann et al. 1999) or homozygous deletions (Pohl et al. 1999) in some oligodendrogliomas. Among recent candidates of interest is *CITED4*, which was found to be differentially expressed between oligodendroglial tumors with and without LOH 1p in an expression microarray (Tews et al. 2006). *CITED4* is not mutated, but carries a hypermethylated promoter in oligodendrogliomas with LOH 1p/19q, and hypermethylation was found to be a significant predictor of longer survival. *CITED4* is an attractive TSG candidate due to the fact that CITED4 protein binds CBP and EP300, is a co-activator of the transcription factor AP-2, blocks binding of HIF1a to EP300, and inhibits HIF1a transactivation as well as hypoxia-mediated reporter gene activation (Tews et al. 2007). Another TSG candidate on 1p31.3 is *DIRAS3* or *ARHI* encoding a RAS-related GTPase that confers growth suppression to breast and ovarian cancer cells (Yu et al. 1999). The promoter region of this gene is significantly hypermethylated in OII and OIII with losses on 1p compared to those tumors without losses. Furthermore, a correlation of *DIRAS3* inactivation with survival was reported (Riemenschneider et al. 2008). The most centromeric gene on 1p is *Notch2*. Mapping may indicate that the translocation breakpoint region maps within this gene (Boulay et al. 2007). Currently, functional data or information about potential translocation partner genes on chromosome 19 is not available. However, the observed translocation breakpoint region defines *Notch2* as the first attractive candidate gene that can be included in the concept of a t(1;19) (q10,p10) translocation.

Fig. 2.4 Typical deletions pattern of 1p and 19q in oligodendroglial and astrocytic tumors by multiplex ligation-dependent probe amplification (MLPA) PCR. The 100% line indicates the presence of two copies of the specific marker; values below the 75% line indicate a loss of one copy. **a1** – OIII, **a2** – corresponding MLPA PCR data for this tumor showing no losses on 1p and 19q. **b1** – OIII, **b2** – nearly all markers on 1p and 19q are below the 75% line indicating a complete loss of both chromosomal arms. **c1** – AIII, **c2** – no losses on 1p and telomeric losses on 19q. **d1** – AIII I, **d2** – telomeric losses on 1p and loss of 19q

2.4.7
Candidate Genes on 19q

Due to the t(1;19)(q10,p10) translocation with a complete loss of 19q in oligodendrogliomas, the mapping studies for identification of the 19q candidate region are likely to have focused on astrocytic tumors with partial deletions. This implies that the suggested 19q13.3 TSG candidate region (Hartmann et al. 2002) is of interest for astrocytic but not for oligodendroglial tumors. Candidates looked at did not reveal mutations in significant numbers (Hartmann et al. 2004). Therefore, attention shifted towards epigenetic silencing of genes by promoter methylation. *PEG3* is imprinted in normal brain and only the paternal allele is expressed. The expression of *PEG* is reduced in some gliomas and glioma cell lines and can be re-expressed by 5-aza-2′-deoxycytidine treatment (Maegawa et al. 2001). However, a link between 19q losses and reduced expression was not shown. In addition, 19q losses exhibited no uniparental deletion pattern suggestive of inactivation of imprinted genes by loss of the active gene copy (Hartmann et al. 2003). These observations further reduce the likelihood of *PEG* being an oligodendroglioma-relevant TSG. *ZNF342* showed frequent promoter methylation in OII and OIII with losses on 19q, expression was reduced in cases with promoter methylation, and expression was restored in cell lines after treatment with a demethylating agent (Hong et al. 2003). However, it remains to be determined whether *ZNF342* promoter methylation did not occur in oligodendrogliomas without 19q losses. Recently, *EMP3* was found to be differentially expressed between low-grade gliomas with and without 19q losses by cDNA microarray expression profiling (Tews et al. 2006). Aberrant methylation in the 5′-region of *EMP3* was significantly associated with reduced mRNA expression and LOH 19q in a similar frequency in OII and OIII, thereby suggesting a role of *EMP3* in the initiation of the majority of oligodendroglial tumors (Kunitz et al. 2007). However, another study did not find a link between *EMP3* promoter methylation and losses on 19q (Li et al. 2007).

2.4.8
IDH1 Mutations in Oligodendroglial Tumors

A whole-genome sequencing project recently identified mutations in the cytosolic NADP+ dependent isocitrate dehydrogenase gene (*IDH1*) in GBM. All mutations were heterozygous and exclusively affected arginine in amino acid position 132 (Parson et al., 2008). We identified *IDH1* mutations in approximately 75% of oligodendrogliomas, oligoastrocytomas and astrocytomas WHO grades II and III (Balss et al., 2008). While that study did not show significant associations between *IDH1* mutations and 1p/19q losses, we now have the impression of a significant association of these lesions (based on a larger series, unpublished data). The mutation frequencies in WHO grade II and anaplastic WHO grade III gliomas were similar, and therefore, *IDH1* mutations might constitute an early role in gliomagenesis.

Isocitrate dehydrogenase catalyzes the oxidative decarboxylation of isocitrate to alpha-ketoglutarate, thereby reducing NADP+ to NADPH. The subcellular localization of the isocitrate dehydrogenase protein is the cytoplasm and the peroxisome (Geisbrecht et al., 1999). In the cytoplasm, the role of the protein might be to provide NADPH under conditions not favorable for generation of NADPH by the hexose monophosphate shunt. In the peroxisome, IDH1 protein is the only known source of NADPH that is required by several enzymes such as hydroxymethyl-CoA-, 2,4-dienoyl-CoS- and acyl-CoA-reductases. An important role of IDH1 in protection from oxidative stress may be concluded from the observation of increased resistance of IDPc, the mouse homolog of IDH1, overexpressing and sensitivity of IDPc deficient

NIH3T3 cells to exposure of hydrogen peroxide (Lee et al., 2002). Further, IDPc negative HL-60 cells exhibited increased caspase-3 activation under oxidative stress, suggesting a role in apoptosis (Kim et al., 2007).

Mutations affected the amino acid arginine in position 132 of the amino acid sequence that belongs to an evolutionary conserved region locating to the binding site of isocitrate. In the vast majority of the cases wild type arginine in position 132 was replaced by histidine. The reported mutations always were heterozygous and alterations suggestive for protein inactivation such as splice site or nonsense mutations were not detected, thus prompting speculations on an activating nature of the mutation (Parson et al., 2008). However, site directed mutagenesis leading to a R132E exchange in rat IDP2 which is homologous to human IDH1 completely abrogated enzyme activity (Jennings et al, 1997). Further, a mutation in porcine NADP-isocitrate dehydrogenase at position 133 (R133Q) corresponding to human position 132, also resulted in downregulation of the enzyme activity (Sounda et al., 2000). Thus, the effect of the R132H mutation on enzyme activity currently is not resolved.

The very high *IDH1* mutation rate implies that besides 1p/19q losses this alteration plays a fundamental role in oligodendrogliomas, oligoastrocytomas and astrocytomas. The functional mechanism of the *IDH1* mutations needs to be clarified in further studies.

2.4.9
Progression-Associated Genetic Alterations

Deletions on the short arm of chromosome 9 occur more frequently in OIII than in OII and can be found in 22–50% of the cases (Reifenberger et al. 1994; Weber et al. 1996; Bigner et al. 1999; Kros et al. 1999; von Deimling et al. 2000; Kitange et al. 2005). *CDKN2A* encoding p16^{INK4a} and *CDKN2B* encoding p15^{INK4b} were identified as major targets of homozygous deletions on 9p21 in OIII (Cairncross et al. 1998; Bigner et al. 1999; Bortolotto et al. 2000; Ino et al. 2001; Watanabe et al. 2001a). Alternatively, these genes are inactivated by promoter hypermethylation in oligodendroglioma (Watanabe et al. 2001a; Wolter et al. 2001). Other genes of the RB1 pathway like *CDK4* (amplification) or *RB1* (promoter hypermethylation) are altered in a lower frequency (Watanabe et al. 2001b).

Losses of chromosome 10 were found in 14–58% of OIII (Reifenberger et al. 1994; Jeuken et al. 1999; Kros et al. 1999; von Deimling et al. 2000; Sanson et al. 2002). Losses on chromosome 10 are inversely associated with losses on 1p/19q (Jeuken et al. 1999; Hoang-Xuan et al. 2001; Ino et al. 2001; Ueki et al. 2002; Thiessen et al. 2003). *PTEN* on 10q23.31 and *MGMT* on 10q26.3 are frequently discussed as target genes for chromosome 10 losses. However, *PTEN* mutations occur only in 3–10% of OIII (Duerr et al. 1998; Jeuken et al. 2000; Sasaki et al. 2001; Sanson et al. 2002). Promoter hypermethylation of *MGMT* was described in most oligodendrogliomas and shows an association with 1p/19q losses.

The inverse association between losses on chromosome 9p and 10 and losses on 1p/19q and the exclusive alteration pattern of *TP53* mutations and 1p/19q losses may suggest genetically different groups of oligodendroglial tumors. On the other hand, 9p and 10q deletions are typical for glioblastoma and anaplastic oligodendroglioma is difficult to distinguish from glioblastoma especially if relaxed criteria are applied for diagnosis.

Several studies have shown the activation of oncogenes in oligodendroglioma (Alonso et al. 2005; Kitange et al. 2005). In analogy to 9p and 10q losses, the activated oncogenes identified are frequently mutated in glioblastoma and, therefore, these findings may also reflect the morphological overlap between anaplastic oligodendroglial tumors with glioblastoma.

2.5
The Origin of Oligodendrogliomas

2.5.1
Phenotype and Genotype of Gliomas

In the rat an O2A precursor cell was identified with the capability to generate both oligodendroglial and astrocytic lineages (Raff et al., 1983). This observation prompted the speculation that oligodendrogliomas and diffuse astrocytomas evolve from the same precursor cell. On the other hand, the nearly mutually exclusive occurrence of 1p/19q losses and *TP53* mutations in oligodendroglial and astrocytic gliomas favoured the existence of different precursor cells for these tumors (Mueller et al., 2002).

However, the observation of *IDH1* mutations in the majority in both, oligodendrogliomas and diffuse astrocytomas may again support the concept of a common precursor cell (Balss et al., 2008). *IDH1* mutations may be a very early tumor-initiating event in the putative human equivalent of the O2A precursor cell. *TP53* mutations and 1p/19q losses may be subsequent lesions. Further studies are necessary to test this hypothesis.

In most cases, human oligoastrocytomas have either an oligodendroglioma genotype (losses on 1p/19q) or an astrocytoma genotype (*TP53* mutations) (Kraus et al. 1995). In only few cases different genetic alterations were observed in the oligodendroglial and astrocytic tumor component (Dong et al. 2002; Qu et al. 2007). If both genetic variants of oligoastrocytomas do have the potential to present an oligodendroglial and an astrocytic phenotype, this might indicate that the morphological appearance of diffuse gliomas is less related to a specific genotype and is more a consequence of local conditions. This concept is supported by a mouse model in which nestin-promoter-driven up-regulation of RCAS-Akt and RCAS-PDGF yielded tumors with features of oligoastrocytoma. In the astrocytic component both pathways were active, in the oligodendroglial component only PDGF-expression was observed. The authors concluded that variant signaling can modify cellular morphology within a tumor (Dai et al. 2005). Both human tumors and murine tumor models demonstrate that molecular parameters more closely characterize oligoastrocytomas than morphology.

2.5.2
Progenitor Cells of Oligodendrocytes and Oligodendroglial Tumors

Recently, $CD133^+$ glioma stem cells were identified in GBM. Another way of identifying stem cells is selection of clones with neurosphere-like growth in defined culture conditions. These cells have the ability of self-renewal and multi-lineage differentiation (Dirks 2008). To date, only limited data are available on glioma stem cells in oligodendrogliomas. In OAIII $CD133^+$/$Nestin^+$ cells were isolated showing neurosphere-like growth and exhibited the ability of self-renewal (Yi et al. 2007). In another study on malignant gliomas with oligodendroglial differentiation, $CD133^+$ cells were identified and displayed neurosphere-like growth, multi-lineage differentiation capability, and tumorigenicity in nude mice. Patients with tumors harboring these $CD133^+$ cells had a less favorable prognosis than patients with $CD133^-$ tumors (Beier et al. 2008). However, it remains unclear if these glioma stem cells are the cells of origin for initiation and progression of glioma, or the results of such processes (Fan et al. 2007).

2.6
Prognosis

Differing values regarding the prognosis of patients with oligodendroglial tumors have been reported. The main reason for these differences is varying criteria for inclusion of patients. The median postoperative survival time of OII ranged from 3.5 to 16.7 years (Shaw et al. 1992; Heegaard et al. 1995; Dehghani et al. 1998; Olson et al. 2000). The 5-year survival rate ranged from 38% to 83% (Sun et al. 1988; Shimizu et al. 1993; Gannett et al. 1994; Heegaard et al. 1995; Dehghani et al. 1998; Wharton et al. 1998; Yeh et al. 2002). Progression to anaplasia occurs in a lower frequency than in astrocytic tumors (Louis et al. 2007).

The median postoperative survival of OIII ranged from 0.9 to 7.3 years (Shaw et al. 1992; Shimizu et al. 1993; Cairncross et al. 1998; Dehghani et al. 1998; van den Bent et al. 1998; Puduvalli et al. 2003).The 5-year survival rate ranged from 23% to 66% (Cairncross et al. 1998; Davis et al. 1998; Dehghani et al. 1998; Puduvalli et al. 2003). Chemotherapy of OIII has prolonged the median time to progression to 25 months for responders (Cairncross et al. 1994; Cairncross et al. 1998). The largest series reported that 50 of 93 patients with OIII who were treated either with chemotherapy or radiation developed tumor progression after a median of 48 months (Puduvalli et al. 2003).

Only few reports exist for OAII. The median postoperative survival times ranged from 3.9 to 6.3 years (Jaskolsky et al. 1987; Shaw et al. 1992) with a 5-year survival rate of 58% (Shaw et al. 1992). One study reported a median duration of survival in OAIII similar to AIII and shorter than in OIII (Winger et al. 1989).

2.6.1
Clinical and Histological/Immunohistological Prognostic Factors

Clinical parameters have been identified for prediction of patient outcome. For example, age at surgery, extent of surgical resection, and postoperative Karnofsky score were associated with survival in both uni- and multivariate analysis. Tumor location and symptoms at presentation showed a significant correlation with survival in uni- but not in multivariate analysis (Schiffer et al. 1997).

The histological features which separate OII from OIIII are based on their relevance for prognosis (Louis et al. 2007). For example, the proliferation index determined by Ki67-positive nuclei correlates with recurrence of oligodendrogliomas (Coleman et al. 2006). In contrast to astrocytic tumors there is no correlation between vascular proliferation or necrosis and clinical outcome in OIII (Schiffer et al. 1999; Smith et al. 2006). However, there seems to be a difference in clinical outcome between OAIII with and without necrosis (Miller et al. 2006; van den Bent et al. 2006). Due to this reason, the WHO 2007 brain tumor classification now separates OAIII from GBM with oligodendroglial features in cases of necrosis (Louis et al. 2007).

2.6.2
Losses on 1p and 19 as a Prognostic Factor

Oligodendrogliomas are the first CNS neoplasm in which a genetic signature was correlated with outcome in phase III trials (Cairncross et al. 2006; van den Bent et al. 2006). Initially, Cairncross et al. identified losses on 1p/19q in OIII to be predictive for chemosensitivity, longer recurrence-free survival after PCV chemotherapy, and longer overall survival (Cairncross et al. 1998). In the meantime multiple studies confirmed these findings (Smith et al. 2000; Van Den Bent et al. 2003; Walker et al. 2005). A correlation of losses on 1p/19q and chemosensitivity to temozolomide was also reported (Chahlavi et al. 2003; Hoang-Xuan et al. 2004; Triebels et al. 2004; Brandes et al. 2006; Kouwenhoven et al. 2006; Levin et al. 2006). Not only losses on 1p/19q correlated with a better outcome. Patients with a t(1;19)(q10,p10) translocation demonstrated a similar response to chemotherapy (Jenkins et al. 2006). An analysis of oligodendroglioma patients with combined losses on 1p/19 which have not been treated by chemotherapy or radiation therapy showed no difference in outcome compared to those without losses. This suggests that combined 1p/19q losses are not prognostic but predictive (Weller et al. 2007).

2.6.3
MGMT as a Prognostic Factor

In GBM, promoter hypermethylation of the *MGMT* gene on chromosome 10q26.3 was identified as a predictor for response to temozolomide treatment (Hegi et al. 2005). Therefore, it appears likely that *MGMT* hypermethylation combined with reduced expression of O6-methylguanine DNA methyltransferase protein could also serve as a prognostic factor in oligodendrogliomas. In fact, one study reported an association between response to temozolomide treatment and MGMT protein expression in OII (Levin et al. 2006). However, in OIII treated by temozolomide, *MGMT* hypermethylation showed only a borderline correlation with overall survival. The authors conclude that further studies on *MGMT* hypermethylation should be performed in randomized trials to test its correlation with survival (Brandes et al. 2006). In OII that were not treated by chemotherapy *MGMT* hypermethylation was not identified as a prognostic marker (Watanabe et al. 2002).

2.6.4
Other Prognostic Molecular Factors

Different molecular markers were identified as prognostic markers for oligodendroglial tumors. Most of them resemble chromosomal areas or are genes that are frequently altered in astrocytic tumors. It should be kept in mind that these markers may indicate an "astrocytic genotype" and, therefore, do not delineate specific oligodendroglial subgroups.

TP53 mutations or LOH 17p13 are rarely found in tumors with an oligodendroglial phenotype and are usually inversely associated with losses on 1p/19q (Ohgaki et al. 1991; Burger et al. 2001; Wolter et al. 2001; Mueller et al. 2002; Ueki et al. 2002). *TP53* mutations or LOH 17p13 were identified as prognostic markers that indicate a reduced progression-free survival (PFS) and total survival (*TP53*) (McLendon et al. 2005) or total survival (LOH 17p13) (Walker et al. 2005). However, in another study focusing on patients with OIII, neither *TP53* mutations nor p53 IHC results were associated with survival (Cairncross et al. 1998).

Losses of chromosome 10 are mostly observed in high-grade gliomas and inversely to losses on 1p/19q (Jeuken et al. 1999; Hoang-Xuan et al. 2001; Ino et al. 2001; Ueki et al. 2002; Thiessen et al. 2003). Different studies reported an association between losses of chromosome 10 and clinical outcome: either progression-free survival (Hoang-Xuan et al. 2001; Sanson et al. 2002) or total survival (Walker et al. 2005) was reduced in patients with oligodendroglial tumors with this chromosomal alteration. However, one study did not find an association between reduced survival and losses of chromosome 10 (Cairncross et al. 1998).

EGFR amplifications are rare events in oligodendroglial tumors inversely associated with losses on 1p/19q (Diedrich et al. 1991; Wong et al. 1994; Reifenberger et al. 1996; Bigner et al. 1999). However, one study identified a few patients with OIII with *EGFR* amplifications that had reduced progression-free survival (Hoang-Xuan et al. 2001).

Prognostic markers that are not inversely linked to 1p/19q losses may be more attractive for identifying specific oligodendroglial subgroups with differing clinical outcome. Homozygous deletions of *CDKN2A* on 9p21 are predominately found in anaplastic oligodendroglial tumors with and without losses on 1p/19q (Reifenberger et al. 1994; Weber et al. 1996; Bigner et al. 1999; Kros et al. 1999; von Deimling et al. 2000; Kitange et al. 2005). Reduced survival was found in patients with OIII with homozygous deletions of *CDKN2A* (Cairncross et al. 1998). Reduced progression-free survival was observed in patients with OIII with homozygous deletions of 9p21 (McLendon et al. 2005). A trend toward an unfavorable outcome was seen in patients with OIII with homozygous deletions of *CDKN2A* (Hoang-Xuan et al. 2001). However, there is an older report that described losses on 9p to be inversely associated with losses on 1p/19q (Weber et al. 1996). In conclusion, deletions of *CDKN2A* on 9p21 may be a prognostic marker to separate different groups of OIII.

Gains on chromosome 8q were identified to be strongly associated with poor outcome in five patients with oligodendroglioma. Three of these patients demonstrated losses on 1p/19q as well. This finding indicates that there may be two subgroups of oligodendroglioma patients with 1p/19q losses that can be separated from each other by the presence or absence of gains on 8q (Kitange et al. 2005). However, these findings need to be confirmed by an independent study.

The fact that *IDH1* is the most frequently mutated gene in oligodendroglial tumors (Balss et al., 2008) raises the question of whether this alteration is of prognostic importance. However, currently no data is available.

2.7
Conclusions

In spite of impressive advances in the diagnostic approach to and therapy of oligodendroglial tumors, many aspects are not yet resolved. Morphological criteria need to be refined with emphasis on more committing guidelines for the diagnosis of oligoastrocytomas. Several aspects render the current concept of a mixed oligoastrocytomas questionable. Amongst them the genetic heterogeneity of this group with hallmarks either typical for astrocytomas or for oligodendrogliomas. Further, there is observation that there is little or no difference between the clinical course of oligodendroglioma and oligoastrocytomas both with combined losses of 1p/19q. We expect molecular analysis to become the major criterion for diagnosis of these tumors in the near future. Whether these analyses will target the t(1;19)(q10,p10) translocation, a putative fusion protein, an associated surrogate marker such as allelic losses, or putative tumor suppressor genes not yet identified will need to be established. The high interobserver variation in the diagnosis of oligodendroglial tumors is also due to the lack of an antigenic profile that clearly distinguishes oligodendroglial from astrocytic tumor cells and that can be used to identify these cells by immunohistochemical analyses on paraffin-embedded tissues. The WHO guidelines for distinction of anaplastic oligoastrocytomas from glioblastoma with oligodendroglial component are controversially discussed among neuropathologists and ongoing studies are expected to alter the current definitions. Given the diagnostic and predictive importance of 1p/19q losses, noninvasive methods for identification of oligodendroglial tumors with 1p/19q losses need to be refined.

References

Aguirre-Cruz L, Mokhtari K, Hoang-Xuan K, Marie Y, Criniere E, Taillibert S, Lopes M, Delattre JY, Sanson M (2004) Analysis of the bHLH transcription factors Olig1 and Olig2 in brain tumors. J Neurooncol 67:265–271

Alonso ME, Bello MJ, Arjona D, Martinez-Glez V, de Campos JM, Isla A, Kusak E, Vaquero J, Gutierrez M, Sarasa JL, Rey JA (2005) Real-time quantitative PCR analysis of gene dosages reveals gene amplification in low-grade oligodendrogliomas. Am J Clin Pathol 123:900–906

Anguelova E, Beuvon F, Leonard N, Chaverot N, Varlet P, Couraud PO, Daumas-Duport C, Cazaubon S (2005) Functional endothelin ET B receptors are selectively expressed in human oligodendrogliomas. Brain Res Mol Brain Res 137:77–88

Azzarelli B, Miravalle L, Vidal R (2004) Immunolocalization of the oligodendrocyte transcription factor 1 (Olig1) in brain tumors. J Neuropathol Exp Neurol 63:170–179

Bailey P, Bucy P (1929) Oligodendrogliomas of the brain. J Pathol Bacteriol 32:735–754

Bailey P, Cushing H (1926) A Classification of Tumors of the Glioma Group on a Histogenetic basis with a Correlation Study of Prognosis. Lippincott, Philadelphia

Balls J, Meyer J, Mueller W, Korshunov A, Hartmann C, von Deimling A (2008) Analysis of the IDH1 codon 132 mutation in brain tumors. Acta Neuropathol. 2008 Dec;116(6):597-602. Epub 2008 Nov 5

Beier D, Wischhusen J, Dietmaier W, Hau P, Proescholdt M, Brawanski A, Bogdahn U, Beier CP (2008) CD133 expression and cancer stem cells predict prognosis in high-grade oligodendroglial tumors. Brain Pathol 18:370–377

Bello MJ, Leone PE, Nebreda P, de Campos JM, Kusak ME, Vaquero J, Sarasa JL, Garcia-Miguel P, Queizan A, Hernandez-Moneo JL, et al. (1995a) Allelic status of chromosome 1 in neoplasms of the nervous system. Cancer Genet Cytogenet 83:160–164

Bello MJ, Leone PE, Vaquero J, de Campos JM, Kusak ME, Sarasa JL, Pestana A, Rey JA (1995b) Allelic loss at 1p and 19q frequently occurs in association and may represent early oncogenic events in oligodendroglial tumors. Int J Cancer 64:207–210

Bello MJ, Vaquero J, de Campos JM, Kusak ME, Sarasa JL, Saez-Castresana J, Pestana A, Rey JA (1994) Molecular analysis of chromosome 1 abnormalities in human gliomas reveals frequent loss of 1p in oligodendroglial tumors. Int J Cancer 57:172–175

Bigner SH, Matthews MR, Rasheed BK, Wiltshire RN, Friedman HS, Friedman AH, Stenzel TT, Dawes DM, McLendon RE, Bigner DD (1999) Molecular genetic aspects of oligodendrogliomas including analysis by comparative genomic hybridization. Am J Pathol 155:375–386

Bortolotto S, Chiado-Piat L, Cavalla P, Bosone I, Chio A, Mauro A, Schiffer D (2000) CDKN2A/p16 inactivation in the prognosis of oligodendrogliomas. Int J Cancer 88:554–557

Boulay JL, Miserez AR, Zweifel C, Sivasankaran B, Kana V, Ghaffari A, Luyken C, Sabel M, Zerrouqi A, Wasner M, Van Meir E, Tolnay M, Reifenberger G, Merlo A (2007) Loss of NOTCH2 positively predicts survival in subgroups of human glial brain tumors. PLoS ONE 2:e576

Brandes AA, Tosoni A, Cavallo G, Reni M, Franceschi E, Bonaldi L, Bertorelle R, Gardiman M, Ghimenton C, Iuzzolino P, Pession A, Blatt V, Ermani M (2006) Correlations between O6-methylguanine DNA methyltransferase promoter methylation status, 1p and 19q deletions, and response to temozolomide in anaplastic and recurrent oligodendroglioma: a prospective GICNO study. J Clin Oncol 24:4746–4753

Burger PC, Minn AY, Smith JS, Borell TJ, Jedlicka AE, Huntley BK, Goldthwaite PT, Jenkins RB, Feuerstein BG (2001) Losses of chromosomal arms 1p and 19q in the diagnosis of oligodendroglioma. A study of paraffin-embedded sections. Mod Pathol 14:842–853

Cairncross G, Berkey B, Shaw E, Jenkins R, Scheithauer B, Brachman D, Buckner J, Fink K, Souhami L, Laperierre N, Mehta M, Curran W (2006) Phase III trial of chemotherapy plus radiotherapy compared with radiotherapy alone for pure and mixed anaplastic oligodendroglioma: Intergroup Radiation Therapy Oncology Group Trial 9402. J Clin Oncol 24:2707–2714

Cairncross G, Macdonald D, Ludwin S, Lee D, Cascino T, Buckner J, Fulton D, Dropcho E, Stewart D, Schold C, Jr., et al. (1994) Chemotherapy for anaplastic oligodendroglioma. National Cancer Institute of Canada Clinical Trials Group. J Clin Oncol 12:2013–2021

Cairncross JG, Ueki K, Zlatescu MC, Lisle DK, Finkelstein DM, Hammond RR, Silver JS, Stark PC, Macdonald DR, Ino Y, Ramsay DA, Louis DN (1998) Specific genetic predictors of chemotherapeutic response and survival in patients with anaplastic oligodendrogliomas. J Natl Cancer Inst 90:1473–1479

Chahlavi A, Kanner A, Peereboom D, Staugaitis SM, Elson P, Barnett G (2003) Impact of chromosome 1p status in response of oligodendroglioma to temozolomide: preliminary results. J Neurooncol 61:267–273

Chin HW, Hazel JJ, Kim TH, Webster JH (1980) Oligodendrogliomas. I. A clinical study of cerebral oligodendrogliomas. Cancer 45:1458–1466

Coleman KE, Brat DJ, Cotsonis GA, Lawson D, Cohen C (2006) Proliferation (MIB-1 expression) in oligodendrogliomas: assessment of quantitative methods and prognostic significance. Appl Immunohistochem Mol Morphol 14:109–114

Cooke HJ (2004) Silence of the centromeres–not. Trends Biotechnol 22:319–321

Coons SW, Johnson PC, Scheithauer BW, Yates AJ, Pearl DK (1997) Improving diagnostic accuracy and interobserver concordance in the classification and grading of primary gliomas. Cancer 79:1381–1393

Dai C, Lyustikman Y, Shih A, Hu X, Fuller GN, Rosenblum M, Holland EC (2005) The characteristics of astrocytomas and oligodendrogliomas are caused by two distinct and interchangeable signaling formats. Neoplasia 7:397–406

Davis FG, Freels S, Grutsch J, Barlas S, Brem S (1998) Survival rates in patients with primary malignant brain tumors stratified by patient age and tumor histological type: an analysis based on Surveillance, Epidemiology, and End Results (SEER) data, 1973–1991. J Neurosurg 88:1–10

de la Monte SM (1989) Uniform lineage of oligodendrogliomas. Am J Pathol 135:529–540

Dehghani F, Schachenmar W, Laun A, Korf HW (1998) Prognostic implication of histopathological, immunohistochemical and clinical features of oligodendrogliomas: a study of 89 cases. Acta Neuropathol (Berl) 95:493–504

Diedrich U, Soja S, Behnke J, Zoll B (1991) Amplification of the c-erbB oncogene is associated with malignancy in primary tumours of neuroepithelial tissue. J Neurol 238:221–224

Dirks PB (2008) Brain tumor stem cells: bringing order to the chaos of brain cancer. J Clin Oncol 26:2916–2924

Dong ZQ, Pang JC, Tong CY, Zhou LF, Ng HK (2002) Clonality of oligoastrocytomas. Hum Pathol 33:528–535

Duerr EM, Rollbrocker B, Hayashi Y, Peters N, Meyer-Puttlitz B, Louis DN, Schramm J, Wiestler OD, Parsons R, Eng C, von Deimling A (1998) PTEN mutations in gliomas and glioneuronal tumors. Oncogene 16:2259–2264

Fan X, Salford LG, Widegren B (2007) Glioma stem cells: Evidence and limitation. Semin Cancer Biol 17:214–218

Ferraresi S, Servello D, De Lorenzi L, Allegranza A (1989) Familial frontal lobe oligodendroglioma. Case report. J Neurosurg Sci 33:317–318

Fuller GN, Hess KR, Rhee CH, Yung WK, Sawaya RA, Bruner JM, Zhang W (2002) Molecular classification of human diffuse gliomas by multidimensional scaling analysis of gene expression profiles parallels morphology-based classification, correlates with survival, and reveals clinically-relevant novel glioma subsets. Brain Pathol 12:108–116

Gadji M, Tsanaclis A-M, Fortin D, Drouin R (2008) Aneuploidy and chromosomal instability in gliomas. Proceedings of the 99th Annual Meeting of the American Association for Cancer Research; Apr 12–16, 2008; Philadelphia (PA): AACR; 2008. Abstract nr 4331

Gannett DE, Wisbeck WM, Silbergeld DL, Berger MS (1994) The role of postoperative irradiation in the treatment of oligodendroglioma. Int J Radiat Oncol Biol Phys 30:567–573

Geisbrecht BV, Gould SJ (1999) The human PICD gene encodes a cytoplasmic and peroxisomal NADP(+)-dependent isocitrate dehydrogenase. J Biol Chem 274:30527–30533

Giannini C, Burger PC, Berkey BA, Cairncross JG, Jenkins RB, Mehta M, Curran WJ, Aldape K (2008) Anaplastic oligodendroglial tumors: refining the correlation among histopathology, 1p 19q deletion and clinical outcome in Intergroup Radiation Therapy Oncology Group Trial 9402. Brain Pathol 18:360–369

Giannini C, Scheithauer BW, Weaver AL, Burger PC, Kros JM, Mork S, Graeber MB, Bauserman S, Buckner JC, Burton J, Riepe R, Tazelaar HD, Nascimento AG, Crotty T, Keeney GL, Pernicone P, Altermatt H (2001) Oligodendrogliomas: reproducibility and prognostic value of histologic diagnosis and grading. J Neuropathol Exp Neurol 60:248–262

Ginsberg LE, Fuller GN, Hashmi M, Leeds NE, Schomer DF (1998) The significance of lack of MR contrast enhancement of supratentorial brain tumors in adults: histopathological evaluation of a series. Surg Neurol 49:436–440

Giordana MT, Mauro A, Soffietti R, Leone M (1981) Association between multiple sclerosis and oligodendroglioma. Case report. Ital J Neurol Sci 2:403–409

Greenfield JG, Graham DI, Lantos PL (2002) Greenfield's neuropathology. Arnold, London/New York

Griffin CA, Burger P, Morsberger L, Yonescu R, Swierczynski S, Weingart JD, Murphy KM (2006) Identification of der(1;19)(q10;p10) in Five Oligodendrogliomas Suggests Mechanism of Concurrent 1p and 19q Loss. J Neuropathol Exp Neurol 65:988–994

Hart MN, Petito CK, Earle KM (1974) Mixed gliomas. Cancer 33:134–140

Hartmann C, Johnk L, Kitange G, Wu Y, Ashworth LK, Jenkins RB, Louis DN (2002) Transcript map of the 3.7-Mb D19S112-D19S246 candidate tumor suppressor region on the long arm of chromosome 19. Cancer Res 62:4100–4108

Hartmann C, Mueller W, Lass U, Kamel-Reid S, von Deimling A (2005) Molecular genetic analysis of oligodendroglial tumors. J Neuropathol Exp Neurol 64:10–14

Hartmann C, Mueller W, Lass U, Stockhammer F, von Eckardstein K, Veelken J, Jeuken J, Wick W, von Deimling A (2003) No preferential loss of paternal 19q alleles in oligodendroglial tumors. Ann Neurol 54:256–258

Hartmann C, Mueller W, von Deimling A (2004) Pathology and molecular genetics of oligodendroglial tumors. J Mol Med 82:638–655

He J, Mokhtari K, Sanson M, Marie Y, Kujas M, Huguet S, Leuraud P, Capelle L, Delattre JY, Poirier J, Hoang-Xuan K (2001) Glioblastomas with an oligodendroglial component: a pathological and molecular study. J Neuropathol Exp Neurol 60:863–871

Heegaard S, Sommer HM, Broholm H, Broendstrup O (1995) Proliferating cell nuclear antigen and Ki-67 immunohistochemistry of oligodendrogliomas with special reference to prognosis. Cancer 76:1809–1813

Hegi ME, Diserens AC, Gorlia T, Hamou MF, de Tribolet N, Weller M, Kros JM, Hainfellner JA, Mason W, Mariani L, Bromberg JE, Hau P, Mirimanoff RO, Cairncross JG, Janzer RC, Stupp R (2005) MGMT gene silencing and benefit from temozolomide in glioblastoma. N Engl J Med 352:997–1003

Herbarth B, Meissner H, Westphal M, Wegner M (1998) Absence of polyomavirus JC in glial brain tumors and glioma-derived cell lines. Glia 22:415–420

Hoang-Xuan K, Aguirre-Cruz L, Mokhtari K, Marie Y, Sanson M (2002) OLIG-1 and 2 gene expression and oligodendroglial tumours. Neuropathol Appl Neurobiol 28:89–94

Hoang-Xuan K, Capelle L, Kujas M, Taillibert S, Duffau H, Lejeune J, Polivka M, Criniere E, Marie Y, Mokhtari K, Carpentier AF, Laigle F, Simon JM, Cornu P, Broet P, Sanson M, Delattre JY (2004) Temozolomide as initial treatment for adults with low-grade oligodendrogliomas or oligoastrocytomas and correlation with chromosome 1p deletions. J Clin Oncol 22:3133–3138

Hoang-Xuan K, He J, Huguet S, Mokhtari K, Marie Y, Kujas M, Leuraud P, Capelle L, Delattre JY, Poirier J, Broet P, Sanson M (2001) Molecular heterogeneity of oligodendrogliomas suggests alternative pathways in tumor progression. Neurology 57:1278–1281

Homma T, Fukushima T, Vaccarella S, Yonekawa Y, Di Patre PL, Franceschi S, Ohgaki H (2006) Correlation among pathology, genotype, and patient outcomes in glioblastoma. J Neuropathol Exp Neurol 65:846–854

Hong C, Bollen AW, Costello JF (2003) The contribution of genetic and epigenetic mechanisms to gene silencing in oligodendrogliomas. Cancer Res 63:7600–7605

Houillier C, Lejeune J, Benouaich-Amiel A, Laigle-Donadey F, Criniere E, Mokhtari K, Thillet J, Delattre JY, Hoang-Xuan K, Sanson M (2006) Prognostic impact of molecular markers in a series of 220 primary glioblastomas. Cancer 106:2218–2223

Huang CI, Chiou WH, Ho DM (1987) Oligodendroglioma occurring after radiation therapy for pituitary adenoma. J Neurol Neurosurg Psychiatry 50:1619–1624

Huang H, Reis R, Yonekawa Y, Lopes JM, Kleihues P, Ohgaki H (1999) Identification in human brain tumors of DNA sequences specific for SV40 large T antigen. Brain Pathol 9:33–42

Husemann K, Wolter M, Buschges R, Bostrom J, Sabel M, Reifenberger G (1999) Identification of two distinct deleted regions on the short arm of chromosome 1 and rare mutation of the CDKN2C gene from 1p32 in oligodendroglial tumors. J Neuropathol Exp Neurol 58:1041–1050

Ichimura K, Vogazianou AP, Liu L, Pearson DM, Backlund LM, Plant K, Baird K, Langford CF, Gregory SG, Collins VP (2008) 1p36 is a preferential target of chromosome 1 deletions in astrocytic tumours and homozygously deleted in a subset of glioblastomas. Oncogene 27:2097–2108

Idbaih A, Marie Y, Pierron G, Brennetot C, Hoang-Xuan K, Kujas M, Mokhtari K, Sanson M, Lejeune J, Aurias A, Delattre O, Delattre JY (2005) Two types of chromosome 1p losses with opposite significance in gliomas. Ann Neurol 58:483–487

Ino Y, Betensky RA, Zlatescu MC, Sasaki H, Macdonald DR, Stemmer-Rachamimov AO, Ramsay DA, Cairncross JG, Louis DN (2001) Molecular subtypes of anaplastic oligodendroglioma: implications for patient management at diagnosis. Clin Cancer Res 7:839–845

Ironside JW, Moss TH, Louis DN, Lowe JS, Well RO (2002) Diagnostic Pathology of Nervous System Tumours. Churchill Livingstone, London

Jaskolsky D, Zawirski M, Papierz W, Kotwica Z (1987) Mixed gliomas. Their clinical course and results of surgery. Zentralbl Neurochir 48:120–123

Jenkins R, Blair H, Flynn H, Passe S, Law M, Ballman K, Giannini C, Buckner JC (2006) A t(1;19)(q10;p10) mediates the combined deletions of 1p and 19q in human oligodendrogliomas. In: 16th Biennial International Brain Tumor Research and Therapy Meeting, Silverado Resort ans Spa, Napa Valley, CA

Jennings GT, Minard KI, McAlister-Henn L (1997) Expression and mutagenesis of mammalian cytosolic NADP+-speciWc isocitrate dehydrogenase. Biochemistry 36:13743–13747

Jeuken JW, Nelen MR, Vermeer H, van Staveren WC, Kremer H, van Overbeeke JJ, Boerman RH (2000) PTEN mutation analysis in two genetic subtypes of high-grade oligodendroglial tumors. PTEN is only occasionally mutated in one of the two genetic subtypes. Cancer Genet Cytogenet 119:42–47

Jeuken JW, Sprenger SH, Wesseling P, Macville MV, von Deimling A, Teepen HL, van Overbeeke JJ, Boerman RH (1999) Identification of subgroups of high-grade oligodendroglial tumors by comparative genomic hybridization. J Neuropathol Exp Neurol 58:606–612

Kashima T, Tiu SN, Merrill JE, Vinters HV, Dawson G, Campagnoni AT (1993) Expression of oligodendrocyte-associated genes in cell lines derived from human gliomas and neuroblastomas. Cancer Res 53:170–175

Kennedy PG, Watkins BA, Thomas DG, Noble MD (1987) Antigenic expression by cells derived from human gliomas does not correlate with morphological classification. Neuropathol Appl Neurobiol 13:327–347

Kim L, Hochberg FH, Thornton AF, Harsh GRt, Patel H, Finkelstein D, Louis DN (1996) Procarbazine, lomustine, and vincristine (PCV) chemotherapy for grade III and grade IV oligoastrocytomas. J Neurosurg 85:602–607

Kim S, Dougherty ER, Shmulevich L, Hess KR, Hamilton SR, Trent JM, Fuller GN, Zhang W (2002) Identification of combination gene sets for glioma classification. Mol Cancer Ther 1:1229–1236

Kim SY, Lee SM, Tak JK et al (2007) Regulation of singlet oxygen-induced apoptosis by cytosolic NADP+-dependent isocitrate dehydrogenase. Mol Cell Biochem 302:27–34

Kitange G, Misra A, Law M, Passe S, Kollmeyer TM, Maurer M, Ballman K, Feuerstein BG, Jenkins RB (2005) Chromosomal imbalances detected by array comparative genomic hybridization in human oligodendrogliomas and mixed oligoastrocytomas. Genes Chromosomes Cancer 42:68–77

Kleihues P, Zulch KJ, Matsumoto S, Radke U (1970) Morphology of malignant gliomas induced in rabbits by systemic application of N-methyl-N-nitrosourea. Z Neurol 198:65–78

Kouwenhoven MC, Kros JM, French PJ, Biemond-Ter Stege EM, Graveland WJ, Taphoorn MJ, Brandes AA, van den Bent MJ (2006) 1p/19q loss within oligodendroglioma is predictive for response to first line temozolomide but not to salvage treatment. Eur J Cancer 42:2499–2503

Kraus JA, Koopmann J, Kaskel P, Maintz D, Brandner S, Schramm J, Louis DN, Wiestler OD, von Deimling A (1995) Shared allelic losses on chromosomes 1p and 19q suggest a common origin of oligodendroglioma and oligoastrocytoma. J Neuropathol Exp Neurol 54:91–95

Kraus JA, Lamszus K, Glesmann N, Beck M, Wolter M, Sabel M, Krex D, Klockgether T, Reifenberger G, Schlegel U (2001) Molecular genetic alterations in glioblastomas with oligodendroglial component. Acta Neuropathol (Berl) 101:311–320

Krex D, Klink B, Hartmann C, von Deimling A, Pietsch T, Simon M, Sabel M, Steinbach J, Heese O, Reifenberger G, Weller M, Schackert G, Network TGG (2007) Long-term survival with glioblastoma multiforme. Brain 130:2596–2606

Kros JM, Lie ST, Stefanko SZ (1994) Familial occurrence of polymorphous oligodendroglioma. Neurosurgery 34:732–736; discussion 736

Kros JM, van Run PR, Alers JC, Beverloo HB, van den Bent MJ, Avezaat CJ, van Dekken H (1999) Genetic aberrations in oligodendroglial tumours: an analysis using comparative genomic hybridization (CGH). J Pathol 188:282–288

Kunitz A, Wolter M, van den Boom J, Felsberg J, Tews B, Hahn M, Benner A, Sabel M, Lichter P, Reifenberger G, von Deimling A, Hartmann C (2007) DNA hypermethylation and Aberrant Expression of the EMP3 Gene at 19q13.3 in Human Gliomas. Brain Pathol 17:363–370

Landry CF, Verity MA, Cherman L, Kashima T, Black K, Yates A, Campagnoni AT (1997) Expression of oligodendrocytic mRNAs in glial tumors: changes associated with tumor grade and extent of neoplastic infiltration. Cancer Res 57:4098–4104

Lebrun C, Fontaine D, Ramaioli A, Vandenbos F, Chanalet S, Lonjon M, Michiels JF, Bourg V, Paquis P, Chatel M, Frenay M (2004) Long-term outcome of oligodendrogliomas. Neurology 62:1783–1787

Lee YY, Van Tassel P (1989) Intracranial oligodendrogliomas: imaging findings in 35 untreated cases. AJR Am J Roentgenol 152:361–369

Lee SM, Koh HJ, Park DC et al (2002) Cytosolic NADP(+)-dependent isocitrate dehydrogenase status modulates oxidative damage to cells. Free Radic Biol Med 32:1185–1196

Levin N, Lavon I, Zelikovitsh B, Fuchs D, Bokstein F, Fellig Y, Siegal T (2006) Progressive low-grade oligodendrogliomas: response to temozolomide and correlation between genetic profile and O6-methylguanine DNA methyltransferase protein expression. Cancer 106:1759–1765

Li KK, Pang JC, Chung NY, Ng YL, Chan NH, Zhou L, Poon WS, Ng HK (2007) EMP3 overexpression is associated with oligodendroglial tumors retaining chromosome arms 1p and 19q. Int J Cancer 120:947–950

Ligon KL, Alberta JA, Kho AT, Weiss J, Kwaan MR, Nutt CL, Louis DN, Stiles CD, Rowitch DH (2004) The oligodendroglial lineage marker OLIG2 is universally expressed in diffuse gliomas. J Neuropathol Exp Neurol 63:499–509

Louis D, Ohgaki H, Wiestler O, Cavenee W (eds) (2007) World Health Organization Classification of Tumours of the Central Nervous System. IARC, Lyon

Lu QR, Park JK, Noll E, Chan JA, Alberta J, Yuk D, Alzamora MG, Louis DN, Stiles CD, Rowitch DH, Black PM (2001) Oligodendrocyte lineage genes (OLIG) as molecular markers for human glial brain tumors. Proc Natl Acad Sci USA 98:10851–10856

Ludwig CL, Smith MT, Godfrey AD, Armbrustmacher VW (1986) A clinicopathological study of 323 patients with oligodendrogliomas. Ann Neurol 19:15–21

Maegawa S, Yoshioka H, Itaba N, Kubota N, Nishihara S, Shirayoshi Y, Nanba E, Oshimura M (2001) Epigenetic silencing of PEG3 gene expression in human glioma cell lines. Mol Carcinog 31:1–9

Magnani I, Moroni RF, Roversi G, Beghini A, Pfundt R, Schoenmakers EF, Larizza L (2005) Identification of oligodendroglioma specific chromosomal copy number changes in the glioblastoma MI-4 cell line by array-CGH and FISH analyses. Cancer Genet Cytogenet 161:140–145

Maintz D, Fiedler K, Koopmann J, Rollbrocker B, Nechev S, Lenartz D, Stangl AP, Louis DN, Schramm J, Wiestler OD, von Deimling A (1997) Molecular genetic evidence for subtypes of oligoastrocytomas. J Neuropathol Exp Neurol 56:1098–1104

Marie Y, Sanson M, Mokhtari K, Leuraud P, Kujas M, Delattre JY, Poirier J, Zalc B, Hoang-Xuan K (2001) OLIG2 as a specific marker of oligodendroglial tumour cells. Lancet 358:298–300

McDonald JM, See SJ, Tremont IW, Colman H, Gilbert MR, Groves M, Burger PC, Louis DN, Giannini C, Fuller G, Passe S, Blair H, Jenkins RB, Yang H, Ledoux A, Aaron J, Tipnis U, Zhang W, Hess K, Aldape K (2005) The prognostic impact of histology and 1p/19q status in anaplastic oligodendroglial tumors. Cancer 104:1468–1477

McLendon RE, Herndon JE, 2nd, West B, Reardon D, Wiltshire R, Rasheed BK, Quinn J, Friedman HS, Friedman AH, Bigner DD (2005) Survival analysis of presumptive prognostic markers among oligodendrogliomas. Cancer 104:1693–1699

Miller CR, Dunham CP, Scheithauer BW, Perry A (2006) Significance of necrosis in grading of oligodendroglial neoplasms: a clinicopathologic and genetic study of newly diagnosed high-grade gliomas. J Clin Oncol 24:5419–5426

Mokhtari K, Paris S, Aguirre-Cruz L, Privat N, Criniere E, Marie Y, Hauw JJ, Kujas M, Rowitch D, Hoang-Xuan K, Delattre JY, Sanson M (2005) Olig2 expression, GFAP, p53 and 1p loss analysis contribute to glioma subclassification. Neuropathol Appl Neurobiol 31:62–69

Mork SJ, Halvorsen TB, Lindegaard KF, Eide GE (1986) Oligodendroglioma. Histologic evaluation and prognosis. J Neuropathol Exp Neurol 45:65–78

Mueller W, Hartmann C, Hoffmann A, Lanksch W, Kiwit J, Tonn J, Veelken J, Schramm J, Weller M, Wiestler OD, Louis DN, von Deimling A (2002) Genetic signature of oligoastrocytomas correlates with tumor location and denotes distinct molecular subsets. Am J Pathol 161:313–319

Mukasa A, Ueki K, Ge X, Ishikawa S, Ide T, Fujimaki T, Nishikawa R, Asai A, Kirino T, Aburatani H (2004) Selective expression of a subset of neuronal genes in oligodendroglioma with chromosome 1p loss. Brain Pathol 14:34–42

Mukasa A, Ueki K, Matsumoto S, Tsutsumi S, Nishikawa R, Fujimaki T, Asai A, Kirino T, Aburatani H (2002) Distinction in gene expression profiles of oligodendrogliomas with and without allelic loss of 1p. Oncogene 21:3961–3968

Nutt CL, Betensky RsA, Brower MA, Batchelor TT, Louis DN, Stemmer-Rachamimov AO (2005) YKL-40 is a differential diagnostic marker for histologic subtypes of high-grade gliomas. Clin Cancer Res 11:2258–2264

Nutt CL, Mani DR, Betensky RA, Tamayo P, Cairncross JG, Ladd C, Pohl U, Hartmann C, McLaughlin ME, Batchelor TT, Black PM, von Deimling A, Pomeroy SL, Golub TR, Louis DN (2003) Gene expression-based classification of malignant gliomas correlates better with survival than histological classification. Cancer Res 63:1602–1607

Ohgaki H, Eibl RH, Wiestler OD, Yasargil MG, Newcomb EW, Kleihues P (1991) p53 mutations in nonastrocytic human brain tumors. Cancer Res 51:6202–6205

Ohnishi A, Sawa H, Tsuda M, Sawamura Y, Itoh T, Iwasaki Y, Nagashima K (2003) Expression of the oligodendroglial lineage-associated markers Olig1 and Olig2 in different types of human gliomas. J Neuropathol Exp Neurol 62:1052–1059

Okamoto H, Li J, Glasker S, Vortmeyer AO, Jaffe H, Robison RA, Bogler O, Mikkelsen T, Lubensky IA, Oldfield EH, Zhuang Z (2007) Proteomic Comparison of Oligodendrogliomas with and without 1pLOH. Cancer Biol Ther 6

Olson JD, Riedel E, DeAngelis LM (2000) Long-term outcome of low-grade oligodendroglioma and mixed glioma. Neurology 54:1442–1448

Parsons DW, Jones S, Zhang X et al (2008) An integrated genomic analysis of human glioblastoma multiforme. Science 321:1807–1812

Perentes E, Rubinstein LJ (1987) Recent applications of immunoperoxidase histochemistry in human neuro-oncology. An update. Arch Pathol Lab Med 111:796–812

Perez-Diaz C, Cabello A, Lobato RD, Rivas JJ, Cabrera A (1985) Oligodendrogliomas arising in the scar of a brain contusion. Report of two surgically verified cases. Surg Neurol 24:581–586

Pohl U, Cairncross JG, Louis DN (1999) Homozygous deletions of the CDKN2C/p18INK4C gene on the short arm of chromosome 1 in anaplastic oligodendrogliomas. Brain Pathol 9:639–643

Puduvalli VK, Hashmi M, McAllister LD, Levin VA, Hess KR, Prados M, Jaeckle KA, Yung WK, Buys SS, Bruner JM, Townsend JJ, Davis R, Sawaya R, Kyritsis AP (2003) Anaplastic oligodendrogliomas: prognostic factors for tumor recurrence and survival. Oncology 65:259–266

Qu M, Olofsson T, Sigurdardottir S, You C, Kalimo H, Nister M, Smits A, Ren ZP (2007) Genetically distinct astrocytic and oligodendroglial components in oligoastrocytomas. Acta Neuropathol (Berl) 113:129–136

RaV MC, Miller RH, Noble M (1983) A glial progenitor cell that develops in vitro into an astrocyte or an oligodendrocyte depending on culture medium. Nature 303:390–396

Reifenberger G, Louis DN (2003) Oligodendroglioma: toward molecular definitions in diagnostic neuro-oncology. J Neuropathol Exp Neurol 62:111–126

Reifenberger J, Reifenberger G, Ichimura K, Schmidt EE, Wechsler W, Collins VP (1996) Epidermal growth factor receptor expression in oligodendroglial tumors. Am J Pathol 149:29–35

Reifenberger J, Reifenberger G, Liu L, James CD, Wechsler W, Collins VP (1994) Molecular genetic analysis of oligodendroglial tumors shows preferential allelic deletions on 19q and 1p. Am J Pathol 145:1175–1190

Riemenschneider MJ, Reifenberger J, Reifenberger G (2008) Frequent biallelic inactivation and transcriptional silencing of the DIRAS3 gene at 1p31 in oligodendroglial tumors with 1p loss. Int J Cancer 122:2503–2510

Rijpkema M, Schuuring J, van der Meulen Y, van der Graaf M, Bernsen H, Boerman R, van der Kogel A, Heerschap A (2003) Characterization of oligodendrogliomas using short echo time 1H MR spectroscopic imaging. NMR Biomed 16:12–18

Rodriguez FJ, Scheithauer BW, Jenkins R, Burger PC, Rudzinskiy P, Vlodavsky E, Schooley A, Landolfi J (2007) Gliosarcoma Arising in Oligodendroglial Tumors ("Oligosarcoma"): A Clinicopathologic Study. Am J Surg Pathol 31:351–362

Sanson M, Leuraud P, Aguirre-Cruz L, He J, Marie Y, Cartalat-Carel S, Mokhtari K, Duffau H, Delattre JY, Hoang-Xuan K (2002) Analysis of loss of chromosome 10q, DMBT1 homozygous deletions, and PTEN mutations in oligodendrogliomas. J Neurosurg 97:1397–1401

Sasaki H, Zlatescu MC, Betensky RA, Ino Y, Cairncross JG, Louis DN (2001) PTEN is a target of chromosome 10q loss in anaplastic oligodendrogliomas and PTEN alterations are associated with poor prognosis. Am J Pathol 159:359–367

Sasaki H, Zlatescu MC, Betensky RA, Johnk LB, Cutone AN, Cairncross JG, Louis DN (2002) Histopathological-molecular genetic correlations in referral pathologist-diagnosed low-grade "oligodendroglioma". J Neuropathol Exp Neurol 61:58–63

Schiffer D, Bosone I, Dutto A, Di Vito N, Chio A (1999) The prognostic role of vessel productive changes and vessel density in oligodendroglioma. J Neurooncol 44:99–107

Schiffer D, Dutto A, Cavalla P, Bosone I, Chio A, Villani R, Bellotti C (1997) Prognostic factors in oligodendroglioma. Can J Neurol Sci 24:313–319

Sega S, Horvat A, Popovic M (2006) Anaplastic oligodendroglioma and gliomatosis type 2 in interferon-beta treated multiple sclerosis patients. Report of two cases. Clin Neurol Neurosurg 108:259–265

Shaw EG, Scheithauer BW, O'Fallon JR, Tazelaar HD, Davis DH (1992) Oligodendrogliomas: the Mayo Clinic experience. J Neurosurg 76:428–434

Shimizu KT, Tran LM, Mark RJ, Selch MT (1993) Management of oligodendrogliomas. Radiology 186:569–572

Shoshan Y, Nishiyama A, Chang A, Mork S, Barnett GH, Cowell JK, Trapp BD, Staugaitis SM (1999) Expression of oligodendrocyte progenitor cell antigens by gliomas: implications for the histogenesis of brain tumors. Proc Natl Acad Sci USA 96:10361–10366

Smith JS, Perry A, Borell TJ, Lee HK, O'Fallon J, Hosek SM, Kimmel D, Yates A, Burger PC, Scheithauer BW, Jenkins RB (2000) Alterations of chromosome arms 1p and 19q as predictors of survival in oligodendrogliomas, astrocytomas, and mixed oligoastrocytomas. J Clin Oncol 18:636–645

Smith SF, Simpson JM, Brewer JA, Sekhon LH, Biggs MT, Cook RJ, Little NS (2006) The presence of necrosis and/or microvascular proliferation does not influence survival of patients with anaplastic oligodendroglial tumours: review of 98 patients. J Neurooncol 80(1):75–82

Soundar S, Danek BL, Colman RF (2000) IdentiWcation by mutagenesis of arginines in the substrate binding site of the porcine NADP-dependent isocitrate dehydrogenase. J Biol Chem 275:5606–5612

Stockhammer F, Thomale U, Plotkin M, Hartmann C, von Deimling A (2007) Association between fluorine-18-labeled fluorodeoxyglucose uptake and 1p and 19q loss of heterozygosity in World Health Organization Grade II gliomas. J Neurosurg 106:633–637

Sun ZM, Genka S, Shitara N, Akanuma A, Takakura K (1988) Factors possibly influencing the prognosis of oligodendroglioma. Neurosurgery 22:886–891

Tanaka J, Hokama Y, Nakamura H (1988) Myelin basic protein as a possible marker for oligodendroglioma. Acta Pathol Jpn 38:1297–1303

Tews B, Felsberg J, Hartmann C, Kunitz A, Hahn M, Toedt G, Neben K, Hummerich L, von Deimling A, Reifenberger G, Lichter P (2006) Identification of novel oligodendroglioma-associated candidate tumor suppressor genes in 1p36 and 19q13 using microarray-based expression profiling. Int J Cancer 119:792–800

Tews B, Roerig P, Hartmann C, Hahn M, Felsberg J, Blaschke B, Sabel M, Kunitz A, Toedt G, Neben K, Benner A, Deimling AV, Reifenberger G, Lichter P (2007) Hypermethylation and transcriptional downregulation of the CITED4 gene at 1p34.2 in oligodendroglial tumours with allelic losses on 1p and 19q. Oncogene

Thiessen B, Maguire JA, McNeil K, Huntsman D, Martin MA, Horsman D (2003) Loss of heterozygosity for loci on chromosome arms 1p and 10q in oligodendroglial tumors: relationship to outcome and chemosensitivity. J Neurooncol 64:271–278

Tice H, Barnes PD, Goumnerova L, Scott RM, Tarbell NJ (1993) Pediatric and adolescent oligodendrogliomas. AJNR Am J Neuroradiol 14:1293–1300

Triebels VH, Taphoorn MJ, Brandes AA, Menten J, Frenay M, Tosoni A, Kros JM, Stege EB, Enting RH, Allgeier A, van Heuvel I, van den Bent MJ (2004) Salvage PCV chemotherapy for temozolomide-resistant oligodendrogliomas. Neurology 63:904–906

Ueki K, Nishikawa R, Nakazato Y, Hirose T, Hirato J, Funada N, Fujimaki T, Hojo S, Kubo O, Ide T, Usui M, Ochiai C, Ito S, Takahashi H, Mukasa A, Asai A, Kirino T (2002) Correlation of histology and molecular genetic analysis of 1p, 19q, 10q, TP53, EGFR, CDK4, and CDKN2A in 91 astrocytic and oligodendroglial tumors. Clin Cancer Res 8:196–201

van den Bent MJ, Carpentier AF, Brandes AA, Sanson M, Taphoorn MJ, Bernsen HJ, Frenay M, Tijssen CC, Grisold W, Sipos L, Haaxma-Reiche H, Kros JM, van Kouwenhoven MC, Vecht CJ, Allgeier A, Lacombe D, Gorlia T (2006) Adjuvant procarbazine, lomustine, and vincristine improves progression-free survival but not overall survival in newly diagnosed anaplastic oligodendrogliomas and oligoastrocytomas: a randomized European Organisation for Research and Treatment of Cancer phase III trial. J Clin Oncol 24:2715–2722

van den Bent MJ, Kros JM, Heimans JJ, Pronk LC, van Groeningen CJ, Krouwer HG, Taphoorn MJ, Zonnenberg BA, Tijssen CC, Twijnstra A, Punt CJ, Boogerd W (1998) Response rate and prognostic factors of recurrent oligodendroglioma treated with procarbazine, CCNU, and vincristine chemotherapy. Dutch Neuro-oncology Group. Neurology 51:1140–1145

Van Den Bent MJ, Looijenga LH, Langenberg K, Dinjens W, Graveland W, Uytdewilligen L, Sillevis Smitt PA, Jenkins RB, Kros JM (2003) Chromosomal anomalies in oligodendroglial tumors are correlated with clinical features. Cancer 97:1276–1284

van Dijk MC, Rombout PD, Boots-Sprenger SH, Straatman H, Bernsen MR, Ruiter DJ, Jeuken JW (2005) Multiplex ligation-dependent probe amplification for the detection of chromosomal gains and losses in formalin-fixed tissue. Diagn Mol Pathol 14:9–16

von Deimling A, Bender B, Jahnke R, Waha A, Kraus J, Albrecht S, Wellenreuther R, Fassbender F, Nagel J, Menon AG, Louis DN, Lenartz D, Schramm J, Wiestler OD (1994) Loci associated with malignant progression in astrocytomas: A candidate on chromosome 19q. Cancer Research 54:1397–1401

von Deimling A, Fimmers R, Schmidt MC, Bender B, Fassbender F, Nagel J, Jahnke R, Kaskel P, Duerr EM, Koopmann J, Maintz D, Steinbeck S, Wick W, Platten M, Muller DJ, Przkora R, Waha A, Blumcke B, Wellenreuther R, Meyer-Puttlitz B, Schmidt O, Mollenhauer J, Poustka A, Stangl AP, Lenartz D, von Ammon K (2000) Comprehensive allelotype and genetic anaysis of 466 human nervous system tumors. J Neuropathol Exp Neurol 59:544–558

von Deimling A, Louis DN, von Ammon K, Petersen I, Wiestler OD, Seizinger BR (1992) Evidence for a tumor suppressor gene on chromosome 19q associated with human astrocytomas, oligodendrogliomas, and mixed gliomas. Cancer Res 52:4277–4279

Walker C, du Plessis DG, Joyce KA, Fildes D, Gee A, Haylock B, Husband D, Smith T, Broome J, Warnke PC (2005) Molecular pathology and clinical characteristics of oligodendroglial neoplasms. Ann Neurol 57:855–865

Watanabe T, Nakamura M, Kros JM, Burkhard C, Yonekawa Y, Kleihues P, Ohgaki H (2002) Phenotype versus genotype correlation in oligodendrogliomas and low-grade diffuse astrocytomas. Acta Neuropathol (Berl) 103:267–275

Watanabe T, Nakamura M, Yonekawa Y, Kleihues P, Ohgaki H (2001a) Promoter hypermethylation and homozygous deletion of the p14ARF and p16INK4a genes in oligodendrogliomas. Acta Neuropathol (Berl) 101:185–189

Watanabe T, Yokoo H, Yokoo M, Yonekawa Y, Kleihues P, Ohgaki H (2001b) Concurrent inactivation of RB1 and TP53 pathways in anaplastic oligodendrogliomas. J Neuropathol Exp Neurol 60:1181–1189

Watson MA, Perry A, Budhjara V, Hicks C, Shannon WD, Rich KM (2001) Gene expression profiling with oligonucleotide microarrays distinguishes World Health Organization grade of oligodendrogliomas. Cancer Res 61:1825–1829

Weber RG, Sabel M, Reifenberger J, Sommer C, Oberstrass J, Reifenberger G, Kiessling M, Cremer T (1996) Characterization of genomic alterations associated with glioma progression by comparative genomic hybridization. Oncogene 13:983–994

Weller M, Berger H, Hartmann C, Schramm J, Westphal M, Simon M, Goldbrunner R, Krex D, Steinbach J, Ostertag C, Loeffler M, Pietsch T, von Deimling A (2007) Combined 1p/19q loss in oligodendroglial tumors: predictive or prognostic biomarker? Clin Cancer Res 13:6933–6937

Wharton SB, Hamilton FA, Chan WK, Chan KK, Anderson JR (1998) Proliferation and cell death in oligodendrogliomas. Neuropathol Appl Neurobiol 24:21–28

Wharton SB, Maltby E, Jellinek DA, Levy D, Atkey N, Hibberd S, Crimmins D, Stoeber K, Williams GH (2007) Subtypes of oligodendroglioma defined by 1p,19q deletions, differ in the proportion of apoptotic cells but not in replication-licensed non-proliferating cells. Acta Neuropathol (Berl) 113:119–127

White ML, Zhang Y, Kirby P, Ryken TC (2005) Can tumor contrast enhancement be used as a criterion for differentiating tumor grades of oligodendrogliomas? AJNR Am J Neuroradiol 26:784–790

Winger MJ, Macdonald DR, Cairncross JG (1989) Supratentorial anaplastic gliomas in adults The prognostic importance of extent of resection and prior low-grade glioma. J Neurosurg 71:487–493

Wolter M, Reifenberger J, Blaschke B, Ichimura K, Schmidt EE, Collins VP, Reifenberger G (2001) Oligodendroglial tumors frequently demonstrate hypermethylation of the CDKN2A (MTS1, p16INK4a), p14ARF, and CDKN2B (MTS2, p15INK4b) tumor suppressor genes. J Neuropathol Exp Neurol 60:1170–1180

Wong AJ, Zoltick PW, Moscatello DK (1994) The molecular biology and molecular genetics of astrocytic neoplasms. Semin Oncol 21:139–148

Xu M, See SJ, Ng WH, Arul E, Back MF, Yeo TT, Lim CC (2005) Comparison of magnetic resonance spectroscopy and perfusion-weighted imaging in presurgical grading of oligodendroglial tumors. Neurosurgery 56:919–926; discussion 919–926

Yeh SA, Lee TC, Chen HJ, Lui CC, Sun LM, Wang CJ, Huang EY (2002) Treatment outcomes and prognostic factors of patients with supratentorial low-grade oligodendroglioma. Int J Radiat Oncol Biol Phys 54:1405–1409

Yi L, Zhou ZH, Ping YF, Chen JH, Yao XH, Feng H, Lu JY, Wang JM, Bian XW (2007) Isolation and characterization of stem cell-like precursor cells from primary human anaplastic oligoastrocytoma. Mod Pathol 20:1061–1068

Yu Y, Xu F, Peng H, Fang X, Zhao S, Li Y, Cuevas B, Kuo WL, Gray JW, Siciliano M, Mills GB, Bast RC, Jr. (1999) NOEY2 (ARHI), an imprinted putative tumor suppressor gene in ovarian and breast carcinomas. Proc Natl Acad Sci USA 96:214–219

Zlatescu MC, TehraniYazdi A, Sasaki H, Megyesi JF, Betensky RA, Louis DN, Cairncross JG (2001) Tumor location and growth pattern correlate with genetic signature in oligodendroglial neoplasms. Cancer Res 61:6713–6715

Zulch K (1986) Brain tumours. Their biology and pathology. Springer, Berlin

Ependymal Tumors

3

Martin Hasselblatt

Abstract Ependymomas represent a heterogeneous group of glial tumors whose biological behavior depends on various histological, molecular, and clinical variables. The scope of this chapter is to review the clinical and histological features as well as the molecular genetics of ependymomas with special emphasis on their influence on tumor recurrence and prognosis. Furthermore, potential molecular targets for therapy are outlined.

3.1
Introduction

Ependymomas are glial tumors originating from the inner surfaces of the ventricles and the spinal cord. Having certain histological features in common, the members of the ependymoma family represent a heterogeneous group of tumors whose biological behavior is dependent on various histological, molecular, and clinical variables. Even though the development of ependymomas has been generally attributed to the neoplastic transformation of ependymal cells, ependymomas exhibit gene expression patterns that resemble those of radial glia cells (Taylor et al. 2005) which give rise to ependymal cells throughout normal development (Spassky et al. 2005).

3.1.1
WHO Classification

According to the WHO classification of central nervous system tumors, ependymoma, and its variants (cellular ependymoma, papillary ependymoma, clear cell ependymoma, and tanycytic ependymoma) correspond to WHO grade II, whereas anaplastic ependymoma corresponds to WHO grade III. Myxopapillary ependymoma, a slow-growing tumor of almost exclusively spinal location, corresponds to WHO grade I (Wiestler et al. 2000; McLendon et al. 2007).

3.1.2
Synonyms

In the older literature ependymomas have also been described as *ependymoblastoma, ependymoglioma,* and *ependymocytoma*. Further historical terms include *glioependymoma, ependymoepithelioma,* and *neuroepithelioma gliomatosum*.

Martin Hasselblatt
Institut für Neuropathologie
Universität Münster
Domagk Str. 19
48129 Münster
E-mail: hasselblatt@uni-muenster.de

3.1.3
Historical Aspects

The attribution of *neuroepithelioma gliomatosum* to ependymal cell origin dates back to the beginning of the last century (Muthmann and Sauerbeck 1903). The concept of ependymal tumors was further refined by Bailey and Cushing, who not only set apart *ependymoma* and *ependymoblastoma* but also acknowledged the worse prognosis in the latter (Bailey and Cushing 1926). In 1932, Roussy and Oberling grouped *ependymocytoma* along with *ependymoblastoma, ependymoglioma*, and *choroid plexus papilloma* (Roussy and Oberling 1932). Soon thereafter, Kernohan and Fletcher-Kernohan recognized epithelial, cellular, and myxopapillary subtypes of ependymoma (Kernohan and Fletcher-Kernohan 1935). In contrast to the above classifications, which had been mainly compiled based on the presumed histogenetic origin rather than biological behavior, Ringertz provided a grading scheme separating benign from malignant ependymomas (Ringertz 1950). Based on postoperative survival data, Zülch developed a clinically meaningful grading concept for gliomas (Zülch 1962), setting the foundation for the current WHO classification of ependymomas.

3.2
Epidemiology and Clinical Features

3.2.1
Incidence

Throughout the last few years, data from large population-based epidemiological studies have become available. According to the Central Brain Tumor Registry of the United States, ependymoma currently accounts for 2.3% of all primary CNS tumors and 5.6% of the 25,539 gliomas diagnosed 1998–2002 in the United States (CBTRUS 2005). The incidence of ependymoma and anaplastic ependymoma in the United States accounts for 0.26 (0.24–0.27) per 100,000 person years. Substantially lower incidence rates in some developing countries are almost certainly due to diagnostic underascertainment (Stiller and Nectoux 1994).

A trend toward an increased incidence of ependymomas from 1988 to 1999 has been reported for the US population (average annual percentage change: + 6.9%) (CBTRUS 2005). In view of an only moderate rise in the incidence of primary brain tumors in general and balancing decreases in the incidence of astrocytomas and unspecified glioma subgroups (average annual percentage change each: −5.7%), however, this observation partly reflects improvements in diagnosis and classification (Hoffman et al. 2006). Incidence rates of pediatric ependymoma in Germany (1990–1999) and Sweden (1973–1992) have remained largely stable (Hjalmars et al. 1999; Kaatsch et al. 2001).

3.2.2
Age and Sex Distribution

Ependymomas occur in all age groups ranging from newborns to the very old (Zülch 1986); a case of fetal ependymoma is on record (Rickert et al. 2002). Median age at diagnosis irrespective of location and histological grade is 39 years (CBTRUS 2005).

As compared to the general population, incidence rates of ependymoma in children are higher both in the United States (0.30/100,000; CBTRUS 2005) and the European Union (0.34/100,000; Peris-Bonet et al. 2006). In children aged 0–14, ependymomas represent 7.0% of all primary CNS tumors in the United States (CBTRUS 2005). Similar percentages apply for Germany (10.4%; Kaatsch et al. 2001),

Taiwan (5.8%; Wong et al. 2005), and Japan (4.6%; Kuratsu et al. 2001). Following astrocytomas and medulloblastomas ependymomas are the third most common neuroepithelial tumor in this age group (CBTRUS 2005; Peris-Bonet et al. 2006). The majority of pediatric ependymomas is of intracranial location.

In adults aged 45–54 years, a second peak in incidence rates of ependymoma and its variants is observed (CBTRUS 2005), which can be mainly attributed to the higher incidence of spinal ependymomas in this age group.

As in other glial tumors, the incidence of ependymoma is slightly higher in males than in females (0.29 vs. 0.22), resulting in a male to female ratio of 1.3:1 and incidence rates are greater in whites (0.27/100,000) than in blacks (0.12/100,000) (CBTRUS 2005).

3.2.3
Environmental Factors

Few population based epidemiological studies have specifically addressed the effect of external factors on the incidence of ependymoma. In pediatric ependymoma, maternal smoking during pregnancy (odds ratio 4.71; 95% CI 1.69–13.1), but not exposure to pesticides and diagnostic X-ray examinations, has been associated with increased risk (Schuz et al. 2001). One recent study reported that in children (< 16 years at age at diagnosis) the risk ratio for individuals with three or more younger siblings as compared to none was more than double (Altieri et al. 2006). Space-time clustering of ependymomas suggesting a role of environmental factors in tumor development has been reported (McNally et al. 2002), but this observation could not be confirmed by others (Hjalmars et al. 1999; Houben et al. 2006). The frequency of simian 40 (SV40), JC, and BK polyomavirus sequences in ependymomas is low (Weggen et al. 2000). Furthermore, in population-based studies exposure to SV40-contaminated poliovirus vaccine was not associated with an increased incidence of ependymoma (Olin and Giesecke 1998; Engels et al. 2003).

3.2.4
Tumor Localization

Ependymomas may occur at any site along the ventricular system and the spinal canal. The fourth ventricle and spinal canal are the most common site of origin, followed by the lateral ventricles and the third ventricle (Prayson 1999). Rarely, ependymomas may arise from heterotopic ependymal cell clusters. In addition to intradural extramedullary ependymoma (Katoh et al. 1995; Robles et al. 2005) and intrasacral ependymoma (Vara-Thorbeck and Sanz-Esponera 1970; Morantz et al. 1979), primary extraneural cases located within the mediastinum (Nobles et al. 1991), retroperitoneum (Morantz et al. 1979), liver (Wiendl et al. 2003), and ovary (Kleinman et al. 1993) are on record.

In adult patients, infratentorial and spinal ependymomas arise with almost equal frequency, whereas supratentorial examples are comparably rare (Schwartz et al. 1999). Ependymomas represent the most common spinal cord tumors in adults (37–47% of intramedullary tumors in neurosurgical series; Guidetti et al. 1981; Cooper 1989; Sandalcioglu et al. 2005). Spinal cord ependymomas most frequently affect the cervical and thoracal segments of the myelon (Schwartz and McCormick 2000), while myxopapillary ependymomas are usually encountered in the conus and cauda region (Sonneland et al. 1985). Dissemination of myxopapillary ependymoma with seeding along the subarachnoid spaces may occur (Davis and Barnard 1985; Rickert et al. 1999; Fassett et al.

2005; Plans et al. 2006). Irrespective of histological subtype, the prognosis of spinal ependymomas is excellent if gross total resection can be achieved (Mork and Loken 1977; Sonneland et al. 1985; McCormick et al. 1990).

In children, spinal ependymomas are far less frequent. In this age group, intracranial ependymomas prevail, the vicinity of the fourth ventricle being the preferred location (Foreman et al. 1996). Ependymomas represent 11–18% of pediatric posterior fossa tumors in neurosurgical series (Chang et al. 1993; Cochrane et al. 1994). Unfortunately, complete resection can less frequently be achieved in infratentorial ependymomas as compared to supratentorially located tumors (Bouffet et al. 1998).

3.2.5
Typical Clinical Presentation

Clinical symptoms depend on tumor location rather than histological grade, even though rapid growth of anaplastic ependymoma may be associated with dramatic clinical deterioration. Supratentorial ependymoma presents with any of the generic expressions of an expanding intraparenchymal mass, i.e., focal neurological deficits, seizures, and intracranial hypertension (Zülch 1986; Burger et al. 2002). In younger children, macrocephaly, failure to thrive, and seizures are unspecific symptoms (Furuta et al. 1998). Infratentorial ependymomas located in the vicinity of the fourth ventricle tend to obstruct the flow of cerebrospinal fluid resulting in hydrocephalus presenting with headache, nausea, and vomiting. Compression and/or infiltration of the cerebellum and brain stem may result in ataxia, nystagmus, and dizziness as well as cranial nerve palsies (Ng 2006). Spinal ependymoma may present with paraparesis, sensual disturbances, bladder dysfunction, as well as low back and radicular pain.

3.2.6
Neuroradiological Imaging

On conventional magnetic resonance imaging studies, ependymomas present as contrast-enhancing solid tumors. Cystic components and hemorrhage may be encountered, especially in supratentorial tumors. Intramedullary ependymoma is often associated with syrinx formation. Diffusion-weighted imaging studies and apparent diffusion coefficient maps might aid in distinguishing ependymoma from pilocytic astrocytomas, medulloblastoma, and supratentorial primitive neuroectodermal tumor (PNET) (Yamasaki et al. 2005; Rumboldt et al. 2006). Postoperative surveillance imaging can reveal early asymptomatic recurrences and improves survival as compared to patients solely identified by recurrent clinical symptoms (Good et al. 2001).

3.3
Pathology

3.3.1
Macroscopic Features

Ependymomas at any site are sharply demarcated soft and fleshy, sometimes nodular and lobulated tumors often resembling a placenta or cauliflower, adjusting themselves in form and size to their surroundings (Zülch 1986; Burger et al. 2002). Intraoperatively, good surgical separation from the surrounding tissues can usually be achieved, especially in spinal ependymomas (Chang et al. 2002; Ng 2006). Posterior fossa tumors are usually firmly attached to the floor of the fourth ventricle. They often protrude into the ventricular lumen extending processes into the lateral recesses, but may also grow to the surface of the brain stem. Through the foraminae of Luschka, ependymoma may also extend towards the cerebellopontine angle (Zülch 1986; Ng 2006).

3.3.2
Histological Features

3.3.2.1
Histological Features of Ependymoma

Ependymoma (grade II WHO) is a well-delineated moderately cellular glioma displaying relatively monomorphic round-to-oval nuclei. Mitoses are rare or absent. The key histological feature is the presence of perivascular pseudorosettes with tumor cells extending fibrillary processes towards centrally located blood vessels and/or ependymal rosettes formed by columnar tumor cells around central lumina (Wiestler et al. 2000; McLendon et al. 2007). Ependymal rosettes are diagnostic for ependymoma, but occur in only a minority of cases. Some ependymomas are predominantly glial in appearance with faint or absent perivascular pseudorosettes. Nevertheless, tumor cells may form tiny intracellular microlumina containing microvilli and cilia, which may be discernible as round intracytoplasmic eosinophilic inclusions even on routine staining (Kawano et al. 2000), but can be more readily identified using immunohistochemistry (see Sect. 3.3.3). The occasional presence of non-palisading necrosis is compatible with a diagnosis of ependymoma grade II WHO (Wiestler et al. 2000; McLendon et al. 2007).

According to the WHO classification, grade II ependymoma can be subdivided into cellular ependymoma, papillary ependymoma, clear cell ependymoma, and tanycytic ependymoma. Cellular ependymoma represents the majority of ependymoma. Distinction of the other far less frequent histopathological variants is not always unequivocal and certainly of limited prognostic impact (Kurt et al. 2006). Nevertheless, because their histological features might mimic those of other tumor entities, recognition of these subtypes represents more than neuropathological folklore.

Papillary ependymoma is characterized by a predominance of papillary structures. Choroid plexus papilloma, papillary meningioma, metastatic carcinoma, and (if located in the vicinity of the third ventricle) papillary tumor of the pineal region (Jouvet et al. 2003) are in the differential diagnosis.

Clear cell ependymoma displays an oligodendroglial appearance with clear perinuclear halos (Kawano et al. 1983). Clear cell ependymoma has a predilection for the supratentorial region in children (Fouladi et al. 2003) and needs to be distinguished from oligodendroglioma, central neurocytoma, clear cell carcinoma, and hemangioblastoma. Anaplastic features compatible with a diagnosis of anaplastic ependymoma (see Sect. 3.3.2.2) are frequent (Fouladi et al. 2003; Rickert et al. 2006).

Tanycytic ependymoma has a predilection for the spinal cord and is composed of stretched tumor cells arranged in fascicles of variable width and cell density (Kawano et al. 2001). As ependymal rosettes are typically absent and pseudorosettes only vaguely delineated, this lesion may be misinterpreted as astrocytoma (Wiestler et al. 2000).

Other rare histological variants of ependymoma include ependymoma with lipomatous (Ruchoux et al. 1998) or neuronal (Rodriguez et al. 2006) differentiation, giant cell ependymoma of the filum terminale (Zec et al. 1996), melanotic ependymoma (McCloskey et al. 1976), as well as signet cell ependymoma with extensive tumor cell vacuolization (Hirato et al. 1997).

3.3.2.2
Histological Features of Anaplastic Ependymoma

The identification of histological parameters predi-cting prognosis in ependymomas remains a controversial issue. According to the WHO classification, anaplastic ependymomas are defined by the presence of increased cellularity and brisk mitotic activity, often associated with microvascular proliferation and pseudopalisading necrosis (Wiestler et al. 2000; McLendon et al. 2007). This somewhat vague definition might partly be responsible for the frequently reported inconstant relationship between histological grade and clinical outcome (Schiffer and Giordana 1998). Nevertheless, ependymomas with two or more of the following features (i.e., mitotic figures, hypercellularity, vascular proliferation, and necrosis) have been shown to be more likely to behave in an aggressive manner (Prayson 1999; Figarella-Branger et al. 2000; Ho et al. 2001).

3.3.2.3
Histological Features of Myxopapillary Ependymoma

Myxopapillary ependymoma is characterized by epithelial-appearing fronds of tumor cells arranged in vague papillary structures around vascularized stromal cores. Mucoid matrix material accumulates between tumor cells and blood vessels also collecting in microcysts, sometimes blurring the papillary growth pattern completely (Zülch 1986; Wiestler et al. 2000; Ng 2006). Only in the rare cases originating from the sacrum or extraspinal soft tissues, may chordoma and myxoid chondrosarcoma enter into the differential diagnosis (Wiestler et al. 2000; Ng 2006).

3.3.3
Immunohistochemistry

As with other glial tumors, the majority of ependymomas display immunoreactivity for GFAP, which is especially prominent in pseudorosettes (Deck et al. 1978; Duffy et al. 1979), and also stain for vimentin and S100 protein (Kimura et al. 1986; Vege et al. 2000). Expression of cytokeratins in ependymoma is rare and usually lacking (Miettinen et al. 1986; Mannoji and Becker 1988; Ang et al. 1990). It is tempting to speculate that papillary ependymomas for which cytokeratin expression has been reported (Mannoji and Becker 1988) might rather have represented papillary tumors of the pineal region, a recently recognized entity thought to arise from the specialized ependymal cells of the subcommisural organ (Jouvet et al. 2003), which stains strongly for cytokeratins (Hasselblatt et al. 2006).

Antibodies directed against epithelial membrane antigen (EMA) serve as valuable tools in the diagnosis of ependymoma (Cruz-Sanchez et al. 1988; Uematsu et al. 1989; Vege et al. 2000; Hasselblatt and Paulus 2003). The distinct punctate and ring-like EMA staining pattern observed in ependymomas represents microlumina of the tumor cells (Kawano et al. 2000) and serves as a sensitive and specific marker of ependymal differentiation (Fig. 3.1). A punctate intracytoplasmic or ring-like EMA staining pattern is observed in 89% and 31% of ependymomas, respectively, but not in the majority of fibrillary astrocytomas, oligodendrogliomas, and glioblastomas (Hasselblatt and Paulus 2003). Apart from the notable absence in

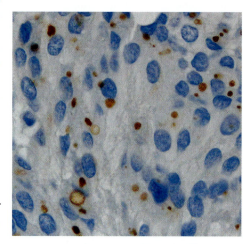

Fig. 3.1 Immunohistochemistry: Typical dot- and ring-like epithelial membrane antigen (EMA) staining pattern in ependymoma

most myxopapillary ependymomas, neither staining pattern is related to tumor grade or localization (Hasselblatt and Paulus 2003).

Of note, in addition to proliferative activity as determined by Ki67/MIB1 labeling indices (Ritter et al. 1998; Prayson 1999; Figarella-Branger et al. 2000; Wolfsberger et al. 2004), some immunohistochemical markers might also serve as predictors of recurrence (see Sect. 3.4.3).

3.4
Genetic Susceptibility and Molecular Genetics

Throughout the last few years, conventional cytogenetic studies such as comparative genomic hybridization (CGH) have been complemented by high-resolution array CGH and microarray approaches, allowing for a more detailed analysis of cytogenetic changes as well as gene expression profiles in ependymomas. The genetic background of ependymomas is complex and partly determined by patient age, tumor localization, and histopathological subtype (Jeuken et al. 2002).

3.4.1
Genetic Susceptibility

Familial occurrence of ependymoma is rare (Savard and Gilchrist 1989; Nijssen et al. 1994; Yokota et al. 2003; Dimopoulos et al. 2006). Of note, genetic alterations affecting chromosome 22 have been reported in most of these families (Savard and Gilchrist 1989; Nijssen et al. 1994; Yokota et al. 2003). Spinal ependymomas manifest in neurofibromatosis type 2, indicating a possible role for the *NF2* tumor suppressor gene in the development of spinal ependymomas (Wiestler et al. 2000) (see Sect. 3.4.2.2). Ependymomas have been described in association with Turcot syndrome (Torres et al. 1997; Mullins et al. 1998), but mutations of the *APC* tumor suppressor gene do not play a role in the pathogenesis of sporadic ependymomas (Onilude et al. 2006).

3.4.2
Molecular Genetics

Irrespective of histological subtype, ependymomas are characterized by frequent gains on chromosomes 1 and 9 as well as losses on chromosomes 22 (Jeuken et al. 2002; Rickert and Paulus 2004).

The fact that monosomy 22 as well as allelic losses on the long arm of chromosome 22 (22q) are among the most frequent genetic changes observed in sporadic ependymomas (Ransom et al. 1992; Lamszus et al. 2001; Carter et al. 2002; Huang et al. 2002; Modena et al. 2006) prompted a quest for potential tumor suppressor genes located on 22q involved in the pathogenesis of ependymomas. In addition to the *NF2* tumor suppressor gene, *SMARCB1* (hSNF5/INI1) is also located on 22q and plays a key role in the pathogenesis of atypical teratoid/rhabdoid tumors (Biegel et al. 1999). However, analysis of a series of 53 ependymomas for mutations and homozygous deletions of *SMARCB1* revealed no alterations (Kraus et al. 2001). The presence of putative tumor suppressor genes at 22q11 (Kraus et al. 2001; Ammerlaan et al. 2005) as well as 22q11.21-12.2 and 22q13.1-13.3 (Huang et al. 2002) has been proposed.

Interestingly, a subset of genes identified by comparison of gene expression profiles of 19 ependymomas and normal brain tissue controls included under-expressed transcripts mapping to 22q12.3-22q13.3, i.e., *FBX7, C22orf2, CBX7*, and the SET domain-binding protein coding gene *SBF1*. Under-expression of one of these genes, the chromobox protein coding gene *CBX7* located at 22q13.1, could be confirmed using RT-PCR in 55% of cases (Suarez-Merino et al. 2005). *CBX7* controls cellular lifespan through regulation of both the p16(Ink4a)/Rb and the Arf/p53 pathways (Gil et al. 2004).

Interestingly, the *SULT4A1* gene located at 22q13.3 has recently been shown to be down-regulated in intracranial ependymomas (Modena et al. 2006). *SULT4A1* codes for a sulphotransferase involved in the metabolism of thyroid hormones, steroids, and neurotransmitters (Falany et al. 2000; Sakakibara et al. 2002) and has not yet been described in association with other brain tumors.

Irrespective of patient age, tumor location, and histological subtype, ependymomas are also characterized by frequent gains on chromosomes 1q and 9 as well as losses on chromosomes 10q, 21, and 16p (Jeuken et al. 2002; Rickert and Paulus 2004). Using array CGH, multiple regions of recurrent gain (including 2q23, 7p21, 12p, 13q21.1, and 20p12) and loss (including 5q31, 6q26, 7q36, 15q21.1, 16q24, 17p13.3, 19p13.2, and 22q13.3) have been identified (Modena et al. 2006).

discriminating patients based on age were identified. Ependymomas in young patients (<3 years) more frequently harbored gains in 9q as well as 11q13 flanking the *CCND1* oncogene, whereas nine clones on chromosome 16 were preferentially lost in infants (Modena et al. 2006).

Gene expression profiles of pediatric ependymomas (children < 16 years) were characterized by over-expression of *HSPB1* (coding for heat-shock protein 27-kd protein 1 located at 7q11.23), *ARHGDIA* (coding for the *RAS* gene member rho GDP-dissociation inhibitor alpha located at 17q25.3), *CDCA5* (coding for cell division cycle associated protein 5 located on chromosome 11), *STAM* (coding for signal-transducing adaptor molecule 1, which is involved in signal transducing pathways of cytokine receptors (Takeshita et al. 1996) and located at 10p14-p13), as well as *LDHB, COL6A1, GPX3*, and *PYCR1* (Korshunov et al. 2003).

3.4.2.1
Patient Age

As compared to the higher incidence in adult samples, monosomy 22 has been reported in only 31% of pediatric ependymomas (Mazewski et al. 1999). Six clones from 22q13 displayed preferential loss in older patients (Modena et al. 2006). Still, loss of 22q is among the most frequent chromosomal abnormalities in pediatric ependymomas (Grill et al. 2002). Gains on 1q have been reported to occur significantly more frequently in children than in adults (Mendrzyk et al. 2006); this result may be partly due to the higher proportion of anaplastic ependymoma in this age group (Hirose et al. 2001). Loss of 17p has been described in up to 50% of sporadic pediatric ependymomas (von Haken et al. 1996), but in contrast to other gliomas, *TP53* mutations appear not to play an important role in the etiology of sporadic ependymomas (Fink et al. 1996; von Haken et al. 1996; Nozaki et al. 1998). On analysis of array CGH hybridization data of intracranial ependymomas, 80 clones

3.2.2.2
Tumor Localization

Spinal ependymomas manifest in neurofibromatosis type 2 indicating a possible role for the *NF2* tumor suppressor gene (Wiestler et al. 2000). Indeed, *NF2* mutations have been detected in a substantial fraction of sporadic intramedullary spinal ependymomas (Birch et al. 1996; Ebert et al. 1999; Hirose et al. 2001), but are rare in intracranial ependymomas (Slavc et al. 1995; von Haken et al. 1996; Ebert et al. 1999). Correspondingly, the *NF2* gene was found to have higher expression in intracranial than in spinal tumors (Korshunov et al. 2003). Other chromosomal alterations observed in spinal ependymomas involve gains on chromosome 7, which have been described in up to 95% of spinal ependymomas (Hirose et al. 2001).

Intracranial location correlated with chromosomal gain of 1q (Mendrzyk et al. 2006). Losses of 9p have been more frequently observed in supratentorial tumors (Modena et al. 2006), whereas 17p13.3 losses have been preferentially observed in infratentorial ependymoma (Modena et al. 2006). Gene expression profiles between supratentorial and infratentorial ependymomas also differ: genes involved in CNS development such as *PAX3, NET1*, and *MSX1* were among the genes up-regulated in supratentorial ependymomas, whereas infratentorial ependymomas were characterized by expression of *NR2E1* (coding for the human drosophila homologue of *tailless*), *PCDH17*, and *GABRB1* (Modena et al. 2006).

3.2.2.3
Histological Subtype

In myxopapillary ependymoma, concurrent gain on chromosomes 9 and 18 is frequent. Other abnormalities include gains of chromosomes 3, 4, 7, 8, 11, 13, 17q, 20, as well as loss of chromosomes 1, 10, and 22 (Mahler-Araujo et al. 2003; Rickert and Paulus 2004; Tamiolakis et al. 2006). On gene expression profiling, myxopapillary ependymomas clustered with spinal ependymomas of other histological subtypes, displaying a common signature with high-expression levels of *HOXB5* (located on 17q21-q22), *PLA2G5* (1p36-p34), and *ITIH2* (10p15), separating them from intracranial ependymoma (Korshunov et al. 2003).

Clear Cell Ependymoma: The most common aberrations in a series of clear cell ependymomas were gains on 1q (38%) as well as losses on chromosomes 9 (77%), 3 (31%), and -22q (23%). Clear cell ependymomas of WHO grade II were characterized by losses on chromosome 9 (40%), whereas WHO grade III cases mainly displayed gains on 1q (63%) and 13q (25%) as well as losses on chromosomes 9 (100%), 3 (38%), and 22q (25%) (Rickert et al. 2006).

Anaplastic Ependymoma: Gains of 1q (Hirose et al. 2001; Mendrzyk et al. 2006) as well as losses on chromosome 9 are preferentially associated with anaplastic ependymomas (Hirose et al. 2001). Because *INK4A* is located on 9p, it has been suggested that the cyclin D/CDK4 pathway might be disrupted more frequently in anaplastic ependymoma (Hirose et al. 2001). Even though mutations of p53 are rare in anaplastic ependymomas (Korshunov et al. 2000), an involvement of p53 pathways has been proposed, because *ARF*, whose product stabilizes p53, is also located on 9p. The role of *ARF* in ependymoma remains controversial: whereas one group failed to detect deletions or promoter hypermethylation of *ARF* (Gaspar et al. 2006), another study reported decreased p14ARF protein expression to be associated with biological aggressiveness (Korshunov et al. 2001). One group suggested that mutations in exon 10 of the *MEN1* gene located on chromosome 11q13 might also be involved in the malignant progression of ependymoma (Lamszus et al. 2001).

Because gene expression patterns of grade II and grade III infratentorial ependymomas are quite similar, it has been suggested that grade III tumors may develop through neoplastic progression (Korshunov et al. 2003).

3.4.3
Tumor Recurrence and Prognosis

The potential influence of genetic alterations on prognosis has clinical implications and therefore has been addressed by several recent studies. Using high-resolution genomic profiling, gains at 1q21.1-32.1 were identified to be associated with tumor recurrence in intracranial ependymomas (Mendrzyk et al. 2006). Highly recurrent gains were also found at 5p15.33, and increased hTERT protein expression was negatively correlated with outcome (Mendrzyk et al. 2006). Furthermore, in addition to frequent gains and high-level amplification of the epidermal growth factor receptor gene (*EGFR*) at 7p11.2, EGFR expression status was significantly correlated with poor prognosis and subdivided intracranial grade II ependymomas into two different risk groups (Mendrzyk et al. 2006).

By comparison of gene expression profiles from seven ependymomas that subsequently recurred and six tumors from patients who remained recurrence-free, a group of three genes was identified that accurately predicted recurrence (Sowar et al. 2006). These genes were *PLEK* (coding for pleckstrin), *NF-kappaB2*, and the PTEN homologous inositol phosphatase pseudogene *LOC374491*.

One study reported that decreased expression of pl4ARF represented an independent prognostic factor (Korshunov et al. 2001) and positive staining for p53 was found to be associated with shorter survival times (Verstegen et al. 2002). In low-grade ependymomas, progression-free survival is significantly shorter in ependymomas displaying tenascin, VEGF, and EGFR immunoreactivity (Korshunov et al. 2002), whereas in anaplastic ependymoma progression-free survival is significantly reduced in tumors displaying low p27 and p14ARF labeling indices as well as positive staining for p53, tenascin, VEGF, and EGFR (Korshunov et al. 2002).

Survivin and topoisomerase IIalpha expression status are also associated with outcome, but seem to be less accurate predictors than proliferative activity as assessed by Ki67/MIB1 labeling (Preusser et al. 2005), which has been shown to represent an excellent predictor of recurrence (Ritter et al. 1998; Prayson 1999; Wolfsberger et al. 2004).

3.4.4
Potential Molecular Targets for Therapy

Members of the tyrosine kinase receptor family and their associated kinase activities represent a novel therapeutic target in the treatment of glioblastoma (Halatsch et al. 2006). Relatively little is known on these pathways in ependymomas.

Over-expression of epidermal growth factor receptor (EGFR) secondary to *EGFR* gene amplification is a common feature of primary malignant gliomas (Libermann et al. 1985) but less frequently encountered in ependymomas (Bijlsma et al. 1995; Marquez et al. 2004; Mendrzyk et al. 2006). Despite the absence of *EGFR* amplification, expression of EGFR protein could be detected in 43% of ependymomas; among EGFR-positive ependymomas, high-grade tumors significantly prevailed (Korshunov et al. 2000). In mice, ZD6474, an inhibitor of the kinase activities associated with EGFR and VEGFR-2, delayed tumor growth of ependymoma xenografts (Rich et al. 2005). A clinical phase I/II trial of the EGFR kinase inhibitor erlotinib for the treatment of young patients with refractory or relapsed malignant brain tumors including anaplastic ependymomas is currently under way (clinicaltrials.gov identifier: NCT00360854).

Other members of the ERBB receptor family may also represent potential therapeutic targets in ependymomas: coexpression of ERBB2 and ERBB4 has been identified in the majority of pediatric ependymomas. High-level coexpression of both receptors was significantly related to proliferative activity and blockade of ERBB2 tyrosine kinase activity using the inhibitor WAY-177820 resulted in reduced AKT phosphorylation and impaired tumor proliferation in vitro (Gilbertson et al. 2002). A multicenter, phase I, dose-escalation study followed by an open-label phase II trial of the EGFR and ERBB2 dual kinase inhibitor lapatinib (Gilbertson 2005) for the treatment of malignant brain tumors including anaplastic ependymomas has been initiated (clinicaltrials.gov identifier: NCT00095940).

PDGF receptor signaling represents another target currently being intensively evaluated for its therapeutic potential in malignant gliomas (Reardon et al. 2005). Expression of both PDGFRα and PDGFRβ has also been described in ependymomas (Black et al. 1996). Interestingly, one patient with recurrent spinal ependymoma experienced partial remission upon imatinib treatment (Fakhrai et al. 2004).

Taken together, currently employed novel therapeutic approaches exploit similarities of ependymomas with other glial tumors rather than addressing pathways specifically associated with ependymoma. Further basic and clinical research into the molecular mechanisms involved in the development of ependymoma is clearly warranted.

References

Altieri A, Castro F, Bermejo JL, Hemminki K (2006) Association between number of siblings and nervous system tumors suggests an infectious etiology. Neurology 67:1979–1983

Ammerlaan AC, de Bustos C, Ararou A, Buckley PG, Mantripragada KK, Verstegen MJ, Hulsebos TJ, Dumanski JP (2005) Localization of a putative low-penetrance ependymoma susceptibility locus to 22q11 using a chromosome 22 tiling-path genomic microarray. Genes Chromosomes Cancer 43:329–338

Ang LC, Taylor AR, Bergin D, Kaufmann JC (1990) An immunohistochemical study of papillary tumors in the central nervous system. Cancer 65:2712–2719

Bailey P, Cushing H (1926) A classification of the tumors of the glioma group on a histogenetic basis with a correlation study of prognosis. Lippincott, Philadelphia

Biegel JA, Zhou JY, Rorke LB, Stenstrom C, Wainwright LM, Fogelgren B (1999) Germ-line and acquired mutations of INI1 in atypical teratoid and rhabdoid tumors. Cancer Res 59:74–79

Bijlsma EK, Voesten AM, Bijleveld EH, Troost D, Westerveld A, Merel P, Thomas G, Hulsebos TJ (1995) Molecular analysis of genetic changes in ependymomas. Genes Chromosomes Cancer 13:272–277

Birch BD, Johnson JP, Parsa A, Desai RD, Yoon JT, Lycette CA, Li YM, Bruce JN (1996) Frequent type 2 neurofibromatosis gene transcript mutations in sporadic intramedullary spinal cord ependymomas. Neurosurgery 39:135–140

Black P, Carroll R, Glowacka D (1996) Expression of platelet-derived growth factor transcripts in medulloblastomas and ependymomas. Pediatr Neurosurg 24:74–78

Bouffet E, Perilongo G, Canete A, Massimino M (1998) Intracranial ependymomas in children: a critical review of prognostic factors and a plea for cooperation. Med Pediatr Oncol 30:319–329; discussion 329–331

Burger PC, Scheithauer BW, Vogel FS (2002) Surgical pathology of the nervous system and its coverings. Churchill Livingstone, New York

Carter M, Nicholson J, Ross F, Crolla J, Allibone R, Balaji V, Perry R, Walker D, Gilbertson R, Ellison DW (2002) Genetic abnormalities detected in ependymomas by comparative genomic hybridisation. Br J Cancer 86:929–939

CBTRUS (2005) Statistical Report: Primary Brain Tumors in the United States, 1998–2002. Central Brain Tumor Registry of the United States, Hinsdale

Chang T, Teng MM, Lirng JF (1993) Posterior cranial fossa tumours in childhood. Neuroradiology 35:274–278

Chang UK, Choe WJ, Chung SK, Chung CK, Kim HJ (2002) Surgical outcome and prognostic factors of spinal intramedullary ependymomas in adults. J Neurooncol 57:133–139

Cochrane DD, Gustavsson B, Poskitt KP, Steinbok P, Kestle JR (1994) The surgical and natural morbidity of aggressive resection for posterior fossa tumors in childhood. Pediatr Neurosurg 20:19–29

Cooper PR (1989) Outcome after operative treatment of intramedullary spinal cord tumors in adults: intermediate and long-term results in 51 patients. Neurosurgery 25:855–859

Cruz-Sanchez FF, Rossi ML, Esiri MM, Reading M (1988) Epithelial membrane antigen expression in ependymomas. Neuropathol Appl Neurobiol 14:197–205

Davis C, Barnard RO (1985) Malignant behavior of myxopapillary ependymoma. Report of three cases. J Neurosurg 62:925–929

Deck JH, Eng LF, Bigbee J, Woodcock SM (1978) The role of glial fibrillary acidic protein in the diagnosis of central nervous system tumors. Acta Neuropathol 42:183–190

Dimopoulos VG, Fountas KN, Robinson JS (2006) Familial intracranial ependymomas. Report of three cases in a family and review of the literature. Neurosurg Focus 20:E8

Duffy PE, Graf L, Huang YY, Rapport MM (1979) Glial fibrillary acidic protein in ependymomas and other brain tumors. Distribution, diagnostic criteria, and relation to formation of processes. J Neurol Sci 40:133–146

Ebert C, von Haken M, Meyer-Puttlitz B, Wiestler OD, Reifenberger G, Pietsch T, von Deimling A (1999) Molecular genetic analysis of ependymal tumors. NF2 mutations and chromosome 22q loss occur preferentially in intramedullary spinal ependymomas. Am J Pathol 155:627–632

Engels EA, Katki HA, Nielsen NM, Winther JF, Hjalgrim H, Gjerris F, Rosenberg PS, Frisch M (2003) Cancer incidence in Denmark following exposure to poliovirus vaccine contaminated with simian virus 40. J Natl Cancer Inst 95:532–539

Fakhrai N, Neophytou P, Dieckmann K, Nemeth A, Prayer D, Hainfellner J, Marosi C (2004) Recurrent spinal ependymoma showing partial remission under Imatimib. Acta Neurochir 146:1255–1258

Falany CN, Xie X, Wang J, Ferrer J, Falany JL (2000) Molecular cloning and expression of novel sulphotransferase-like cDNAs from human and rat brain. Biochem J 346 Pt 3:857–864

Fassett DR, Pingree J, Kestle JR (2005) The high incidence of tumor dissemination in myxopapillary ependymoma in pediatric patients. Report of five cases and review of the literature. J Neurosurg 102:59–64

Figarella-Branger D, Civatte M, Bouvier-Labit C, Gouvernet J, Gambarelli D, Gentet JC, Lena G, Choux M, Pellissier JF (2000) Prognostic factors in intracranial ependymomas in children. J Neurosurg 93:605–613

Fink KL, Rushing EJ, Schold SC Jr, Nisen PD (1996) Infrequency of p53 gene mutations in ependymomas. J Neurooncol 27:111–115

Foreman NK, Love S, Thorne R (1996) Intracranial ependymomas: analysis of prognostic factors in a population-based series. Pediatr Neurosurg 24:119–125

Fouladi M, Helton K, Dalton J, Gilger E, Gajjar A, Merchant T, Kun L, Newsham I, Burger P, Fuller C (2003) Clear cell ependymoma: a clinicopathologic and radiographic analysis of 10 patients. Cancer 98:2232–2244

Furuta T, Tabuchi A, Adachi Y, Mizumatsu S, Tamesa N, Ichikawa T, Tamiya T, Matsumoto K, Ohmoto T (1998) Primary brain tumors in children under age 3 years. Brain Tumor Pathol 15:7–12

Gaspar N, Grill J, Geoerger B, Lellouch-Tubiana A, Michalowski MB, Vassal G (2006) p53 Pathway dysfunction in primary childhood ependymomas. Pediatr Blood Cancer 46:604–613

Gil J, Bernard D, Martinez D, Beach D (2004) Polycomb CBX7 has a unifying role in cellular lifespan. Nat Cell Biol 6:67–72

Gilbertson RJ (2005) ERBB2 in pediatric cancer: innocent until proven guilty. Oncologist 10:508–517

Gilbertson RJ, Bentley L, Hernan R, Junttila TT, Frank AJ, Haapasalo H, Connelly M, Wetmore C, Curran T, Elenius K, Ellison DW (2002) ERBB receptor signaling promotes ependymoma cell proliferation and represents a potential novel therapeutic target for this disease. Clin Cancer Res 8:3054–3064

Good CD, Wade AM, Hayward RD, Phipps KP, Michalski AJ, Harkness WF, Chong WK (2001) Surveillance neuroimaging in childhood intracranial ependymoma: how effective, how often, and for how long? J Neurosurg 94:27–32

Grill J, Avet-Loiseau H, Lellouch-Tubiana A, Sevenet N, Terrier-Lacombe MJ, Venuat AM, Doz F, Sainte-Rose C, Kalifa C, Vassal G (2002) Comparative genomic hybridization detects specific cytogenetic abnormalities in pediatric ependymomas and choroid plexus papillomas. Cancer Genet Cytogenet 136:121–125

Guidetti B, Mercuri S, Vagnozzi R (1981) Long-term results of the surgical treatment of 129 intramedullary spinal gliomas. J Neurosurg 54:323–330

Halatsch ME, Schmidt U, Behnke-Mursch J, Unterberg A, Wirtz CR (2006) Epidermal growth factor receptor inhibition for the treatment of glioblastoma multiforme and other malignant brain tumours. Cancer Treat Rev 32:74–89

Hasselblatt M, Paulus W (2003) Sensitivity and specificity of epithelial membrane antigen staining patterns in ependymomas. Acta Neuropathol 106:385–388

Hasselblatt M, Blümcke I, Jeibmann A, Rickert CH, Jouvet A, van de Nes JA, Kuchelmeister K, Brunn A, Fevre-Montange M, Paulus W (2006) Immunohistochemical profile and chromosomal imbalances in papillary tumours of the pineal region. Neuropathol Appl Neurobiol 32:278–283

Hirato J, Nakazato Y, Iijima M, Yokoo H, Sasaki A, Yokota M, Ono N, Hirato M, Inoue H (1997) An unusual variant of ependymoma with extensive tumor cell vacuolization. Acta Neuropathol 93:310–316

Hirose Y, Aldape K, Bollen A, James CD, Brat D, Lamborn K, Berger M, Feuerstein BG (2001) Chromosomal abnormalities subdivide ependymal tumors into clinically relevant groups. Am J Pathol 158:1137–1143

Hjalmars U, Kulldorff M, Wahlqvist Y, Lannering B (1999) Increased incidence rates but no space-time clustering of childhood astrocytoma in Sweden, 1973–1992: a population-based study of pediatric brain tumors. Cancer 85:2077–2090

Ho DM, Hsu CY, Wong TT, Chiang H (2001) A clinicopathologic study of 81 patients with ependymomas and proposal of diagnostic criteria for anaplastic ependymoma. J Neurooncol 54:77–85

Hoffman S, Propp JM, McCarthy BJ (2006) Temporal trends in incidence of primary brain tumors in the United States, 1985–1999. Neurooncol 8:27–37

Houben MP, Aben KK, Teepen JL, Schouten-Van Meeteren AY, Tijssen CC, Van Duijn CM, Coebergh JW (2006) Stable incidence of childhood and adult glioma in The Netherlands, 1989–2003. Acta Oncol 45:272–279

Huang B, Starostik P, Kuhl J, Tonn JC, Roggendorf W (2002) Loss of heterozygosity on chromosome 22 in human ependymomas. Acta Neuropathol 103:415–420

Jeuken JW, Sprenger SH, Gilhuis J, Teepen HL, Grotenhuis AJ, Wesseling P (2002) Correlation between localization, age, and chromosomal imbalances in ependymal tumours as detected by CGH. J Pathol 197:238–244

Jouvet A, Fauchon F, Liberski P, Saint-Pierre G, Didier-Bazes M, Heitzmann A, Delisle MB, Biassette HA, Vincent S, Mikol J, Streichenberger N, Ahboucha S, Brisson C, Belin MF, Fevre-Montange M (2003) Papillary tumor of the pineal region. Am J Surg Pathol 27:505–512

Kaatsch P, Rickert CH, Kuhl J, Schuz J, Michaelis J (2001) Population-based epidemiologic data on brain tumors in German children. Cancer 92:3155–3164

Katoh S, Ikata T, Inoue A, Takahashi M (1995) Intradural extramedullary ependymoma. A case report. Spine 20:2036–2038

Kawano N, Ohba Y, Nagashima K (2000) Eosinophilic inclusions in ependymoma represent microlumina: a light and electron microscopic study. Acta Neuropathol 99:214–218

Kawano N, Yada K, Aihara M, Yagishita S (1983) Oligodendroglioma-like cells (clear cells) in ependymoma. Acta Neuropathol 62:141–144

Kawano N, Yagishita S, Oka H, Utsuki S, Kobayashi I, Suzuki S, Tachibana S, Fujii K (2001) Spinal tanycytic ependymomas. Acta Neuropathol 101:43–48

Kernohan JW, Fletcher-Kernohan EM (1935) Ependymomas. A study of 109 cases. Assoc Res Nerv Ment Dis 16:182–209

Kimura T, Budka H, Soler-Federsppiel S (1986) An immunocytochemical comparison of the glia-associated proteins glial fibrillary acidic protein (GFAP) and S-100 protein (S100P) in human brain tumors. Clin Neuropathol 5:21–27

Kleinman GM, Young RH, Scully RE (1993) Primary neuroectodermal tumors of the ovary. A report of 25 cases. Am J Surg Pathol 17:764–778

Korshunov A, Golanov A, Timirgaz V (2000) Immunohistochemical markers for intracranial ependymoma recurrence. An analysis of 88 cases. J Neurol Sci 177:72–82

Korshunov A, Golanov A, Timirgaz V (2001) p14ARF protein (FL-132) immunoreactivity in intracranial ependymomas and its prognostic significance: an analysis of 103 cases. Acta Neuropathol 102:271–277

Korshunov A, Golanov A, Timirgaz V (2002) Immunohistochemical markers for prognosis of ependymal neoplasms. J Neurooncol 58:255–270

Korshunov A, Neben K, Wrobel G, Tews B, Benner A, Hahn M, Golanov A, Lichter P (2003) Gene expression patterns in ependymomas correlate with tumor location, grade, and patient age. Am J Pathol 163:1721–1727

Kraus JA, de Millas W, Sorensen N, Herbold C, Schichor C, Tonn JC, Wiestler OD, von Deimling A, Pietsch T (2001) Indications for a tumor suppressor gene at 22q11 involved in the pathogenesis of ependymal tumors and distinct from hSNF5/INI1. Acta Neuropathol 102:69–74

Kuratsu J, Takeshima H, Ushio Y (2001) Trends in the incidence of primary intracranial tumors in Kumamoto, Japan. Int J Clin Oncol 6:183–191

Kurt E, Zheng PP, Hop WC, van der Weiden M, Bol M, van den Bent MJ, Avezaat CJ, Kros JM (2006) Identification of relevant prognostic histopathologic features in 69 intracranial ependymomas, excluding myxopapillary ependymomas and subependymomas. Cancer 106:388–395

Lamszus K, Lachenmayer L, Heinemann U, Kluwe L, Finckh U, Hoppner W, Stavrou D, Fillbrandt R, Westphal M (2001) Molecular genetic alterations on chromosomes 11 and 22 in ependymomas. Int J Cancer 91:803–808

Libermann TA, Nusbaum HR, Razon N, Kris R, Lax I, Soreq H, Whittle N, Waterfield MD, Ullrich A, Schlessinger J (1985) Amplification, enhanced expression and possible rearrangement of EGF receptor gene in primary human brain tumours of glial origin. Nature 313:144–147

Mahler-Araujo MB, Sanoudou D, Tingby O, Liu L, Coleman N, Ichimura K, Collins VP (2003) Structural genomic abnormalities of chromosomes 9 and 18 in myxopapillary ependymomas. J Neuropathol Exp Neurol 62:927–935

Mannoji H, Becker LE (1988) Ependymal and choroid plexus tumors. Cytokeratin and GFAP expression. Cancer 61:1377–1385

Marquez A, Wu R, Zhao J, Tao J, Shi Z (2004) Evaluation of epidermal growth factor receptor (EGFR) by chromogenic in situ hybridization (CISH) and immunohistochemistry (IHC) in archival gliomas using bright-field microscopy. Diagn Mol Pathol 13:1–8

Mazewski C, Soukup S, Ballard E, Gotwals B, Lampkin B (1999) Karyotype studies in 18 ependymomas with literature review of 107 cases. Cancer Genet Cytogenet 113:1–8

McCloskey JJ, Parker JC, Jr., Brooks WH, Blacker HM (1976) Melanin as a component of cerebral gliomas: the melanotic cerebral ependymoma. Cancer 37:2373–2379

McCormick PC, Torres R, Post KD, Stein BM (1990) Intramedullary ependymoma of the spinal cord. J Neurosurg 72:523–532

McLendon RE, Wiestler OD, Kros JM, Korshunov A, Ng HK (2007) Ependymal tumours. In: Louis DN, Ohgaki H, Wiestler OD, Cavenee W (eds) Pathology and genetics of tumours of the nervous system. IARC Press, Lyon

McNally RJ, Cairns DP, Eden OB, Alexander FE, Taylor GM, Kelsey AM, Birch JM (2002) An infectious aetiology for childhood brain tumours? Evidence from space-time clustering and seasonality analyses. Br J Cancer 86:1070–1077

Mendrzyk F, Korshunov A, Benner A, Toedt G, Pfister S, Radlwimmer B, Lichter P (2006) Identification of gains on 1q and epidermal growth factor receptor overexpression as independent prognostic markers in intracranial ependymoma. Clin Cancer Res 12:2070–2079

Miettinen M, Clark R, Virtanen I (1986) Intermediate filament proteins in choroid plexus and ependyma and their tumors. Am J Pathol 123:231–240

Modena P, Lualdi E, Facchinetti F, Veltman J, Reid JF, Minardi S, Janssen I, Giangaspero F, Forni M, Finocchiaro G, Genitori L, Giordano F, Riccardi R, Schoenmakers EF, Massimino M, Sozzi G (2006) Identification of tumor-specific molecular signatures in intracranial ependymoma and association with clinical characteristics. J Clin Oncol 24:5223–5233

Morantz RA, Kepes JJ, Batnitzky S, Masterson BJ (1979) Extraspinal ependymomas. Report of three cases. J Neurosurg 51:383–391

Mork SJ, Loken AC (1977) Ependymoma: a follow-up study of 101 cases. Cancer 40:907–915

Mullins KJ, Rubio A, Myers SP, Korones DN, Pilcher WH (1998) Malignant ependymomas in a patient with Turcot's syndrome: case report and management guidelines. Surg Neurol 49:290–294

Muthmann A, Sauerbeck E (1903) Über eine Gliageschwulst des 4. Ventrikels. Neuroepithelioma gliomatosum. Beitr pathol Anat 34:445

Ng HK (2006) Ependymoma, subependymoma and myxopapillary ependymoma. In: McLendon RE, Rosenblum MK and Bigner DD (eds) Russell and Rubinstein's pathology of tumors of the nervous system. Hodder Arnold, London

Nijssen PC, Deprez RH, Tijssen CC, Hagemeijer A, Arnoldus EP, Teepen JL, Holl R, Niermeyer MF (1994) Familial anaplastic ependymoma: evidence of loss of chromosome 22 in tumour cells. J Neurol Neurosurg Psychiatry 57:1245–1248

Nobles E, Lee R, Kircher T (1991) Mediastinal ependymoma. Hum Pathol 22:94–96

Nozaki M, Tada M, Matsumoto R, Sawamura Y, Abe H, Iggo RD (1998) Rare occurrence of inactivating p53 gene mutations in primary non-astrocytic tumors of the central nervous system: reappraisal by yeast functional assay. Acta Neuropathol (Berl) 95:291–296

Olin P, Giesecke J (1998) Potential exposure to SV40 in polio vaccines used in Sweden during 1957: no impact on cancer incidence rates 1960 to 1993. Dev Biol Stand 94:227–233

Onilude OE, Lusher ME, Lindsey JC, Pearson AD, Ellison DW, Clifford SC (2006) APC and CTNNB1 mutations are rare in sporadic ependymomas. Cancer Genet Cytogenet 168:158–161

Peris-Bonet R, Martinez-Garcia C, Lacour B, Petrovich S, Giner-Ripoll B, Navajas A, Steliarova-Foucher E (2006) Childhood central nervous system tumours–incidence and survival in Europe (1978–1997): report from Automated Childhood Cancer Information System project. Eur J Cancer 42:2064–2080

Plans G, Brell M, Cabiol J, Villa S, Torres A, Acebes JJ (2006) Intracranial retrograde dissemination in filum terminale myxopapillary ependymomas. Acta Neurochir 148:343–346; discussion 346

Prayson RA (1999) Clinicopathologic study of 61 patients with ependymoma including MIB-1 immunohistochemistry. Ann Diagn Pathol 3:11–18

Preusser M, Wolfsberger S, Czech T, Slavc I, Budka H, Hainfellner JA (2005) Survivin expression in intracranial ependymomas and its correlation with tumor cell proliferation and patient outcome. Am J Clin Pathol 124:543–549

Ransom DT, Ritland SR, Kimmel DW, Moertel CA, Dahl RJ, Scheithauer BW, Kelly PJ, Jenkins RB (1992) Cytogenetic and loss of heterozygosity studies in ependymomas, pilocytic astrocytomas, and oligodendrogliomas. Genes Chromosomes Cancer 5:348–356

Reardon DA, Egorin MJ, Quinn JA, Rich JN, Gururangan S, Vredenburgh JJ, Desjardins A, Sathornsumetee S, Provenzale JM, Herndon JE 2nd, Dowell JM, Badruddoja MA, McLendon RE, Lagattuta TF, Kicielinski KP, Dresemann G, Sampson JH, Friedman AH, Salvado AJ, Friedman HS (2005) Phase II study of imatinib mesylate plus hydroxyurea in adults with recurrent glioblastoma multiforme. J Clin Oncol 23:9359–9368

Rich JN, Sathornsumetee S, Keir ST, Kieran MW, Laforme A, Kaipainen A, McLendon RE, Graner MW, Rasheed BK, Wang L, Reardon DA, Ryan AJ, Wheeler C, Dimery I, Bigner DD, Friedman HS (2005) ZD6474, a novel tyrosine kinase inhibitor of vascular endothelial growth factor receptor and epidermal growth factor receptor, inhibits tumor growth of multiple nervous system tumors. Clin Cancer Res 11:8145–8157

Rickert CH, Paulus W (2004) Comparative genomic hybridization in central and peripheral nervous system tumors of childhood and adolescence. J Neuropathol Exp Neurol 63:399–417

Rickert CH, Kedziora O, Gullotta F (1999) Ependymoma of the cauda equina. Acta Neurochir 141:781–782

Rickert CH, Gocke H, Paulus W (2002) Fetal ependymoma associated with Down's syndrome. Acta Neuropathol 103:78–81

Rickert CH, Korshunov A, Paulus W (2006) Chromosomal imbalances in clear cell ependymomas. Mod Pathol 19:958–962

Ringertz N (1950) Grading of Gliomas. Acta Pathol Microbiol Scand 27:51–64

Ritter AM, Hess KR, McLendon RE, Langford LA (1998) Ependymomas: MIB-1 proliferation index and survival. J Neurooncol 40:51–57

Robles SG, Saldana C, Boto GR, Martinez A, Zamarron AP, Jorquera M, Mata P (2005) Intradural extramedullary spinal ependymoma: a benign pathology? Spine 30:E251–254

Rodriguez FJ, Scheithauer BW, Robbins PD, Burger PC, Hessler RB, Perry A, Abell-Aleff PC, Mierau GW (2006) Ependymomas with neuronal differentiation: a morphologic and immunohistochemical spectrum. Acta Neuropathol 113(3):313–324

Roussy G, Oberling C (1932) Histologic classification of tumours of the central nervous system. Arch Neurol Psychiatr 27:1281–1289

Ruchoux MM, Kepes JJ, Dhellemmes P, Hamon M, Maurage CA, Lecomte M, Gall CM, Chilton J (1998) Lipomatous differentiation in ependymomas: a report of three cases and comparison with similar changes reported in other central nervous system neoplasms of neuroectodermal origin. Am J Surg Pathol 22:338–346

Rumboldt Z, Camacho DL, Lake D, Welsh CT, Castillo M (2006) Apparent diffusion coefficients for differentiation of cerebellar tumors in children. AJNR Am J Neuroradiol 27:1362–1369

Sakakibara Y, Suiko M, Pai TG, Nakayama T, Takami Y, Katafuchi J, Liu MC (2002) Highly conserved mouse and human brain sulfotransferases: molecular cloning, expression, and functional characterization. Gene 285:39–47

Sandalcioglu IE, Gasser T, Asgari S, Lazorisak A, Engelhorn T, Egelhof T, Stolke D, Wiedemayer H (2005) Functional outcome after surgical treatment of intramedullary spinal cord tumors: experience with 78 patients. Spinal Cord 43:34–41

Savard ML, Gilchrist DM (1989) Ependymomas in two sisters and a maternal male cousin with mosaicism with monosomy 22 in tumour. Pediatr Neurosci 15:80–84

Schiffer D, Giordana MT (1998) Prognosis of ependymoma. Childs Nerv Syst 14:357–361

Schuz J, Kaletsch U, Kaatsch P, Meinert R, Michaelis J (2001) Risk factors for pediatric tumors of the central nervous system: results from a German population-based case-control study. Med Pediatr Oncol 36:274–282

Schwartz TH, McCormick PC (2000) Intramedullary ependymomas: clinical presentation, surgical treatment strategies and prognosis. J Neurooncol 47:211–218

Schwartz TH, Kim S, Glick RS, Bagiella E, Balmaceda C, Fetell MR, Stein BM, Sisti MB, Bruce JN (1999) Supratentorial ependymomas in adult patients. Neurosurgery 44:721–731

Slavc I, MacCollin MM, Dunn M, Jones S, Sutton L, Gusella JF, Biegel JA (1995) Exon scanning for mutations of the NF2 gene in pediatric ependymomas, rhabdoid tumors and meningiomas. Int J Cancer 64:243–247

Sonneland PR, Scheithauer BW, Onofrio BM (1985) Myxopapillary ependymoma. A clinicopathologic and immunocytochemical study of 77 cases. Cancer 56:883–893

Sowar K, Straessle J, Donson AM, Handler M, Foreman NK (2006) Predicting which children are at risk for ependymoma relapse. J Neurooncol 78:41–46

Spassky N, Merkle FT, Flames N, Tramontin AD, Garcia-Verdugo JM, Alvarez-Buylla A (2005) Adult ependymal cells are postmitotic and are derived from radial glial cells during embryogenesis. J Neurosci 25:10–18

Stiller CA, Nectoux J (1994) International incidence of childhood brain and spinal tumours. Int J Epidemiol 23:458–464

Suarez-Merino B, Hubank M, Revesz T, Harkness W, Hayward R, Thompson D, Darling JL, Thomas DG, Warr TJ (2005) Microarray analysis of pediatric ependymoma identifies a cluster of 112 candidate genes including four transcripts at 22q12.-q13.3. Neurooncol 7:20–31

Takeshita T, Arita T, Asao H, Tanaka N, Higuchi M, Kuroda H, Kaneko K, Munakata H, Endo Y, Fujita T, Sugamura K (1996) Cloning of a novel signal-transducing adaptor molecule containing an SH3 domain and ITAM. Biochem Biophys Res Commun 225:1035–1039

Tamiolakis D, Papadopoulos N, Venizelos I, Lambropoulou M, Nikolaidou S, Bolioti S, Kiziridou A, Manavis J, Alexiadis G, Simopoulos C (2006) Loss of chromosome 1 in myxopapillary ependymoma suggests a region out of chromosome 22 as critical for tumour biology: a FISH analysis of four cases on touch imprint smears. Cytopathology 17:199–204

Taylor MD, Poppleton H, Fuller C, Su X, Liu Y, Jensen P, Magdaleno S, Dalton J, Calabrese C, Board J, Macdonald T, Rutka J, Guha A, Gajjar A, Curran T, Gilbertson RJ (2005) Radial glia cells are candidate stem cells of ependymoma. Cancer Cell 8:323–335

Torres CF, Korones DN, Pilcher W (1997) Multiple ependymomas in a patient with Turcot's syndrome. Med Pediatr Oncol 28:59–61

Uematsu Y, Rojas-Corona RR, Llena JF, Hirano A (1989) Distribution of epithelial membrane antigen in normal and neoplastic human ependyma. Acta Neuropathol 78:325–328

Vara-Thorbeck R, Sanz-Esponera J (1970) Intrasacral ependymoma. Case report. J Neurosurg 32:589–592

Vege KD, Giannini C, Scheithauer BW (2000) The immunophenotype of ependymomas. Appl Immunohistochem Mol Morphol 8:25–31

Verstegen MJ, Leenstra DT, Ijlst-Keizers H, Bosch DA (2002) Proliferation- and apoptosis-related proteins in intracranial ependymomas: an immunohistochemical analysis. J Neurooncol 56:21–28

von Haken MS, White EC, Daneshvar-Shyesther L, Sih S, Choi E, Kalra R, Cogen PH (1996) Molecular genetic analysis of chromosome arm 17p and chromosome arm 22q DNA sequences in sporadic pediatric ependymomas. Genes Chromosomes Cancer 17:37–44

Weggen S, Bayer TA, von Deimling A, Reifenberger G, von Schweinitz D, Wiestler OD, Pietsch T (2000) Low frequency of SV40, JC and BK polyomavirus sequences in human medulloblastomas, meningiomas and ependymomas. Brain Pathol 10:85–92

Wiendl H, Feiden W, Scherieble H, Renz T, Dichgans J, Weller M (2003) March 2003: a 41-year-old female with a solitary lesion in the liver. Brain Pathol 13:421–423

Wiestler OD, Schiffer D, Coons SW, Prayson RA, Rosenblum MK (2000) Ependymal tumours. In: Kleihues P, Cavenee WK (eds) Pathology and genetics of tumours of the nervous system. IARC Press, Lyon

Wolfsberger S, Fischer I, Hoftberger R, Birner P, Slavc I, Dieckmann K, Czech T, Budka H, Hainfellner J (2004) Ki-67 immunolabeling index is an accurate predictor of outcome in patients with intracranial ependymoma. Am J Surg Pathol 28:914–920

Wong TT, Ho DM, Chang KP, Yen SH, Guo WY, Chang FC, Liang ML, Pan HC, Chung WY (2005) Primary pediatric brain tumors: statistics of Taipei VGH, Taiwan (1975–2004). Cancer 104:2156–2167

Yamasaki F, Kurisu K, Satoh K, Arita K, Sugiyama K, Ohtaki M, Takaba J, Tominaga A, Hanaya R, Yoshioka H, Hama S, Ito Y, Kajiwara Y, Yahara K, Saito T, Thohar MA (2005) Apparent diffusion coefficient of human brain tumors at MR imaging. Radiology 235:985–991

Yokota T, Tachizawa T, Fukino K, Teramoto A, Kouno J, Matsumoto K, Emi M (2003) A family with spinal anaplastic ependymoma: evidence of loss of chromosome 22q in tumor. J Hum Genet 48:598–602

Zec N, De Girolami U, Schofield DE, Scott RM, Anthony DC (1996) Giant cell ependymoma of the filum terminale. A report of two cases. Am J Surg Pathol 20:1091–1101

Zülch KJ (1962) Die Gradeinteilung (Grading) der Malignität der Hirngeschwülste. Acta Neurochir 10:639–645

Zülch KJ (1986) Brain tumors. Their biology and pathology. Springer, Berlin

Pediatric Gliomas

4

Stefan Pfister and Olaf Witt

Abstract Pediatric gliomas comprise a clinically, histologically, and molecularly very heterogeneous group of CNS tumors. In addition, these tumors are largely different from their counterparts occurring in adults, although they are histologically indistinguishable and uniformly classified by the current WHO classification for CNS tumors. Pilocytic astrocytoma (WHO grade I), mainly arising in the posterior fossa, is the most common representative in children, whereas glioblastoma multiforme (WHO grade IV) predominates in adults. When radical surgical resection is possible in low-grade gliomas, it will likely cure the patient. If complete surgical resection is not possible, however, for example in brainstem gliomas, which are defined by their anatomic localization rather than by their histological or molecular features, therapeutic options are limited and prognosis is usually poor. Recent genome-wide analyses applying different microarray-based methods to investigate DNA copy-number aberrations, mRNA expression signatures, and methylation patterns have shed some light on the pathways involved in the pathogenesis of pediatric gliomas. Mitogen-activated protein kinase (MAPK) and PI3K/AKT signaling were identified as prominent oncogenic pathways in astrocytic tumors in several studies, whereas NOTCH signaling was implicated in the pathogenesis of a subset of intracranial ependymomas. Future therapeutic strategies targeting these (and other) pathways or conferring epigenetic modifications in the tumor might contribute to a better treatment outcome of patients with unresectable or disseminated tumors at diagnosis. Consideration of reliable molecular markers for outcome prediction will most likely result in a better stratification of patients into different risk groups with adjusted treatment intensity in the future.

4.1 Introduction

Brain tumors, together with leukemias, are the leading cause of cancer-related mortality in children, despite being only half as frequent as leukemias in this age group (Pollack et al. 2008). According to a population-based study by Kaatsch and colleagues (Kaatsch et al. 2001), gliomas comprise approximately 60% of cases among pediatric brain tumors, whereas the remaining

Stefan Pfister (✉)
Department of Pediatric Hematology and Oncology
Heidelberg University Hospital
Im Neuenheimer Feld 153
D – 69120 Heidelberg
Germany
E-mail: stefan.pfister@med.uniheidelberg.de/
s.pfister@dkfz.de

40% are heterogeneous and consist of medulloblastomas and other embryonal tumors (26%), craniopharyngiomas (4%), pineal tumors (1%), meningiomas (1%), and others (11%; Table 4.1).

All glial cells in the central nervous system (CNS) (e.g., astrocytes, oligodendrocytes, ependymocytes) may give rise to benign as well as malignant neoplasms (gliomas): astrocytes may give rise to astrocytomas of various grades or glioblastoma multiforme, oligodendrocytes may give rise to oligodendrogliomas, and ependymocytes may develop into ependymomas and choroid plexus tumors. Pediatric gliomas may be further sub-classified by their localization and histological subtype. Since the localization of an individual brain tumor plays an important role for the overall prognosis of the patient, pediatric gliomas are separated into the following groups according to their anatomic site: supratentorial gliomas, brainstem gliomas, and cerebellar gliomas.

Histologically, CNS tumors are uniformly diagnosed and graded according to the World Health Organization (WHO) classification (Louis et al. 2007) as described in other chapters of this book. The 2007 WHO classification distinguishes 22 different glioma subtypes with various tumor grades. The frequencies of these entities in pediatric patients are summarized in Table 4.2. Following the frequency of occurrence in children, this chapter will focus on pilocytic and diffuse astrocytoma, ependymoma, anaplastic astrocytoma (AA), and glioblastoma (GBM).

4.2 Epidemiology and Clinical Features

The incidence of CNS tumors in children seems to be the highest in Scandinavian countries with an incidence rate of approximately four CNS tumors per 100,000 children per year (Kaatsch et al. 2001). Particularly low overall incidence rates of 1.7 were found in Hong Kong and in Costa Rica. Male patients are over-represented in the same population-based study, with a male to female ratio of about 1.3:1. An increase in brain tumor incidence of about 1–2% per year, which has been reported in adults, was not observed in US American children in a population-based study (Linabery and Ross 2008). Pilocytic astrocytomas comprise the most frequent brain tumor in children older than 3 years of age, whereas in infants, embryonal tumors (medulloblastoma, supratentorial primitive neuroectodermal tumor) are most common.

Certain hereditary cancer syndromes confer a genetic susceptibility for the development of

Table 4.1 Main histologic subtypes, WHO grade, and frequency of central nervous system tumors in children (From Kaatsch et al. 2001)

	Tumor entity	Who grade	Frequency(%)
Gliomas	Astrocytomas	I–IV	41.7
	Ependymomas	I–III	10.4
	Gangliogliomas[a]	I	3.2
	Oligodendrogliomas	II–III	1.1
Non-glial tumors	Medulloblastomas and other embryonal tumors	IV	25.7
	Craniopharyngiomas	I	4.4
	Pineal tumors	I–IV	1.3
	Meningiomas	I–III	1.2
	Others (e.g., lymphomas, germ cell tumors, metastases)	n/a	11.0

[a]Gangliogliomas are mixed neuronal-glial tumors

Table 4.2 Gliomas, tumor grades, and frequency according to the WHO classification of CNS tumors (Louis et al. 2007 and Kaatsch et al. 2001)

Tumor entity	Who grade I	II	III	IV	Frequency(%)
Astrocytic tumors					38.8
Subependymal giant cell astrocytoma	X				0.4
Pilocytic astrocytoma	X				14.8
Pilomyxoid astrocytoma		X			n/a
Diffuse astrocytoma		X			2.2
Pleomorphic xanthoastrocytoma		X			0.4
Anaplastic astrocytoma			X		1.9
Glioblastoma				X	2.8
Giant cell sarcoma				X	0.1
Gliosarcoma				X	0.1
Astrocytoma, not otherwise specified					15.6
Oligodendroglial tumors					1.5
Oligodendroglioma		X			1.4
Anaplastic oligodendroglioma			X		0.1
Oligoastrocytic tumors					0.6
Oligoastrocytoma		X			n/a
Anaplastic oligoastrocytoma			X		n/a
Ependymal tumors					8.9
Subependymoma	X				0.1
Myxopapillary ependymoma	X				0.3
Ependymoma		X			5.3
Anaplastic ependymoma			X		3.3
Choroid plexus tumors					1.8
Choroid plexus papilloma	X				1.2
Atypical choroids plexus papilloma		X			n/a
Choroid plexus carcinoma			X		0.6

ªFrequency among pediatric CNS tumors excluding germ cell tumors

various glial tumors in childhood. Approximately 15% of patients with neurofibromatosis type 1 (NF1) develop pilocytic astrocytomas, particularly of the optic nerve. Conversely, up to one third of patients with a pilocytic astrocytoma of the optic tract have NF1. Patients with neurofibromatosis type 2 (NF2) may typically develop spinal ependymomas, whereas diffuse and pilocytic astrocytomas are less common in these patients. Astrocytomas, glioblastomas, and choroid plexus carcinomas are also observed in patients with Li-Fraumeni syndrome (*TP53*) and Turcot syndrome type 1 (*MLH1, MSH2, PMS2*). Hereditary cancer syndromes are discussed in more detail in a separate chapter of this book.

Pilocytic astrocytoma (WHO grade I) comprises the most frequent brain tumor in children with an age-adjusted incidence of 0.8 per 100,000 children per year (Ohgaki and Kleihues 2005). In the pediatric cohort, about two-thirds of pilocytic astrocytomas arise in the cerebellum. Clinical symptoms typically develop slowly, as reflected by a slowly growing lesion. Signs and symptoms may include focal neurological deficits, but also non-localizing signs, such as chronic headache, macrocephaly, or endocrinological deficits. In the case of optical tract involvement, loss of visual acuity and narrowing of visual fields may be presenting symptoms. In patients with NF1, an asymptomatic pilocytic astrocytoma may be detected during routine diagnostic work-up. Seizures are uncommon in pilocytic astrocytomas because these tumors typically do not arise in the cerebral cortex. On neuroimaging, pilocytic astrocytomas appear well circumscribed and contrast enhancing, often exophytic and cystic. Although sensitive medical imaging may suggest extensive infiltration, this might in part be due to peritumoral edema and Wallerian degeneration of surrounding tissue. Surprisingly, pilocytic astrocytomas very occasionally may metastasize to the neuroaxis, which is not a negative prognostic marker per se.

Diffuse astrocytoma (WHO grade II) is about 6–7 times less common in children than pilocytic astrocytoma. These tumors may be located in any region of the CNS with the most frequent location being the frontal and temporal lobes in around one third of cases, whereas the cerebellum comprises an uncommon location. Seizures are a common presenting symptom, sometimes proceeded by more subtle signs, e.g., sensomotor changes or speech difficulties. Frontal lobe tumors often present with changes in behavior or personality. In contrast to pilocytic astrocytomas, diffuse astrocytomas typically do not show contrast enhancement on neuroimaging and present as a homogeneous mass with low density. Contrast enhancement characteristically appears upon malignant progression to anaplastic astrocytoma or secondary glioblastoma. Malignant progression, however, which in adults eventually occurs in a majority of cases with diffuse astrocytoma (60–70%), is only observed in around 10% of children with this tumor (Broniscer et al. 2007; Ohgaki and Kleihues 2005; Watanabe et al. 1997).

The usual first-line treatment of pilocytic and diffuse astrocytomas in children consists of surgical tumor resection. Macroscopically completely resected tumors have an excellent long-term prognosis. In nonresectable situations, radiation therapy is indicated. Chemotherapy is currently evaluated in patients with tumors refractory to radiation, in young infants or patients with NF1 harboring a high risk for secondary malignancies following radiation therapy. The overall 10-year survival rate of children with pilocytic or diffuse astrocytomas exceeds 80%.

Anaplastic astrocytoma (WHO grade III) occurs at about the same frequency in children as diffuse astrocytoma (Kaatsch et al. 2001). Anaplastic astrocytomas predominantly occur in the cerebral hemispheres, but may also occur in deep midline structures of the cerebrum, and occasionally in the posterior fossa. Clinical presentation largely resembles that of diffuse astrocytoma. Anaplastic astrocytomas typically display contrast enhancement on neuroimaging; however, a subset of grade III astrocytomas lack uptake of contrast medium rendering it indistinguishable from grade II lesions radiologically.

Glioblastoma multiforme (WHO grade IV) occurs about 1.5 times more often than anaplastic astrocytoma in children, but is about 100 times less common in children than in adults. A combined frontotemporal location is particularly typical; however, parietal and occipital lobes may also be affected. On neuroimaging, glioblastomas typically show ring enhancement of the tumor margin with central necrosis and marked peritumoral edema.

First-line treatment of pediatric anaplastic astrocytomas and glioblastomas generally involves radical surgical resection whenever possible and wide local radiotherapy (in children > 3 years of age). Despite attempts of therapy intensification by adding toxic chemotherapy regimens to surgery and radiation, the overall prognosis of anaplastic astrocytoma and glioblastoma remains the poorest in pediatric oncology. Unresectable glioblastomas have a 5-year event-free survival rate of 5%, grossly resected tumors of 30% (Finlay et al. 1995). Temozolomide, which has been demonstrated to be beneficial in adult patients with GBM, is currently evaluated in pediatric high-grade gliomas. However, preliminary results in small noncontrolled series demonstrate marginal efficacy only (Barone et al. 2006). The role of intense chemotherapy in the treatment of high-grade gliomas in children is still controversial. However, infants younger than 3 years with anaplastic astrocytoma and glioblastoma appear to have a much better prognosis and may respond well to intensive chemotherapy protocols. Hopefully, novel treatment strategies such as targeted therapies, immunotherapy, or oncolytic viruses will help to improve the outcome of this challenging brain tumor entity in the future.

Brainstem gliomas comprise a histologically very heterogeneous group of glial tumors in the pediatric cohort arising in the midbrain, pons, or medulla oblongata. Brainstem gliomas account for approximately 10–20% of pediatric CNS tumors (Hargrave et al. 2006; Recinos et al. 2007), and share the dismal characteristic that they are often not accessible to surgical resection. Brainstem gliomas are better subcategorized biologically than histologically as diffusely infiltrating and focal brainstem tumors. Diffusely infiltrating tumors have an extremely poor prognosis (10-year survival < 10%) due to their nonresectable location involving the pons. Focal brainstem tumors are typically located in the midbrain or medulla rather than in the pons and characteristically display AN exophytic growth behavior. The latter tumors have a much better prognosis, especially if the tumor is accessible to surgical resection. Novel treatment strategies in pediatric pons glioma involving targeting of the EGFR pathway are underway (Finlay and Zacharoulis 2005).

Ependymomas (WHO grade II) originate from the lining epithelium of the ventricles or spinal canal. Ependymomas of the pediatric age group are typically localized in the fourth ventricle, whereas spinal ependymomas are uncommon in children (with the exception of patients with neurofibromatosis type 2). The incidence peaks in the under 4 years age group (5.2 cases per 1,000,000), and males are twice as commonly affected as females (Ries et al. 1999). **Anaplastic features** (defining WHO grade III ependymomas) are far more frequent in intracranial than in spinal tumors, particularly in ependymomas of the posterior fossa. Anaplastic ependymomas are typically contrast enhancing on magnetic resonance (MR) imaging, and are accompanied by microvascular proliferation and pseudopalisading necrosis histologically. The single most important prognostic factor is the extent of tumor resection: Survival rates are approximately 70% in patients after gross tumor resection, whereas patients with incomplete resection have a very poor outcome (overall survival of < 30%).

4.3
Histopathology

Since histopathological characteristics and diagnostic criteria according to the WHO classification of CNS tumors (Louis et al. 2007) uniformly apply for pediatric and adult tumors, we will herein focus on the histopathological features of pilocytic astrocytoma, which is not covered by other chapters of this book.

Pilocytic astrocytoma is a tumor of low-to-moderate cellularity and typically shows a biphasic pattern with varying proportions of compacted bipolar cells with characteristic Rosenthal fibers and loose-textured multipolar cells with microcysts and PAS-positive granular bodies. Nuclei have a hyperchromatic and pleomorphic appearance, and mitosis is rarely observed. Infiltration of the leptomeninges is compatible with pilocytic astrocytoma and is a priori not a sign of malignancy. As evidenced by their contrast enhancement in medical imaging, pilocytic astrocytomas are highly vascularized typically displaying glomeruloid vascular proliferations. Regressive changes, such as markedly hyalinized, sometimes ecstatic vessels, calcifications, infarct-like necrosis, and lymphocytic infiltrates are frequently observed. Like other astrocytic tumors, pilocytic astrocytomas stain positive for "glial fibrillary acid protein" (GFAP). As described in Chap. 1, expression of vimentin, S-100 protein, microtubule-associated protein 2 (MAP2), and alpha B-crystallin is also commonly observed in pediatric astrocytic tumors; however, these antigens are less specific than GFAP and also expressed in most other glial tumors and many non-glial neoplasms. Labeling indices for the proliferation-associated antigen Ki-67 (MIB-1) typically range from 0% to 3.9% (mean 1.1%) in pilocytic astrocytomas.

4.4
Molecular Genetics

Pilocytic Astrocytoma. Autosomal dominantly inherited neurofibromatosis type 1 (NF1) is associated with a predisposition to the development of low-grade astrocytomas. In particular, pilocytic astrocytoma of the optic nerve and chiasm, but also diffuse astrocytoma, occurs with increased frequency in NF1 patients (Listernick et al. 2007). Neurofibromin, the gene product of the NF1 gene, physiologically contributes to growth arrest of astrocytic cells and neuronal differentiation by down-regulation of the mitogen-activated protein kinase (MAPK) signaling pathway via its GTPase-activating domain. Loss of neurofibromin expression conversely leads to increased Ras activity and astrocyte proliferation (Yunoue et al. 2003).

Interestingly, MAPK signaling was also shown to be activated in virtually all sporadic pilocytic astrocytomas (Sharma et al. 2005). Furthermore, gene expression profiles of NF1-associated pilocytic astrocytomas and sporadic pilocytic astrocytomas showed similar activation of MAPK pathway target genes, indicating that constitutive activation of the MAPK pathway is commonly involved in the pathogenesis of sporadic and hereditary astrocytomas (Rorive et al. 2006; Sharma et al. 2007). We and others identified activating mutations in *KRAS* (Fig. 4.1a), which result in activation of MAPK signaling, in a minor fraction of sporadic pilocytic astrocytomas (Janzarik et al. 2007; Sharma et al. 2005). Comprising by far the most

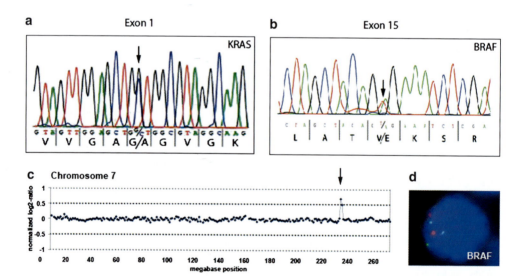

Fig. 4.1a–d Genetic aberrations in pilocytic astrocytomas involving the MAPK pathway. Activating mutations of *KRAS* (**a**) and *BRAF* (**b**) in pediatric pilocytic astrocytomas. Gene-duplication of *BRAF* as assessed by array-CGH (**c**) or fluorescence in situ hybridization (FISH) (**d**). For FISH, *red signals* represent a centromeric probe from chromosome 7, and *green signals* represent the *BRAF*-specific probe

frequent genetic event in pilocytic astrocytoma identified to date, we were recently able to characterize *BRAF* as a centrally important oncogene in the pathogenesis of pediatric pilocytic astrocytoma (Pfister et al. 2008). More that 50% of pilocytic astrocytomas in this age group display a duplication of the *BRAF* locus and consecutive expression of a fusion transcript involving the kinase domain of BRAF and the 5´part of the uncharacterized gene KIAA1549. (David TW Jones et al. 2008). Approximately 6% of the remaining tumors show an activating mutation of *BRAF* at hotspot codon 600 in exon 15 (Fig. 4.1b–d). Previous studies investigating DNA copy-number changes in more than 160 pilocytic and diffuse astrocytomas had revealed normal karyotypes in the vast majority of cases. (Bigner et al. 1997; Jenkins et al. 1989; Jones et al. 2006; Orr et al. 2002; Sanoudou et al. 2000; Zattara-Cannoni et al. 1998). However, these studies employed a variety of technologies with generally inferior resolution. The most frequent aberrations detected in these studies involved trisomy of chromosome 5 and of chromosome 7 or gains of 7q.

Diffuse Astrocytoma. Mutations of *TP53*, which comprise the most frequent molecular genetic alteration in low-grade astrocytomas of otherwise healthy adults, are not a frequent event in the pediatric age group (Felix et al. 1995; Litofsky et al. 1994). *BRAF* gene duplications were only observed in a minority of diffuse astrocytoma cases (approximately 15%) in our array-CGH study (Pfister et al. 2008). The frequency of epigenetically silenced *MGMT*, another frequent event in adult diffuse astrocytomas (Watanabe et al. 1997), is not known for pediatric cases at present as is the frequency of IDH1 mutations (Balss et al. 2008)

Anaplastic Astrocytoma. Due to the infrequency of occurrence, anaplastic astrocytomas and glioblastomas are often summarized as "high-grade" gliomas in pediatric studies, which sometimes prohibits a more specific data analysis.

In a CGH study investigating ten anaplastic astrocytomas in children, a significantly shorter survival was found for tumors showing a gain of chromosomal material at chromosome arm 1q (Rickert et al. 2001). In the same study, gains of 5q, and losses of 6q, 9q, 12q, and 22q, were identified to be characteristic genomic aberrations in anaplastic astrocytomas in children. In contrast to adult high-grade gliomas, in which microsatellite instability appears generally absent, approximately 25% of pediatric anaplastic astrocytomas display a microsatellite instability phenotype as a result of mutations in various DNA mismatch repair genes (Alonso et al. 2001; Cheng et al. 1999). Similar to the situation in adults, mutations in the *PTEN* tumor suppressor gene at 10q23 are rarely observed in pediatric anaplastic astrocytoma (6%). If present, however, *PTEN* mutations are associated with poor prognosis (Raffel et al. 1999).

Pediatric Glioblastoma. Although histologically indistinguishable from adult glioblastomas, the molecular signatures of pediatric glioblastomas are very different from their adult counterparts. *TP53* mutations, which comprise a hallmark genetic lesion in secondary, but not in primary glioblastomas in adults, frequently occur in de novo (primary) pediatric glioblastomas. Genomic amplification of the *EGFR* gene, which comprises the most frequent genetic change in adult primary glioblastoma, is rarely ($<10\%$) observed in pediatric tumors (Bredel et al. 1999; Sung et al. 2000). However, elevated immunoreactivity for *EGFR* is observed in 80% of pediatric tumors indicating a different mechanism for the activation of this gene (Bredel et al. 1999). Similarly, whereas adult primary glioblastomas display a high frequency of mutations of the *PTEN* tumor suppressor gene at 10q23, pediatric glioblastomas rarely harbor such mutations. Although LOH at 10q23 may be present in as many as 80% of cases, homozygous deletions are only seen in a minority (approx. 8%) of pediatric glioblastomas. If mutations of *PTEN* are observed, these seem to be associated with poor prognosis in the pediatric cohort (Cheng et al. 1999; Raffel et al. 1999). In a CGH study comparing pediatric with adult glioblastomas, + 1q, + 3q, + 16p, –8q, and –17p were more frequent in the pediatric age group than in adult glioblastomas (Rickert et al. 2001). In a recent mRNA expression profiling study comparing pediatric and adult glioblastomas, two prognostically different subsets of pediatric glioblastomas were defined: one subset with MAPK and AKT pathway activation associated with very poor prognosis, and a second subset with better prognosis, which did not show activated MAPK and AKT signaling. This second set of pediatric glioblastomas, in turn, did not share the genomic fingerprint characterizing long-term survivors in adult glioblastomas (Faury et al. 2007). In the same study, over-expression of *YBX1* was specific for pediatric glioblastomas and might comprise a novel mechanism for *EGFR* over-expression in these tumors. In a study by Pollack and colleagues, p53 immunostaining was identified as an independent prognostic marker for patient outcome in a large patient cohort of pediatric malignant gliomas (Pollack et al. 2002).

Ependymoma and Anaplastic Ependymoma. Neurofibromatosis type 2 is associated with spinal ependymomas in about 5% of cases (Parry et al. 1994), indicating a role of the *NF2* tumor suppressor gene at 22q12.2 in these tumors (Ebert et al. 1999; Lamszus et al. 2001). Cytogenetic studies by conventional comparative genomic hybridization (CGH) revealed numerous chromosomal aberrations in pediatric ependymoma, such as a 30–50% incidence of chromosome 22 changes, including monosomy 22 and deletions of 22q (Carter et al. 2002; Hirose et al. 2001; Mazewski et al. 1999). About 40% of pediatric ependymomas have been reported to display balanced profiles by CGH in comparison to only 10% in adults (Carter et al. 2002; Dyer et al. 2002; Hirose et al. 2001), and it has been suggested that the development of ependymomas at younger age might often be independent of chromosomal instability. However, with increased resolution using array-CGH, we found DNA copy-number aberrations in 93% of pediatric ependymomas (Mendrzyk et al. 2006). In the same study, we identified gains at 1q and over-expression of EGFR protein as novel molecular markers for poor patient outcome. Furthermore, increased hTERT protein expression was associated with adverse outcome (Mendrzyk et al. 2006). This finding is exactly in line with another study published at the same date investigating hTERT expression in 65 children with intracranial ependymoma. In this study, hTERT protein expression comprised the most important single predictor of survival amongst all known pathological clinical markers (Tabori et al. 2006). By investigating consecutive tumor samples of a patient with several relapses from an anaplastic ependymoma, we were recently able to show that molecular progression occurs in these tumors in a similar way as that described in other brain tumors (Milde et al. 2008). Furthermore, we were able to identify SHREW1 as a candidate gene for tumor dissemination in ependymoma (Milde et al. 2008).

RNA expression profiling using cDNA microarrays identified differences in ependymoma subgroups and potential candidate genes on chromosome 22q (Korshunov et al. 2003; Suarez-Merino et al. 2005). More recently, deletions at 6q25.3 were identified as a potential prognostic marker for favorable outcome in intracranial ependymomas, which mostly occur in children (Monoranu et al. 2008). In a CGH study investigating a relatively small cohort of pediatric patients with intracranial tumors, combined loss of 6p22-pter and 13q14.3-qter was identified as a potential predictor for reduced survival (Pezzolo et al. 2008).

4.5
Molecular Diagnostics

Routine molecular diagnostics have unfortunately not yet been established in pediatric neuropathology. However, *MGMT* methylation status may be analyzed prior to temozolomide treatment of high-grade astrocytomas to predict treatment response to alkylating chemotherapy (Donson et al. 2007). As previously described, *MGMT* promoter methylation can be easily assessed by methylation-specific polymerase chain reaction (MSP) analysis or bisulfite genomic sequencing.

Furthermore, there is good evidence that the phosphorylation status of ERK can serve as a good surrogate marker for MAPK activation in astrocytomas (Faury et al. 2007; Pfister et al. 2007). Therefore, MAPK pathway activation should be prospectively evaluated to determine its potential role in developing novel targeted therapies in future trials.

In ependymoma, hTERT protein expression was identified as a predictive marker in two large independent pediatric patient cohorts indicating that assessment of hTERT expression by immunohistochemistry warrants prospective evaluation in these tumors.

4.6 Pathways to Pediatric Astrocytoma

MAPK Signaling and the PI3K/AKT Pathway. As previously discussed, subsets of pediatric astrocytomas of different WHO grades show activation of MAPK and/or PI3K/AKT signaling. Interestingly, tumors with combined activation of MAPK and PI3K/AKT signaling, which supposedly have an activation upstream or at the level of EGFR (Fig. 4.2), are typically highly

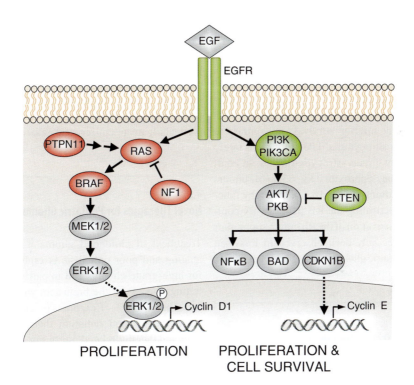

Fig. 4.2 Activation of MAPK and AKT signaling in low-grade and high-grade astrocytic tumors. Schematic representation of genes that have been implicated in the pathogenesis of pediatric low-grade astrocytomas (in *red*) all belonging to the MAPK pathway. Proteins carrying mutations in a majority of adult primary glioblastomas and associated with poor prognosis when present in pediatric glioblastomas are indicated in *green*

malignant, express a gene signature that resembles a neuronal stem-cell phenotype, and are associated with particularly poor outcome (Faury et al. 2007). A second subset of high-grade astrocytomas, which is not associated with activation of MAPK and PI3K signaling, may in contrast originate from astroglial precursors (Faury et al. 2007). Importantly, gene expression signatures from both subgroups do not overlap with their adult counterparts. In low-grade astrocytic tumors, MAPK signaling without concomitant activation of the PI3K/AKT pathway (downstream of EGFR) seems to be the leading molecular characteristic for a majority of tumors (Pfister et al. 2008; Sharma et al. 2005).

The Cell-Cycle Regulatory Pathways pRB and p53. Mutations and concomitant accumulation of (non-functional) TP53 protein are the only frequent genetic aberration that occur at the same frequency in pediatric and adult glioblastomas affecting approximately one third of these tumors (Pollack et al. 2001; Pollack et al. 2002). In the pediatric population, high p53 expression was associated with significantly inferior survival. In contrast to high-grade astrocytoma, TP53 mutations rarely occur in low-grade astrocytic tumors. In adult glioblastoma, approximately 85% of tumors carry alterations of the p16 gene, thereby functionally inactivating the RB pathway. By comparison, inactivation of the Rb tumor-suppressor pathway has only been observed in less than 25% of pediatric glioblastomas (Sung et al. 2000).

4.7
Pathways to Pediatric Ependymoma

Combining array-CGH and mRNA expression profiling analyses in ependymomas from supratentorial, infratentorial (posterior fossa), and spinal localizations, Taylor and colleagues postulated that these histologically identical tumors are derived from different populations of radial glia stem cells (Taylor et al. 2005). Furthermore, the authors demonstrated that tumors from different localizations harbor characteristic genomic aberrations, namely, deletion of 9p21.3 (CDKN2A/B) in supratentorial tumors, gain of 1q (among others) in infratentorial ependymoma, and 22q deletions in spinal tumors. Each of these subgroups was additionally associated with a distinct gene expression signature: NOTCH and Ephrin signaling was predominant in supratentorial cases, HOX genes and IGF1 signaling components were up-regulated in spinal tumors, whereas infratentorial ependymomas showed over-expression of aquaporin- and ID (inhibitor of DNA binding) genes. Identification of such characteristic signaling pathways for clinically distinct subsets of ependymomas might contribute to the development of more tailored therapeutic approaches in the future. Furthermore, and this is discussed in more detail in Chap. 1, understanding brain tumors as a stem cell disease might move the focus of future treatment strategies towards the eradication of these relatively small populations of slow-dividing and particularly treatment-resistant cells.

4.8
Novel Therapies for Pediatric Gliomas

Treatment of childhood glioma is still challenging and poor prognosis is especially true for high-grade gliomas and in particular infiltrating gliomas of the brainstem with survival rates below 10%. Response to conventional chemotherapy and radiation therapy is often poor and therapy-related morbidity is a significant problem in children with gliomas. Thus, novel treatment strategies are urgently required.

Temozolomide, which is currently the gold standard for adjuvant chemotherapy in adult patients with glioblastoma (Stupp et al. 2005), has not shown convincing efficacy in children

Table 4.3 Clinical trials involving targeted therapies for treating children with gliom (selected from clinical trials)

Targets	Entity	Phase I	Phase II	Phase III	Compound
EGF-Pathway					
EGF-Receptor	Pons Glioma			X	Nimotuzumab
EGF-Receptor tyrosine kinase	High grade glioma, pons glioma	X			Erlotinib
EGF-Receptor tyrosine kinase	Brain stem glioma	X	X		Gefitinib
EGFR/ErbB2 tyrosine kinase	Malignant glioma, ependymoma		X		Lapatinib
Ras/Farnesyltransferase	High grade glioma, pons glioma		X		Tipifarnib
VEGFR/EGFR tyrosine kinase	Brain stem glioma	X			Vandetanib
Other Kinases					
ABL tyrosine kinase	Brain stem glioma, High grade glioma		X		Imatinib
PKC/AKT serine/threonine kinase	CNS tumors	X			Enzastaurin
VEGF/Angiogenesis					
VEGF	Brain stem glioma, malignant glioma, ependymoma		X		Bevacizumab
VEGF-receptor	CNS tumors	X			Cediranib (AZD2171)
Angiogenesis?	Brain tumors		X		Thalidomide
Angiogenesis?	CNS tumors	X			Lenalidomide
Immune system					
Glioma cell/MHC class	Malignant glioma	X			Autologous dendritic cell immunotherapy
IL13-receptor	Malignant glioma	X	X		IL13-PE38QQR immunotoxin
TGF-receptor	High grade glioma	X	X		TGFa-PE38 immunotoxin
HDACs					
Class I HDACs	Solid tumors	X			Depsipeptide
Class I HDACs	CNS tumors	X			Valproic acid
Class I + II HDACs	Solid tumors	X			Vorinostat
Miscellaneous					
Alpha/beta 3,5 integrin	Brain tumors	X			Cilengitide
Retinoic acid receptor	Malignant glioma			X	Isotretinoin
COX-2	Brainstem glioma	X			Rofecoxib

ABL, Abelson tyrosine kinase; ErbB2, erythroblastic leukemia viral oncogene homolog 2; EGF, epidermal growth factor; COX-2, cyclooxygenase 2; HDAC, histone deacetylase; IL13, interleukin 13; MHC, major histocompatibility class; PKC, protein kinase C; TGF, transforming growth factor; VEGF, vascular epithelial growth factor

so far (Barone et al. 2006). However, silencing of the DNA repair gene MGMT resulted in prolonged survival of children with glioblastoma in a small series (Donson et al. 2007) as it has been demonstrated in adults (Hegi et al. 2005). Therefore, this molecular information should be included in treatment decisions on the use of temozolomide in children with gliomas in clinical trials as previously mentioned.

Significant progress in understanding the molecular and genetic biology of gliomas has been made in recent years. Several pathways and key proteins involved in glioma tumor growth are now available for selective drug targeting. For example, activation of the EGFR, MAPK, and AKT pathways, or inactivation of PTEN, has been identified in pediatric high-grade gliomas (Bredel et al. 1999; Faury et al. 2007; Raffel et al. 1999) and antibodies or small molecule compounds are now available to target these pathways. In pediatric low-grade astrocytomas, aberrant activation of the MAPK pathway was found (Pfister et al. 2008). Again, pharmacological tools are available to block aberrant signal transduction through this pathway and to exert antitumoral effects in vitro (Pfister et al. 2008). Other promising novel compounds include anti-angiogenic agents blocking signal transduction via the VEGF pathway, histone-deacetylase inhibitors targeting the epigenetic repression machinery, and differentiation-inducing compounds. In addition, immunotherapy approaches using dendritic cell vaccines are underway and feasibility has been demonstrated in young patients with relapsed high-grade astrocytoma and glioblastoma (Rutkowski et al. 2004). Finally, biological agents such as oncolytic viruses are being evaluated for the treatment of glioma, although they has not been systematically studied in children so far.

Several of these novel targeted therapies are now being evaluated in clinical studies, some of which have recently been completed. Table 4.3 provides an overview of phase I and II clinical trials, including drugs given alone or in combination with chemotherapy in pediatric glioma patients. Because these trials focus on dose finding, toxicity, and pharmacokinetics, no conclusion on the efficacy of these novel targeted therapies can be drawn at present.

4.9 Conclusion

This review describes the advances in our understanding of the molecular pathogenesis of pediatric gliomas in the last 2 decades, which is largely based on the availability of genome-wide screening methods that help to establish characteristic molecular "fingerprints" for certain tumor entities or subsets thereof. Translating this molecular knowledge into clinical application should help clinicians to improve tailoring therapy intensity to disease risk and to develop more specific "targeted" therapies in order to improve the unsatisfactory treatment results of children with high-grade gliomas.

References

Alonso M, Hamelin R, Kim M, Porwancher K, Sung T, Parhar P, Miller DC, Newcomb EW (2001) Microsatellite instability occurs in distinct subtypes of pediatric but not adult central nervous system tumors. vol 61, pp 2124–2128

Balss J, Meyer J, Mueller W, Korshunov A, Hartmann C, von Deimling A (2008) Analysis of the IDH1 codon 132 mutation in brain tumors 116(6):597–602.

Barone G, Maurizi P, Tamburrini G, Riccardi R (2006) Role of temozolomide in pediatric brain tumors. Childs Nerv Syst 22: 652–61

Bigner SH, McLendon RE, Fuchs M, McKeever PE, Friedman HS (1997) Chromosomal characteristics of childhood brain tumors. Cancer Genetics Cytogenetics 97: 125–134

Bredel M, Pollack IF, Hamilton RL, James CD (1999) Epidermal growth factor receptor expression and gene amplification in high-grade non-brainstem gliomas of childhood. Clin Cancer Res 5:1786–1792

Broniscer A, Baker SJ, West AN, Fraser MM, Proko E, Kocak M, Dalton J, Zambetti GP, Ellison DW, Kun LE, Gajjar A, Gilbertson RJ, Fuller CE (2007) Clinical and molecular characteristics of malignant transformation of low-grade glioma in children. vol 25, pp 682–689

Carter M, Nicholson J, Ross F, Crolla J, Allibone R, Balaji V, Perry R, Walker D, Gilbertson R, Ellison DW (2002) Genetic abnormalities detected in ependymomas by comparative genomic hybridisation. Br J Cancer 86:929–939

Cheng Y, Ng H, Zhang S, Ding M, Pang J, Zheng J, Poon W (1999) Genetic alterations in pediatric high-grade astrocytomas. Hum Pathol 30:1284–1290

David TW Jones, Kocialkowski S, Liu L, Pearson DM, Baecklund LM, Ichimura K, Collins P (2008) Tandem duplication producing a novel oncogenic BRAF fusion gene defines the majority of filocyctic astrocytonas. Cancer Res 68(21)

Donson A, Addo-Yobo S, Handler M, Gore L, Foreman N (2007) MGMT promoter methylation correlates with survival benefit and sensitivity to temozolomide in pediatric glioblastoma. Pediatr Blood Cancer 48:403–407

Dyer S, Prebble E, Davison V, Davies P, Ramani P, Ellison D, Grundy R (2002) Genomic imbalances in pediatric intracranial ependymomas define clinically relevant groups. Am J Pathol 161:2133–2141

Ebert C, von Haken M, Meyer-Puttlitz B, Wiestler OD, Reifenberger G, Pietsch T, von Deimling A (1999) Molecular genetic analysis of ependymal tumors. NF2 mutations and chromosome 22q loss occur preferentially in intramedullary spinal ependymomas. Am J Pathol 155: 627–632

Faury D, Nantel A, Dunn SE, Guiot M-C, Haque T, Hauser P, Garami M, Bognar L, Hanzely Z, Liberski PP, Lopez-Aguilar E, Valera ET, Tone LG, Carret A-S, Del Maestro RF, Gleave M, Montes J-L, Pietsch T, Albrecht S, Jabado N (2007) Molecular profiling identifies prognostic subgroups of pediatric glioblastoma and shows increased YB-1 expression in tumors. J Clin Oncol 25: 1196–1208

Felix C, Slavc I, Dunn M, Strauss E, Phillips P, Rorke L, Sutton L, Bunin G, Biegel J (1995) p53 gene mutations in pediatric brain tumors. Med Pediatr Oncol 25:431–436

Finlay JL, Boyett JM, Yates AJ, Wisoff JH, Milstein JM, Geyer JR, Bertolone SJ, McGuire P, Cherlow JM, Tefft M, et al. (1995) Randomized phase III trial in childhood high-grade astrocytoma comparing vincristine, lomustine, and prednisone with the eight-drugs-in-1-day regimen. Childrens Cancer Group. J Clin Oncol 13:112–123

Finlay JL, Zacharoulis S (2005) The treatment of high grade gliomas and diffuse intrinsic pontine tumors of childhood and adolescence: a historical - and futuristic - perspective. J Neurooncol 75:253–266

Hargrave D, Bartels U, Bouffet E (2006) Diffuse brainstem glioma in children: critical review of clinical trials. Lancet Oncol 7: 241–248

Hegi ME, Diserens AC, Gorlia T, Hamou MF, de Tribolet N, Weller M, Kros JM, Hainfellner JA, Mason W, Mariani L, Bromberg JE, Hau P, Mirimanoff RO, Cairncross JG, Janzer RC, Stupp R (2005) MGMT gene silencing and benefit from temozolomide in glioblastoma. N Engl J Med 352: 997–1003

Hirose Y, Aldape K, Bollen A, James CD, Brat D, Lamborn K, Berger M, Feuerstein BG (2001) Chromosomal abnormalities subdivide ependymal tumors into clinically relevant groups. Am J Pathol 158: 1137–1143

Janzarik W, Kratz C, Loges N, Olbrich H, Klein C, Schaefer T, Scheurlen W, Roggendorf W, Weiller C, Niemeyer C, Korinthenberg R, Pfister S, Omran H (2007) Further evidence for a somatic KRAS Mutation in a low-grade Astrocytoma. Neuropediatrics 38:1–3

Jenkins RB, Kimmel DW, Moertel CA, Schultz CG, Scheithauer BW, Kelly PJ, Dewald GW (1989) A cytogenetic study of 53 human gliomas. Cancer Genetics and Cytogenetics 39:253–279

Jones D, Ichimura K, Liu L, Pearson D, Plant K, Collins V (2006) Genomic analysis of pilocytic astrocytomas at 0.97 Mb resolution shows an increasing tendency toward chromosomal copy number change with age. J Neuropathol Exp Neurol 65:1049–1058

Kaatsch P, Rickert C, Kühl J, Schüz J, Michaelis J (2001) Population-based epidemiologic data on brain tumors in German children. Cancer 92:3155–3164

Korshunov A, Neben K, Wrobel G, Tews B, Benner A, Hahn M, Golanov A, Lichter P (2003) Gene expression patterns in ependymomas correlate with tumor location, grade, and patient age. Am J Pathol 163:1721–1727

Lamszus K, Lachenmayer L, Heinemann U, Kluwe L, Finckh U, Hoppner W, Stavrou D, Fillbrandt R, Westphal M (2001) Molecular genetic alterations on chromosomes 11 and 22 in ependymomas. Int J Cancer 91:803–808

Linabery A, Ross J (2008) Trends in childhood cancer incidence in the U.S. (1992–2004). Cancer 112:416–432

Listernick R, Ferner R, Liu G, Gutmann D (2007) Optic pathway gliomas in neurofibromatosis-1:

Controversies and recommendations. Ann Neurol 61:189–198

Litofsky N, Hinton D, Raffel C (1994) The lack of a role for p53 in astrocytomas in pediatric patients. Neurosurgery 34:967–972

Louis D, Ohgaki H, Wiestler O, Cavenee W, Burger P, Jouvet A, Scheithauer B, Kleihues P (2007) The 2007 WHO Classification of tumours of the central nervous system. Acta Neuropathologica 114:97–109

Mazewski C, Soukup S, Ballard E, Gotwals B, Lampkin B (1999) Karyotype studies in 18 ependymomas with literature review of 107 cases. Cancer Genet Cytogenet 113:1–8

Mendrzyk F, Korshunov A, Benner A, Toedt G, Pfister S, Radlwimmer B, Lichter P (2006) Identification of gains on 1q and epidermal growth factor receptor overexpression as independent prognostic markers in intracranial ependymoma. Clin Cancer Res 12:2070–2079

Milde T, Pfister S, Korshunov A, Deubzer H, Oehme I, Ernst A, Starzinski-Powitz A, Seitz A, Lichter P, von Deimling A, Witt O (2008) Stepwise accumulation of distinct genomic aberrations in a patient with progressively metastasizing ependymoma. Genes Chromosomes Cancer, *2008 Nov 21*.

Monoranu C-M, Huang B, Zangen IL v, Rutkowski S, Vince GH, Gerber NU, Puppe B, Roggendorf W (2008) Correlation between 6q25.3 deletion status and survival in pediatric intracranial ependymomas. Cancer Genetics Cytogenetics 182:18–26

Ohgaki H, Kleihues P (2005) Population-based studies on incidence, survival rates, and genetic alterations in astrocytic and oligodendroglial gliomas. J Neuropathol Exp Neurol 64:479–489

Orr L, Fleitz J, McGavran L, Wyatt-Ashmead J, Handler M, Foreman N (2002) Cytogenetics in pediatric low-grade astrocytomas. vol 38, pp 173–177

Parry DM, Eldridge R, Kaiser-Kupfer MI, Bouzas EA, Pikus A, Patronas N (1994) Neurofibromatosis 2 (NF2): clinical characteristics of 63 affected individuals and clinical evidence for heterogeneity. Am J Med Genet 52: 450–461

Pezzolo A, Capra V, Raso A, Morandi F, Parodi F, Gambini C, Nozza P, Giangaspero F, Cama A, Pistoia V, Garre ML (2008) Identification of novel chromosomal abnormalities and prognostic cytogenetics markers in intracranial pediatric ependymoma. Cancer Lett 261:235–243

Pfister S, Janzarik W, Remke M, Ernst A, Werft W, Becker N, Toedt G, Wittmann A, Kratz C, Olbrich H, Ahmadi R, Thieme B, Joos S, Radlwimmer B, Kulozik A, Pietsch T, Herold-Mende C, Gnekow A, Reifenberger G, Korshunov A, Scheurlen W, Omran H, Lichter P (2008) BRAF gene duplication constitutes a mechanism of MAPK pathway activation in low-grade astrocytomas. J Clin Invest. 2008; May 1;118(5):1739–1749.

Pfister S, Schlaeger C, Mendrzyk F, Wittmann A, Benner A, Kulozik A, Scheurlen W, Radlwimmer B, P L (2007) Array-based profiling of reference-independent methylation status (aPRIMES) identifies frequent promoter methylation and consecutive downregulation of ZIC2 in pediatric medulloblastoma. Nucleic Acids Res 35:e51

Pollack IF, Finkelstein SD, Burnham J, Holmes EJ, Hamilton RL, Yates AJ, Finlay JL, Sposto R (2001) Age and TP53 mutation frequency in childhood malignant gliomas: results in a multi-institutional cohort. Cancer Res 61: 7404–7407

Pollack IF, Finkelstein SD, Woods J, Burnham J, Holmes EJ, Hamilton RL, Yates AJ, Boyett JM, Finlay JL, Sposto R (2002) Expression of p53 and prognosis in children with malignant gliomas. N Engl J Med 346:420–427

Pollack L, Stewart S, Thompson T, Li J (2008) Stat Bite: childhood cancer deaths by site, 2004. J Natl Cancer Inst 100:165

Raffel C, Frederick L, O'Fallon JR, Atherton-Skaff P, Perry A, Jenkins RB, James CD (1999) Analysis of oncogene and tumor suppressor gene alterations in pediatric malignant astrocytomas reveals reduced survival for patients with PTEN mutations. Clin Cancer Res 5:4085–4090

Recinos PF, Sciubba DM, Jallo GI (2007) Brainstem tumors: where are we today? Pediatr Neurosurg 43:192–201

Rickert CH, Strater R, Kaatsch P, Wassmann H, Jurgens H, Dockhorn-Dworniczak B, Paulus W (2001) Pediatric high-grade astrocytomas show chromosomal imbalances distinct from adult cases. Am J Pathol 158:1525–1532

Ries L, Smith M, Gurney J (1999) Cancer incidence and survival among children and adolescents: United States SEER program 1975–1995, National Cancer Institute, SEER Program, Bethesda, MD

Rorive S, Maris C, Debeir O, Sandras F, Vidaud M, Bièche I, Salmon I, Decaestecker C (2006) Exploring the distinctive biological characteristics of pilocytic and low-grade diffuse astrocytomas using microarray gene expression profiles. J Neuropathol Exp Neurol 65:794–807

Rutkowski S, De Vleeschouwer S, Kaempgen E, Wolff JE, Kuhl J, Demaerel P, Warmuth-Metz M, Flamen P, Van Calenbergh F, Plets C, Sorensen N,

Opitz A, Van Gool SW (2004) Surgery and adjuvant dendritic cell-based tumour vaccination for patients with relapsed malignant glioma, a feasibility study. Br J Cancer 91:1656–1662

Sanoudou D, Tingby O, Ferguson-Smith M, Collins V, Coleman N (2000) Analysis of pilocytic astrocytoma by comparative genomic hybridization. Brit J Cancer 82:1218–1222

Sharma M, Zehnbauer B, Watson M, Gutmann D (2005) RAS pathway activation and an oncogenic RAS mutation in sporadic pilocytic astrocytoma. Neurology 65:1335–1336

Sharma MK, Mansur DB, Reifenberger G, Perry A, Leonard JR, Aldape KD, Albin MG, Emnett RJ, Loeser S, Watson MA, Nagarajan R, Gutmann DH (2007) Distinct genetic signatures among pilocytic astrocytomas relate to their brain region origin. Cancer Res 67:890–900

Stupp R, Mason WP, van den Bent MJ, Weller M, Fisher B, Taphoorn MJ, Belanger K, Brandes AA, Marosi C, Bogdahn U, Curschmann J, Janzer RC, Ludwin SK, Gorlia T, Allgeier A, Lacombe D, Cairncross JG, Eisenhauer E, Mirimanoff RO (2005) Radiotherapy plus concomitant and adjuvant temozolomide for glioblastoma. N Engl J Med 352: 987–996

Suarez-Merino B, Hubank M, Revesz T, Harkness W, Hayward R, Thompson D, Darling JL, Thomas DG, Warr TJ (2005) Microarray analysis of pediatric ependymoma identifies a cluster of 112 candidate genes including four transcripts at 22q12.1-q13.3. Neurooncol 7: 20–31

Sung T, Miller D, Hayes R, Alonso M, Yee H, Newcomb E (2000) Preferential inactivation of the p53 tumor suppressor pathway and lack of EGFR amplification distinguish de novo high grade pediatric astrocytomas from de novo adult astrocytomas. Brain Pathol 10:249–259

Tabori U, Ma J, Carter M, Zielenska M, Rutka J, Bouffet E, Bartels U, Malkin D, Hawkins C (2006) Human telomere reverse transcriptase expression predicts progression and survival in pediatric intracranial ependymoma. J Clin Oncol 24:1522–1528

Taylor MD, Poppleton H, Fuller C, Su X, Liu Y, Jensen P, Magdaleno S, Dalton J, Calabrese C, Board J, MacDonald T, Rutka J, Guha A, Gajjar A, Curran T, Gilbertson RJ (2005) Radial glia cells are candidate stem cells of ependymoma. Cancer Cell 8:323–335

Watanabe K, Sato K, Biernat W, Tachibana O, von Ammon K, Ogata N, Yonekawa Y, Kleihues P, Ohgaki H (1997) Incidence and timing of p53 mutations during astrocytoma progression in patients with multiple biopsies. Clin Cancer Res 3:523–530

Yunoue S, Tokuo H, Fukunaga K, Feng L, Ozawa T, Nishi T, Kikuchi A, Hattori S, Kuratsu J, Saya H, Araki N (2003) Neurofibromatosis type I tumor suppressor neurofibromin regulates neuronal differentiation via its GTPase-activating protein function toward Ras. vol 278, pp 26958–26969

Zattara-Cannoni H, Gambarelli D, Lena G, Dufour H, Choux M, Grisoli F, Vagner-Capodano AM (1998) Are juvenile pilocytic astrocytomas benign tumors? A cytogenetic study in 24 cases. Cancer Genetics Cytogenetics 104:157–160

Hereditary Tumor Syndromes and Gliomas

David Reuss and Andreas von Deimling

Abstract Several congenital syndromes caused by germline mutations in tumor suppressor genes predispose to the development of glial tumors. In the last few decades our knowledge about the molecular functions of these genes and the pathogenesis of hereditary tumor syndromes has greatly increased. The most common syndromes are the neurofibromatoses (type 1 and type 2) and the tuberous scleroses complex. There are interesting overlaps in the molecular pathogenesis. Deregulation of Ras or downstream Ras pathways including MEK/ERK and AKT/mTOR plays an important role in these three syndromes. Other rare syndromes include Li-Fraumeni, melanoma-astrocytoma, and Turcot syndrome involving cell cycle regulators and DNA repair genes. The genes and pathways involved in the pathogenesis of these syndromes also play an important role in the development of sporadic tumors. Therefore research on hereditary syndromes contributes substantially to our understanding of tumor formation.

David Reuss (✉)
Department of Neuropathology
Institute of Pathology and
Clinical Cooperation Unit Neuropathology,
German Cancer Research Center
Im Neuenheimer Feld 220/221
69120 Heidelberg
Germany
E-mail: David.Reuss@med.uni-heidelberg.de

5.1 Neurofibromatosis

5.1.1 Historic Aspects

Descriptions of patients with characteristic features of neurofibromatosis go back to the second century (Huson and Hughes 1994). Friedrich Daniel von Recklinghausen coined the term "neurofibromatosis" (1882). In the second half of the twentieth century the clinical difference between a "peripheral" (NF1) and a "central" (NF2) form of neurofibromatosis was established. After the identification of the *NF1* and the *NF2* genes in the early 1990s, the two forms were recognized as distinct genetic entities.

5.1.2 Neurofibromatosis Type 1

Synonyms: von Recklinghausen's disease, Watson disease, peripheral neurofibromatosis.

Neurofibromatosis type 1 (NF1) is an autosomal dominant familial tumor syndrome affecting 1 in 3,500 individuals. It is characterized by multiple benign tumors and a predisposition to malignant neoplasms. The most consistent features of NF1 are café-au-lait spots and dermal and plexiform neurofibromas. Furthermore, patients develop different tumors of the

Table 5.1 Diagnostic criteria for NF1

The presence of two or more of the following signs identify the NF1 patient:
1. Six or more café-au-lait patches, diameter greater than 5 mm in prepubertal and over 15 mm in postpubertal individuals
2. Two or more neurofibromas of any type or one plexiform neurofibroma
3. Axillary and/or inguinal freckling
4. Glioma of the n. opticus
5. A distinctive osseous lesion, such as dysplasia of the sphenoid wing, thinning of the long bone cortex, with or without pseudarthrosis
6. A first-degree relative (parent, sibling, or offspring) with NF1 according to the above criteria 1–5

central nervous system (pilocytic astrocytomas WHO grade I, but also glioblastomas WHO grade IV). Additional manifestations of NF1 are bone deformities (scoliosis, macrocephaly, pseudarthrosis), small stature, encroachment of central nervous system functions such as intellectual properties, changes of personality structure, and vascular malformations particularly fibromuscular hyperplasia (Bader 1986).

The variable expressivity of the symptoms results in a complex clinical picture. The guidelines for the diagnosis of NF1 have been established by an NIH consensus development conference statement and are listed in Table 5.1. The frequency of selected NF1-associated symptoms is given in Table 5.2.

The increased risk for malignancies is of special clinical importance because these tumors are the major cause of early death in NF1 patients (Friedman 1999). Malignancies include malignant peripheral nerve sheath tumor (MPNST), triton tumor, rhabdomyosarcoma, acute myeloid leukemia, and malignant astrocytoma (Huson and Hughes 1994).

5.1.2.1
Molecular Genetics

The basis of inheritance in NF1 is a germline mutation in the *NF1* tumor suppressor gene. The *NF1* gene was isolated using positional cloning

Table 5.2 Frequency of characteristic symptoms in NF1-patients

Symptoms	Frequency
Neurofibromas postpubertal	90%
thereof leading to neurological deficits	10%
Cognitive and social problems	50%
Plexiform neurofibromas	30%
Scoliosis	30%
Pilocytic astrocytomas	15%

(Cawthon et al. 1990b; Viskochil et al. 1990). It maps to the chromosomal region 17q11.2. Germline alterations in both parental alleles have never been seen and the intrauterine lethality of mouse embryos with biallelic germline mutation suggests prenatal lethality of biallelic *NF1* deficiency in humans too (Jacks et al. 1994).

The *NF1* gene spans at least 335 kb containing 60 exons with an 8,457-bp open reading frame that codes for 2,818 amino acids (neurofibromin type I). It belongs to the group of giant genes according to the classification of McKusick. Exon 27b of *NF1* carries three embedded genes: *EVI2A* (ecotropic viral integration site 2A), *EVI2B* (ecotropic viral integration site 2B), and *OMG* (oligodendrocyte myelin glycoprotein). All three genes are encoded in reverse direction to the *NF1* sense strand (Cawthon et al. 1990a, 1991; Viskochil et al. 1991; Shen et al. 1996; Habib et al. 1998). At least 12 *NF1* pseudogenes are distributed on different human chromosomes; however, none of these pseudogenes contains sequences beyond exon 29. The extensive size of the *NF1* gene may contribute to the high rate of spontaneous mutations being the cause of disease in approximately 50% of the patients. *NF1* mutations affect all regions of the gene without significant hotspots. The majority of the mutations lead to a truncated protein (about 80%) and only a small proportion code for missense mutations (10%). With respect to genotype–phenotype correlation, it has been reported that large deletions (up to 1.5 Mb genomic DNA) of the *NF1* gene are associated with an earlier age of onset of cutaneous neurofibromas, learning disability, dysmorphic features, and developmental delay (Castle et al. 2003). In addition, a recent study reported on 21 unrelated probands with the same *c.*2970–2972 delAAT (p.990delM) germline mutation but without cutaneous or plexiform neurofibromas (Upadhyaya et al. 2007).

5.1.2.2
Molecular Pathogenesis

The *NF1* gene product, neurofibromin, is expressed ubiquitously with the highest levels in the central and peripheral nervous systems, in leukocytes, and the adrenal gland (DeClue et al. 1991; Gutmann et al. 1991; Daston et al. 1992). There are at least five human isoforms. All but neurofibromin type I are generated by alternative splicing of four exons: 9a, 10a-2, 23a, and 48a. Neurofibromin type I does not contain any of these exons (Nishi et al. 1991; Gutman et al. 1993; Danglot et al. 1995; Kaufmann et al. 2002). The molecular weight of human neurofibromin is 250–280 kDa in SDS page. Neurofibromin localizes mainly to the cytoplasm, but it has been found in the nucleus and a nuclear localization signal of neurofibromin encoded by exon 43 of the *NF1* gene has been reported (Vandenbroucke et al. 2004).

There are only a few putative functional domains within neurofibromin: RasGAP, SEC14-like, and a pleckstrin homology (PH)-like domain. Beside these, a cysteine/serine-rich domain (CSRD) upstream of RasGAP has been described (Fahsold et al. 2000).

5.1.2.3
Neurofibromin and Ras Proteins

The monomeric GTP/GDP-binding proteins of the Ras superfamily are functionally active in the GTP-bound form. Guanine exchange factors (GEFs) promote the switch from the inactive GDP-form to the active GTP-form. The active GTP form is localized in the membrane and has a low intrinsic GTPase activity. The physiological inactivation is enhanced by up to five orders of magnitude by GTPase-activating proteins (GAPs). Neuro-fibromin belongs to the specific GAPs of the subfamily of Ras proteins. Due to its function the corresponding domain of neurofibromin is called the "GAP-related domain" (GRD). This is the best studied region of the *NF1* gene. The domain shares high homology to related domains of other GAPs and to IRA1 and IRA2, proteins with inhibitory effect on Ras in *Saccharomyces cerevisiae*. Significant homology can be observed between *NF1* and *IRA1* in regions that extend beyond the GAP-related domain. Neurofibromin exerts its activity on H-Ras, K-Ras (viral Harvey and Kirsten murine sarcoma oncogenes), N-Ras (human neuroblastoma oncogene), R-Ras, as well as Tc21 (R-Ras2). Multiple activators such as hormones, cytokines, growth factors, extracellular matrix proteins, or antigens in T-cell activation can affect GTP-Ras formation. Some heterotrimeric G proteins are also able to activate Ras proteins. There are at least seven different effectors of GTP-Ras proteins initiating different signal cascades, which in the end lead to differences in gene expression. One major signal cascade which has been shown to play a critical role in cell proliferation is activated by interaction of active Ras with Raf serine/threonine kinase. Raf serine/threonine-kinase phosphorylates a second kinase, the MAP kinase/ERK kinase (MEK). MEK phosphorylates ERK family members. Phosphorylated ERK phosphorylates a number of other proteins like other kinases (S6 kinase) and transcription factors, such as CREB (Grand and Owen 1991; Boguski and McCormick 1993; Macara et al. 1996).

Loss of functional neurofibromin can favor the active status of Ras and therefore continuously stimulate the Raf-MEK-ERK pathway leading to cell proliferation.

Another cascade which is triggered by activated Ras leads to the activation of phosphoinositide 3-kinase (PI3K), followed by phosphorylation of protein kinase AKT (also known as protein kinase B). AKT has the ability to inactivate the hamartin/tuberin complex by phosphorylation. The consequence of hamartin/tuberin inhibition is the activation of the small GAP Rheb (Ras homologue enriched in brain) which activates the kinase serine/threonine target of rapamycin (TOR or mTOR) (Pan et al. 2004). Evidence for an activation of mTOR in NF1-associated tumors has been reported and neurofibromin-dependency of the mTOR pathway could be demonstrated in cell culture systems (Dasgupta et al. 2005; Johannessen et al. 2005).

Thus, Ras proteins influence in a cell type-specific manner a diversity of cell processes such as proliferation, migration, differentiation, apoptosis, and senescence.

The SEC14 domain is found in secretory proteins and in lipid-regulated proteins and may play a role in co-regulating Ras GTPase activity (Aravind et al. 1999; D'Angelo et al. 2006; Welti et al. 2007). There is evidence that neurofibromin may exhibit Ras-modulating effects independent of its GAP activity by participating in the rearrangement of cytoskeletal components (Corral et al. 2003). A recent publication reveals the ability of neurofibromin to bind caveolin (Cav-1), a membrane protein, which is known to regulate signaling molecules like Ras, protein kinase C, and growth factor receptors. The fact that missense mutations occur in potential caveolin-binding sites speaks in favor of a role of caveolin in neurofibromin function (Boyanapalli et al. 2006).

5.1.2.4
Neurofibromin and Adenylate Cyclases

Neurofibromin function seems to be involved in the cAMP protein kinase A (PKA-) pathway. There is evidence from *Drosophila* models that neurofibromin is involved in activation of adenylate cyclases (AC) (Guo et al. 1997, 2000; The et al. 1997). Lower neuropeptide- and G protein-stimulated AC activity in $NF1^{-/-}$ than in $NF1^{+/-}$ mouse brains has been found, indicating that neurofibromin regulates AC activity also in mammals (Tong et al. 2002). Recently two *NF1*-dependent adenylate cyclase pathways in *Drosophila* brain have been described (Hannan et al. 2006). On the other hand, a threefold increase of cAMP levels in Schwann cells from *NF1*-null mice compared to wild-type has been found arguing for an antagonistic role of neurofibromin at cAMP accumulation (Kim et al. 2001). An increased baseline level of cAMP has also been seen in neurofibromin-deficient astrocytes, but it could be demonstrated that inactivation of neurofibromin in astrocytes results in reduced cAMP generation in response to pituitary adenylate cyclase-activating polypeptide (PACAP), attenuated calcium influx, and Rap1 activation (Dasgupta et al. 2003). In this context is has to be noted that cAMP exhibits mitogenic effects in Schwann cells, whereas increased cAMP levels in astrocytes lead to a growth inhibitory signal (Dugan et al. 1999; Kim, Ratner et al. 2001). Thus the role of neurofibromin in AC activity seems to be cell type specific and coupled to an antiproliferative effect.

5.1.2.5
NF1 and Astrocytomas

NF1 is associated with a highly increased occurrence of pilocytic astrocytomas (PA) WHO grade I (15–20% of patients). Preferential localizations are the optic tracts (opticus glioma) and the brainstem.

According to the classical "two-hit" hypothesis for the inactivation of tumor suppressor genes, several studies could prove that NF1-associated PA harbor a somatic mutation ("second hit") in the NF1 gene (von Deimling et al. 1993; Gutmann et al. 2000; Kluwe et al. 2001). Furthermore, lack of neurofibromin expression has been found along with elevated levels of Ras-GTP and activation of the Raf/MAPK and PI3K/AKT pathways in an NF1-associated PA (Lau et al. 2000). The suggested role of neurofibromin in NF1-associated PA gave rise to the question of whether it is of same importance in the pathogenesis of histological identical sporadic pilocytic astrocytomas. It has been shown that NF1 gene mutations occur at low frequency in sporadic PA and that the NF1 expression is increased (approximately 10- to 20-fold) in sporadic PA compared to normal brain (Platten et al. 1996; Wimmer et al. 2002). These data argue against neurofibromin loss of function as a typical molecular event in the pathogenesis of sporadic PA. PAs were analyzed for activation of Ras and Ras mutations. While only 1 of 21 tumors harbored an oncogenic K-Ras mutation, all tumors demonstrated activation of the Ras pathway (Sharma et al. 2005). Recently a gene expression profile in NF1-accociated PA distinct to that of sporadic cases has been found (Sharma et al. 2007).

Thus, it can be concluded that NF1-associated and sporadic pilocytic astrocytomas both share a hyperactivation of the Ras pathway, but that the underlying molecular events are different. The increased expression of *NF1* in sporadic PA is most probably the result of a positive feedback regulation by activated Ras.

Using a mouse model in which the mice lack *NF1* function in the central nervous system (CNS), global reactive gliosis in the adult murine brain and an increased proliferation of glial progenitor cells could be determined. Additionally, the mice developed enlarged optic nerves and some of them developed optic pathway gliomas (Zhu et al. 2005b).

The results of epidemiological studies revealed that NF1 patients also have an increased risk for malignant gliomas (Blatt et al. 1986; Rasmussen et al. 2001). In a mouse model of NF1-associated malignant gliomas all mice lacking *TP53* in the germline and *NF1* function in CNS cells and all mice with compound heterozygosity for *TP53* and *NF1* in CNS cells developed malignant astrocytomas (grade II astrocytomas to grade IV glioblastomas). Mice lacking *NF1* in CNS cells and heterozygosity for *TP53* rarely developed CNS tumors (1/18). It can be concluded that *TP53* loss prior to or concomitant with *NF1* loss (Ras activation) is required for effective malignant tumor formation (Zhu et al. 2005a) in this model.

5.1.3
Neurofibromatosis Type 2

Neurofibromatosis type 2 (NF2) is a dominantly inherited familial tumor syndrome affecting 1 in 40,000 individuals predisposing to benign and, less frequently, malignant neoplasms. The most important diagnostic feature of NF2 is the development of bilateral vestibular schwannomas. Further frequent tumors include meningiomas, astrocytomas, and ependymomas. Due to the multiplicity and the unfavorable tumor sites in patients with NF2, schwannomas in the cerebellopontine angle, and spinal ependymomas, the clinical presentation is often much more severe than might be anticipated from the histological analysis of the lesions.

The guidelines for the diagnosis of NF2 are listed in Table 5.3. The frequency of selected NF2-associated symptoms is given in Table 5.4.

5.1.3.1
Molecular Genetics

The basis of inheritance in NF2 is a germline mutation in the *NF2* tumor suppressor gene, located in chromosome region 22q12.2 (Rouleau et al. 1993; Trofatter et al. 1993). It is phylo-

Table 5.3 Diagnostic criteria for NF2

The following are diagnostic:		
1.		Bilateral vestibular schwannomas; or
2.		A first-degree relative with NF2, and either
	(a)	A unilateral vestibular schwannoma or
	(b)	Two of the following: meningioma, schwannoma, glioma, posterior subcapsular lens opacity, or cerebral calcification; or
3.		Two of the following
	(a)	Unilateral vestibular schwannoma
	(b)	Multiple meningiomas
	(c)	Either schwannoma, glioma, neurofibroma, posterior subcapsular lens opacity, or cerebral calcification

Table 5.4 Frequency of characteristic symptoms in NF2 patients

Tumors or symptoms	Frequency
Spinal tumors	92%
Bilateral vestibular schwannomas	81%
Ophthalmologic abnormalities	62%
Skin schwannomas	59%
Cerebral meningiomas	58%
Cranial nerve tumors	48%
Abdominal calcification	10%
Peripheral neuropathy	10%

genetically highly conserved. Mice with homozygous *NF2* germline mutations are not viable (McClatchey et al. 1997). The *NF2* gene spans 119 kb containing 17 exons. Most of the mutations lead to a truncated protein due to a high rate of nonsense mutations (34%). Missense mutations occur in about 7% of cases (http://neurosurgery.mgh.harvard.edu/NFclinic/NFresearch.htm). There is no direct correlation between geno- and phenotype, but statistically protein truncating mutations are more often associated with a severe clinical course than missense mutations. Remarkably big deletions of the *NF2* gene have been observed in patients with a milder phenotype (Bourn et al. 1994; Parry et al. 1996; Ruttledge et al. 1996; Evans et al. 1998; Lopez-Correa et al. 2000).

5.1.3.2
Molecular Pathogenesis

The *NF2* gene product, merlin or schwannomin, is expressed in most human tissues including the brain. Two isoforms spanning either exons 1–15 and 17 or exons 1–16 are known. Isoform I or "NF2–17" lacks exon 16 and isoform II or "NF2–16" contains exon 16. Merlin exhibits homology to the protein 4.1 family including ezrin, moesin, and radixin (ERM proteins). These proteins share the FERM (four-point one, ezrin, radixin, moesin) domain at the amino terminus (Rouleau et al. 1993; Trofatter et al. 1993). There are two other obvious functional domains, a coiled-coil region and a short carboxy terminal domain. Merlin isoform I and the ERM proteins might exist in two different conformations. The amino- and the carboxy terminus can bind to each other (folded conformation). Phosphorylation near the carboxy terminus inhibits head-to-tail folding and thereby leads to an open configuration (Gary and Bretscher 1995; Matsui et al. 1998). Merlin isoform II is not able to form an intramolecular association and exists in a constitutively open conformation (Sherman et al. 1997; Gonzalez-Agosti et al. 1999). Merlin has many properties in common with the ERM proteins, but shows a unique tumor suppressor function. Finding specific interaction partners of merlin, which do not interact in the same manner with ERM proteins, could be a way to understand its tumor suppressor function. The fact that missense mutations occur in the FERM domain of merlin argues for merlin-specific protein–protein interactions and specific functions. In addition the FERM domain of merlin shows significant differences to ERM proteins. Beside structural similarities, merlin's C-terminal domain lacks the F-actin-binding ability of the ERM proteins. However, merlin can instead bind F-actin with its FERM domain (Xu and Gutmann 1998; Brault et al. 2001; James et al. 2001). Several other merlin-interacting proteins have been identified: examples are beta-spectrin II (Scoles et al. 1998; Neill and Crompton 2001), solute carrier family 9 (sodium/hydrogen exchanger) (Murthy et al. 1998), schwannomin-interacting protein 1 (Goutebroze et al. 2000), beta 1 integrin (Obremski et al. 1998), CD44 (Sainio et al. 1997; Morrison et al. 2001), hepatocyte growth factor-regulated tyrosine kinase substrate (Scoles et al. 2000), Rho GDP dissociation inhibitor (Maeda et al. 1999), syndecan-binding protein (Jannatipour et al. 2001), paxillin (Fernandez-Valle et al. 2002), and RIb subunit of the PKA (Bretscher et al. 2002; Gronholm et al. 2003). Many of these proteins are plasma membrane-associated proteins or proteins with adaptor function connecting membrane proteins to cytoskeletal components.

Merlin was found to mediate contact inhibition of cell proliferation. At high cell density, merlin is hypo-phosphorylated and active in inhibiting cell growth in response to hyaluronate (HA), a component of the extracellular matrix. This function is dependent on interactions with CD44, a transmembrane HA receptor. At low cell density, merlin is phosphorylated, forms a complex with ezrin and moesin, which is associated with CD44, and does not show growth inhibitory activity (Morrison et al. 2001).

Mitogen-activated protein kinases (MAPK or ERKs), which are downstream targets of active Ras, play a well-known role in regulation of cell proliferation and differentiation (Winston and Hunter 1995; Marshall 1996). Merlin was shown to exert anti-Ras activity (Tikoo et al. 1994; Kim et al. 2002; Lim et al. 2003). The exact mechanism mediating this effect is not known. In recent years there has been progress in understanding by which means merlin is able to influence these signaling pathways. Adaptor protein paxillin binds directly to merlin and mediates the localization of merlin to the plasma membrane, where it associates with beta 1 integrin and erbB2. Paxillin allows the binding of Rho-GTPase regulators and effectors as well as kinases and phosphatases at beta 1 integrin-dependent contacts. It recruits PAK to focal complexes (Fernandez-Valle, Tang et al. 2002). Merlin has an inhibitory function on activated kinase PAK1, a critical mediator of the Rac/Cdc42 signaling pathway. The inhibitory function is mediated by a direct interaction between merlin and PAK1 (Kissil et al. 2003). It was observed that merlin is able to inhibit the Ral guanine nucleotide dissociation stimulator (RalGDS), a downstream molecule of Ras, via direct interaction (Ryu et al. 2005). In a recent study it has been shown that merlin displays an inhibitory effect on the growth hormone-stimulated activation of the Raf-ERKs pathway by binding to growth factor receptor-bound protein 2 (Grb2) (Lim et al. 2006). The nucleotide exchange factor son of sevenless homolog (Sos) may bind the Grb2 SH3 domain, and the formation of an EGFR/Sos/Grb2 complex is associated with Ras activation (Buday 1999). The protein magicin is able to interact with merlin as well as Grb2 and is capable of forming a complex with these proteins (Wiederhold et al. 2004). Another recent study reports evidence for an inhibitory role of merlin in activation of Ras and Rac (Morrison et al. 2007). Merlin was found to bind PIKE-L (PI3K enhancer), a GTPase that binds to PI3K and triggers its activation. Merlin was shown to compete with PI3K for binding to PIKE-L, thereby inhibiting activation of the PI3K-AKT pathway (Rong et al. 2004). It has been shown that the protein kinase AKT directly binds to and phosphorylates merlin on residues Thr 230 and Ser 315, thereby abolishing merlin's head-to-tail folding and promoting its degradation by ubiquitination (Tang et al. 2007). Another study describes the direct interaction of merlin with the eukaryotic initiation factor 3 (eIF3) p110 subunit (eIF3c). The FERM domain of merlin was shown to bind the C-terminal half of eIF3c. Increased expression of eIF3c elevated cell proliferation and merlin was effective at inhibiting cellular proliferation when eIF3c levels were at their highest (Scoles et al. 2006).

These observations show that merlin plays a role in modulating receptor–cytoskeleton linkage as well as in signaling to the cytoskeleton affecting cell growth and adhesion.

5.1.3.3
NF2 and Tumors

Merlin is nearly absent in tumors from NF2 patients. In addition to the inherited defect, the second allele of the *NF2* gene has been inactivated – usually by a deletion including major portions of chromosome 22. This is consistent with the "two-hit" hypothesis by Knudson explaining the high incidence of tumors in patients who have inherited a mutation in a tumor suppressor gene. Somatic *NF2* gene mutations are observed to a high degree in those sporadic tumor types that characterize the NF2 tumor syndrome. Sporadic tumors with *NF2* mutations include schwannoma, meningioma (with transitional and fibroblastic variants being more often affected than meningotheliomatous meningiomas), and ependymomas in spinal localization usually in adult patients. NF2 patients typically develop multiple meningiomas and the tumors occur at a younger age than in the general population. Meningiomas in NF2 are often recurrent but the frequency of atypical or anaplastic meningiomas is not increased in NF2 (Antinheimo et al. 1997).

5.2
Tuberous Sclerosis Complex

Tuberous sclerosis complex (TSC) is an autosomal-dominant inherited syndrome affecting 1 in 6,000 to 10,000 individuals. The disease is characterized by the development of different types of benign hamartomas involving the CNS, skin, kidney, and heart. The majority of hamartomas associated with TSC are extremely rare in the general population and are therefore highly diagnostic for TSC (Table 5.5). The clinical picture is variable, making a clinical diagnosis difficult in some cases.

Criteria for TSC have been established. Criteria for definite TSC: either two major features or one major feature plus two minor features. Criteria for probable TSC: One major plus one minor feature. Criteria suggestive of TSC: either one major or two or more minor features (Roach et al. 1998). CNS manifestations are cortical tubera, subependymal nodules, and subependymal giant cell astrocytomas and the majority of patients (78–92%) have epileptic seizures. Mental retardation can be part of the syndrome (Kwiatkowski and Short 1994). An increased risk for malignancies exists only for kidney tumors (malignant angiolipoma or renal cell carcinoma) with a lifetime risk of 2–3% (Cook et al. 1996; Al-Saleem et al. 1998).

5.2.1
Molecular Genetics

TSC is caused by mutations in one of two different genes: *TSC1* located on chromosome 9q34 and *TSC2* on chromosome 16p13.3 (European Chromosome 16 Tubererous Sclerosis Consortium 1993; van Slegtenhorst et al. 1997). Families with TSC carry germline mutations in *TSC1* and *TSC2* in 50% of cases. There is a high rate of spontaneous mutations representing 65–85% of all cases. Spontaneous cases are more often due to a *TSC2* germline mutation (65%). The *TSC1* gene has 23 exons and encodes

Table 5.5 Diagnostic criteria for TSC

Major features	Minor features
Facial angiofibromas or forehead plaque	Multiple randomly distributed pits in dental enamel
Nontraumatic ungual or periungual fibroma	Hamartomatous rectal polyps
Hypomelanotic macules (3 or more)	Bone cysts
Shagreen patch (connective tissue nevus)	Cerebral white matter radial migration lines[a]
Cortical tuber[a]	Gingival fibromas
Subependymal nodule	Nonrenal hamartoma
Subependymal giant cell astrocytoma	Retinal achromic patch
Multiple retinal nodular hamartomas	"Confetti" skin lesions
Cardiac rhabdomyoma, single or multiple	Multiple renal cysts
Lymphangioleiomyomatosis[b]	
Renal angiomyolipoma[b]	

[a] When cerebral cortical tuber and cerebral white matter migration lines occur together, they should be counted as one rather than two features of TSC (**Adapted from Tuberous Sclerosis Consensus Conference; Roach et al. 1998**)

[b] When both lymphangioleiomyomatosis and renal angiomyolipomas are present, other features of tuberous sclerosis are required for definite diagnosis

for the 130-kDa protein hamartin. The *TSC2* gene has 42 exons and encodes for the 198-kDa protein tuberin. Nearly all germline mutations of *TSC1* are protein truncating, whereas 20% of those in *TSC2* are missense mutations (Cheadle et al. 2000).

5.2.2
Molecular Pathogenesis

Hamartin and tuberin bind to each other and form a stable complex. This explains the similarity of clinical symptoms in two genetically distinct diseases. Hamartin/tuberin interacts with the AKT and the mTOR pathway. Upon growth factor simulation, receptor tyrosine kinases recruit type Ia phosphoinositide 3-kinase (PI3K) to the cell membrane followed by the formation of phosphatidylinositol-3,4,5-trisphosphate. Thereby the kinase AKT (PKB) localizes to the membrane where it is phosphorylated and activated amongst others by the mTOR-rictor complex at S473 and by PDK1 at T308 (Vanhaesebroeck and Alessi 2000; Sarbassov et al. 2005). Active AKT phosphorylates several proteins (e.g., the FOXO family of transcription factors, BAD, GSK3) including tuberin. At least five sites of tuberin can be phosphorylated by AKT (Dan et al. 2002; Manning and Cantley 2003; Downward 2004). In analogy to neurofibromin and Ras, the hamartin/tuberin complex acts as a specific GAP for Rheb (Ras homolog enriched in brain). Loss of hamartin/tuberin function results in increased levels of Rheb-GTP which in turn plays a central role in the activation of mTOR (mammalian target of rapamycin) kinase (Garami et al. 2003; Inoki et al. 2003a; Zhang et al. 2003). mTOR forms two complexes: mTORC1 (with raptor and GβL) and mTORC2 (with rictor and GβL). mTORC1 phosphorylates ribosomal S6 kinases (S6K1 and S6K2) and the eukaryotic initiation factor 4E (eIF4E)-binding protein (4E-BP1), which is (upon other events) necessary for their activation. These targets affect cell growth, proliferation, and survival (Raught et al. 2004; Richardson et al. 2004). Both hamartin and tuberin have multiple phosphorylation sites and phosphorylation of the different sites has different effects on the activity of the hamartin/tuberin complex. Whereas phosphorylation by AKT has an inhibitory influence, the phosphorylation by the energy-sensitive AMP-activated protein kinase (AMPK) results in an enhanced Rheb-GAP activity of hamartin/tuberin (Inoki et al. 2003b). Mutations in the tumor suppressor gene *LKB1* are associated with the Peutz-Jeghers syndrome, for which gastrointestinal hamartomas are characteristic. *LKB1* encodes for an AMPK-activating kinase. Its loss also leads to elevated mTOR activity (Corradetti et al. 2004; Shaw et al. 2004).

It has been demonstrated that the MAPK/ERK1/2 pathway can activate mTOR via hamartin/tuberin inhibition by phosphorylation (Roux et al. 2004; Ma et al. 2005).

5.2.3
Subependymal Giant Cell Astrocytomas

Subependymal giant cell astrocytomas (SEGA) are tumors with large cells exhibiting morphological and immunohistochemical properties of astrocytes and neurons. Mutational analysis revealed that cells in SEGA harbor "two-hits" in *TSC1* or *TSC2* consistent with Knudson's theory. An activation of the mTOR pathway can be found by immunohistochemical staining of phosphorylated S6 (Chan et al. 2004). Furthermore, in SEGA high levels of AKT and ERK1/2 phosphorylation have been found indicating an involvement of these pathways in tumor formation (Han et al. 2004).

5.3
Li-Fraumeni and Li-Fraumeni-Like Syndrome

This rare cancer-predisposing syndrome was described by Li and Fraumeni in 1969. A wide range of tumors may occur, with typical entities being premenopausal breast cancer (24%), sarcomas (bone sarcomas 12.6%; soft tissue sarcomas 11.6%), brain tumors (12%), adrenal cortex cancer, and acute leukemia (Kleihues et al. 1997). Two different syndromes are distinguished. The classic Li-Fraumeni syndrome (LFS) and the Li-Fraumeni-like syndrome (LFL) (Table 5.6)

The mean age of onset of brain tumors in LFS is 25 years. Brain tumors are mainly astrocytic tumors (64%) followed by medulloblastomas/PNET and choroid plexus tumors (together 25%). Other entities occur at a lower frequency (Kleihues, Schauble et al. 1997). There are different descriptions of LFS families with a high incidence of CNS tumors (Dockhorn-Dworniczak et al. 1996; Lynch et al. 2000). In 71–77% of classic LFS and in 22–40% of LFL the underlying molecular genetic event is a germline mutation of the *TP53* gene. The majority of the mutations are missense mutations and occur within exons 5–8 (Institute Curie Database). The gene encodes for the p53 protein, which is a central checkpoint protein in the cell cycle and has an essential role in promoting DNA damage repair and apoptosis thereby possessing tumor suppressor function (Vousden and Lu 2002). Furthermore some p53 mutants are believed to acquire oncogenic properties (Frazier et al. 1998; Sigal and Rotter 2000; Vikhanskaya et al. 2007). Despite intensive efforts in mutation analysis it is not possible to detect a *TP53* germline mutation in all LFS or LFL patients, indicating that there are alternative molecular alterations. Heterozygous germline mutations in the *hCHK2* gene, which encodes a G_2 checkpoint control protein, were found in patients with LFS/LFL (Bell et al.

Table 5.6 Diagnostic criteria for LFS and LFL

Li-Fraumeni syndrome is defined as:
Proband with a sarcoma < 45 years of age plus a first-degree relative with any cancer < 45 years of age plus an additional first- or second-degree relative in the same lineage with any cancer < 45 years of age or a sarcoma at any age.
The Li-Fraumeni-like syndrome is defined as:
Proband with any childhood tumor or a sarcoma, brain tumor or adrenocortical tumor < 45 years of age plus a first- or second-degree relative in the same lineage with a typical LFS tumor at any age and an additional first- or second-degree relative in the same lineage with any cancer < 60 years of age.

1999; Varley 2003). However, there are numerous LFS/LFL families for which the underlying germline mutation remains unidentified. Some candidate genes like *MDM2* (Birch et al. 1994), *PTEN, CDKN2* (Burt et al. 1999) (Brown et al. 2000; Portwine et al. 2000), *Bcl10* (Stone et al. 1999), and *TP63* (Bougeard et al. 2001) could be excluded.

5.4
Melanoma–Astrocytoma Syndrome

In 1990 Kaufman et al. described a family with cutaneous malignant melanoma or cerebral astrocytoma, or both, in eight members over three generations (Kaufman et al. 1993). Others reported on families in which several members developed malignant melanoma, dysplastic nevi, astrocytoma in all grades, benign, or malignant schwannoma, neurofibroma, or meningioma (Azizi et al. 1995; Bahuau et al. 1997). The chromosomal region 9p21 has been identified as a locus for predisposition to malignant melanoma (Kamb et al. 1994a). There are three candidate genes in this region: *CDKN2A* (encodes p16 protein), *CDKN2B* (encodes p15 protein), and the gene encoding p14ARF. The protein p14ARF is encoded by an alternative exon 1 (1ß) and exon 2 of the *CDKN2A* gene. Controlled by its own promoter, exon 1ß is spliced to *CDKN2A* exon 2 in an alternate reading frame to that of the p16 protein (Kamb et al. 1994b; Stone et al. 1995).

The function of both p15 and p16 is to prevent progression in the cell cycle through the G_1 restriction point through inhibition of CDK4/CDK6 in the retinoblastoma pathway (Roussel 1999). MDM2 binds to p53 and promotes its degradation by the ubiquitin pathway (Oliner et al. 1992; Weber et al. 1999). MDM2 is also able to inactivate the retinoblastoma protein (Rb) (Xiao et al. 1995). P14ARF binds to MDM2 triggering the sequestering of MDM2. Thereby, no binding of MDM2 to p53 or Rb is possible, resulting in p53 activation.

In two melanoma–astrocytoma families large germline deletions of 9p21 which involve *CDKN2A* and *CDKN2A* exon 1ß have been described (Bahuau et al. 1998). In a family with melanomas, neurofibromas, and multiple dysplastic nevi, splice site mutations were detected. The mutations appear to result in transcripts which lack exon 2, encoding for both p16 and p14 proteins (Petronzelli et al. 2001; Prowse et al. 2003). Other families showed some features of the melanoma–astrocytoma syndrome and a germline deletion of exon 1ß of the *CDKN2A* gene. The deletion identified did not appear to disrupt the function of the p16 protein (Randerson-Moor et al. 2001).

It may be assumed that functional loss of both the p16 and p14ARF tumor suppressor genes or of p14ARF alone might be the predisposing factor in these families.

5.5
Turcot Syndrome

Turcot syndrome is defined as the occurrence of multiple colorectal adenomas and/or colorectal adenocarcinoma in combination with a primary brain tumor. Most cases of Turcot syndrome occur in patients with the familial adenomatous polyposis or hereditary non-polyposis colorectal carcinoma syndromes. Brain tumors are typically astrocytomas including glioblastomas or medulloblastomas (together 95% of brain tumors). Two main phenotypes can be distinguished. One involves development of thousands of polyps in the colon and medulloblastoma, and the other one shows few polyps but development of colorectal carcinoma and glial brain tumors. These two groups seem to be associated with different genetical alterations. The group of patients with numerous polyps and medulloblastomas often harbor a germline mutation in the adenomatous polyposis coli (*APC*) gene on chromosome 5q21 (Hamilton et al. 1995). The other group of patients with occurrence of glial brain tumors (mainly glioblastomas) has mutations in the DNA mismatch repair (MMR) genes *hMSH2, hMLH1*, or *hPMS2* (Lucci-Cordisco et al. 2003). Indeed there are also reports about patients with Turcot syndrome who developed both glioblastoma and medulloblastoma (McLaughlin et al. 1998).

5.6
Familial Gliomas

Families have been described that do not suffer from one of the discussed syndromes, but in which the frequency of gliomas is increased.

The pattern of tumor occurrence is different from most familial cancers. There is no involvement of multiple generations or occurrence at an unusually early age. The prognosis for affected patients is as for typical high-grade astrocytomas (Grossman et al. 1999).

Using segregation analysis, both autosomal recessive as well as multifactorial mendelian models have been proposed, while a model postulating a purely environmental cause was rejected (de Andrade et al. 2001; Malmer et al. 2001). Investigations of candidate genes for familial gliomas included *TP53, PTEN, CDKN2A*, and *CDK4. TP53* was found to harbor a germline mutation in a patient with familial glioma that did not meet all the criteria of Li-Fraumeni syndrome (Tachibana et al. 2000; Paunu et al. 2001).

References

Al-Saleem T, Wessner LL, Scheithauer BW, Patterson K, Roach ES, Dreyer SJ, Fujikawa K, Bjornsson J, Bernstein J, Henske EP (1998) Malignant tumors of the kidney, brain, and soft tissues in children and young adults with the tuberous sclerosis complex. Cancer 83(10):2208–2216

Antinheimo J, Haapasalo H, Haltia M, Tatagiba M, Thomas S, Brandis A, Sainio M, Carpen O, Samii M, Jaaskelainen J (1997) Proliferation potential and histological features in neurofibromatosis 2-associated and sporadic meningiomas. J Neurosurg 87(4):610–614

Aravind L, Neuwald AF, Ponting CP (1999) Sec14p-like domains in NF1 and Dbl-like proteins indicate lipid regulation of Ras and Rho signaling. Curr Biol 9(6):R195–197

Azizi E, Friedman J, Pavlotsky F, Iscovich J, Bornstein A, Shafir R, Trau H, Brenner H, Nass D (1995) Familial cutaneous malignant melanoma and tumors of the nervous system. A hereditary cancer syndrome. Cancer 76(9):1571–1578

Bader JL (1986) Neurofibromatosis and cancer. Ann N Y Acad Sci 486:57–65

Bahuau M, Vidaud D, Jenkins RB, Bieche I, Kimmel DW, Assouline B, Smith JS, Alderete B, Cayuela JM, Harpey JP, Caille B, Vidaud M (1998) Germ-line deletion involving the INK4 locus in familial proneness to melanoma and nervous system tumors. Cancer Res 58(11):2298–2303

Bahuau M, Vidaud D, Kujas M, Palangie A, Assouline B, Chaignaud-Lebreton M, Prieur M, Vidaud M, Harpey JP, Lafourcade J, Caille B (1997) Familial aggregation of malignant melanoma/dysplastic naevi and tumours of the nervous system: an original syndrome of tumour proneness. Ann Genet 40(2):78–91

Bell DW, Varley JM, Szydlo TE, Kang DH, Wahrer DC, Shannon KE, Lubratovich M, Verselis SJ, Isselbacher KJ, Fraumeni JF, Birch JM, Li FP, Garber JE, Haber DA (1999) Heterozygous germ line hCHK2 mutations in Li-Fraumeni syndrome. Science 286(5449):2528–2531

Birch JM, Heighway J, Teare MD, Kelsey AM, Hartley AL, Tricker KJ, Crowther D, Lane DP, Santibanez-Koref MF (1994) Linkage studies in a Li-Fraumeni family with increased expression of p53 protein but no germline mutation in p53. Br J Cancer 70(6):1176–1181

Blatt J, Jaffe R, Deutsch M, Adkins JC (1986) Neurofibromatosis and childhood tumors. Cancer 57(6):1225–1229

Boguski MS, McCormick F (1993) Proteins regulating Ras and its relatives. Nature 366(6456):643–654

Bougeard G, Limacher JM, Martin C, Charbonnier F, Killian A, Delattre O, Longy M, Jonveaux P, Fricker JP, Stoppa-Lyonnet D, Flaman JM, Frebourg T (2001) Detection of 11 germline inactivating TP53 mutations and absence of TP63 and HCHK2 mutations in 17 French families with Li-Fraumeni or Li-Fraumeni-like syndrome. J Med Genet 38(4):253–257

Bourn D, Carter SA, Mason S, Gareth D, Evans R, Strachan T (1994) Germline mutations in the neurofibromatosis type 2 tumour suppressor gene. Hum Mol Genet 3(5):813–816

Boyanapalli M, Lahoud OB, Messiaen L, Kim B, Anderle de Sylor MS, Duckett SJ, Somara S, Mikol DD (2006) Neurofibromin binds to caveolin-1 and regulates ras, FAK, and Akt. Biochem Biophys Res Commun 340(4):1200–1208

Brault E, Gautreau A, Lamarine M, Callebaut I, Thomas G, Goutebroze L (2001) Normal membrane localization and actin association of the NF2 tumor suppressor protein are dependent on folding of its N-terminal domain. J Cell Sci 114(Pt 10):1901–1912

Bretscher A, Edwards K, Fehon RG (2002) ERM proteins and merlin: integrators at the cell cortex. Nat Rev Mol Cell Biol 3(8):586–599

Brown LT, Sexsmith E, Malkin D (2000) Identification of a novel PTEN intronic deletion in Li-Fraumeni syndrome and its effect on RNA processing. Cancer Genet Cytogenet 123(1):65–68

Buday L (1999) Membrane-targeting of signalling molecules by SH2/SH3 domain-containing adaptor proteins. Biochim Biophys Acta 1422(2):187–204

Burt EC, McGown G, Thorncroft M, James LA, Birch JM, Varley JM (1999) Exclusion of the genes CDKN2 and PTEN as causative gene defects in Li-Fraumeni syndrome. Br J Cancer 80(1–2):9–10

Castle B, Baser ME, Huson SM, Cooper DN, Upadhyaya M (2003) Evaluation of genotype-phenotype correlations in neurofibromatosis type 1. J Med Genet 40(10):e109

Cawthon RM, O'Connell P, Buchberg AM, Viskochil D, Weiss RB, Culver M, Stevens J, Jenkins NA, Copeland NG, White R (1990a) Identification and characterization of transcripts from the neurofibromatosis 1 region: the sequence and genomic structure of EVI2 and mapping of other transcripts. Genomics 7(4):555–565

Cawthon RM, Weiss R, Xu GF, Viskochil D, Culver M, Stevens J, Robertson M, Dunn D, Gesteland R, O'Connell P, et al. (1990b) A major segment of the neurofibromatosis type 1 gene: cDNA sequence, genomic structure, and point mutations. Cell 62(1):193–201

Cawthon RM, Andersen LB, Buchberg AM, Xu GF, O'Connell P, Viskochil D, Weiss RB, Wallace MR, Marchuk DA, Culver M, et al. (1991) cDNA sequence and genomic structure of EV12B, a gene lying within an intron of the neurofibromatosis type 1 gene. Genomics 9(3):446–60

Chan JA, Zhang H, Roberts PS, Jozwiak S, Wieslawa G, Lewin-Kowalik J, Kotulska K, Kwiatkowski DJ (2004) Pathogenesis of tuberous sclerosis subependymal giant cell astrocytomas: biallelic inactivation of TSC1 or TSC2 leads to mTOR activation. J Neuropathol Exp Neurol 63(12):1236–42

Cheadle JP, Reeve MP, Sampson JR, Kwiatkowski DJ (2000) Molecular genetic advances in tuberous sclerosis. Hum Genet 107(2):97–114

Cook JA, Oliver K, Mueller RF, Sampson J (1996) A cross sectional study of renal involvement in tuberous sclerosis. J Med Genet 33(6):480–484

Corradetti MN, Inoki K, Bardeesy N, DePinho RA, Guan KL (2004) Regulation of the TSC pathway by LKB1: evidence of a molecular link between tuberous sclerosis complex and Peutz-Jeghers syndrome. Genes Dev 18(13):1533–1538

Corral T, Jimenez M, Hernandez-Munoz I, Perez de Castro I, Pellicer A (2003) NF1 modulates the effects of Ras oncogenes: evidence of other NF1 function besides its GAP activity. J Cell Physiol 197(2):214–224

D'Angelo I, Welti S, Bonneau F, Scheffzek K (2006) A novel bipartite phospholipid-binding module in the neurofibromatosis type 1 protein. EMBO Rep 7(2):174–179

Dan HC, Sun M, Yang L, Feldman RI, Sui XM, Ou CC, Nellist M, Yeung RS, Halley DJ, Nicosia SV, Pledger WJ, Cheng JQ (2002) Phosphatidylinositol 3-kinase/Akt pathway regulates tuberous sclerosis tumor suppressor complex by phosphorylation of tuberin. J Biol Chem 277(38):35364–35370

Danglot G, Regnier V, Fauvet D, Vassal G, Kujas M, Bernheim A (1995) Neurofibromatosis 1 (NF1) mRNAs expressed in the central nervous system are differentially spliced in the 5' part of the gene. Hum Mol Genet 4(5):915–920

Dasgupta B, Dugan LL, Gutmann DH The neurofibromatosis 1 gene product neurofibromin regulates pituitary adenylate cycase-activating polypeptide-mediated signaling in astrocytes. J Neurosci 23(26):8949–8954.

Dasgupta B, Yi Y, Chen DY, Weber JD, Gutmann DH (2005) Proteomic analysis reveals hyperactivation of the mammalian target of rapamycin pathway in neurofibromatosis 1-associated human and mouse brain tumors. Cancer Res 65(7):2755–2760

Daston MM, Scrable H, Nordlund M, Sturbaum AK, Nissen LM, Ratner N (1992) The protein product of the neurofibromatosis type 1 gene is expressed at highest abundance in neurons, Schwann cells, and oligodendrocytes. Neuron 8(3):415–428

de Andrade M, Barnholtz JS, Amos CI, Adatto P, Spencer C, Bondy ML (2001) Segregation analysis of cancer in families of glioma patients. Genet Epidemiol 20(2):258–270

DeClue JE, Cohen BD, Lowy DR (1991) Identification and characterization of the neurofibromatosis type 1 protein product. Proc Natl Acad Sci USA 88(22):9914–9918

Dockhorn-Dworniczak B, Wolff J, Poremba C, Schafer KL, Ritter J, Gullotta F, Jurgens H, Bocker W (1996) A new germline TP53 gene mutation in a family with Li-Fraumeni syndrome. Eur J Cancer 32A(8):1359–1365

Downward J (2004) PI 3-kinase, Akt and cell survival. Semin Cell Dev Biol 15(2):177–182

Dugan LL, Kim JS, Zhang Y, Bart RD, Sun Y, Holtzman DM, Gutmann DH (1999) Differential effects of cAMP in neurons and astrocytes. Role of B-raf. J Biol Chem 274(36):25842–25848

Europen Chromosome 16 Tuberous Sclerosis Consortium (1993) Identification and characterization of the tuberous sclerosis gene on chromosome 16. The European Chromosome 16 Tuberous Sclerosis Consortium. Cell 75(7):1305–1315

Evans DG, Trueman L, Wallace A, Collins S, Strachan T (1998) Genotype/phenotype correlations in type 2 neurofibromatosis (NF2): evidence for more severe disease associated with truncating mutations. J Med Genet 35(6):450–455

Fahsold R, Hoffmeyer S, Mischung C, Gille C, Ehlers C, Kucukceylan N, Abdel-Nour M, Gewies A, Peters H, Kaufmann D, Buske A, Tinschert S, Nurnberg P (2000) Minor lesion mutational spectrum of the entire NF1 gene does not explain its high mutability but points to a functional domain upstream of the GAP-related domain. Am J Hum Genet 66(3):790–818

Fernandez-Valle C, Tang Y, Ricard J, Rodenas-Ruano A, Taylor A, Hackler E, Biggerstaff J, Iacovelli J (2002) Paxillin binds schwannomin and regulates its density-dependent localization and effect on cell morphology. Nat Genet 31(4):354–362

Frazier MW, He X, Wang J, Gu Z, Cleveland JL, Zambetti GP (1998) Activation of c-myc gene expression by tumor-derived p53 mutants requires a discrete C-terminal domain. Mol Cell Biol 18(7):3735–3743

Friedman JM (1999) Epidemiology of neurofibromatosis type 1. Am J Med Genet 89(1):1–6

Garami A, Zwartkruis FJ, Nobukuni T, Joaquin M, Roccio M, Stocker H, Kozma SC, Hafen E, Bos JL, Thomas G (2003) Insulin activation of Rheb, a mediator of mTOR/S6K/4E-BP signaling, is inhibited by TSC1 and 2. Mol Cell 11(6):1457–1466

Gary R, Bretscher A (1995) Ezrin self-association involves binding of an N-terminal domain to a normally masked C-terminal domain that includes the F-actin binding site. Mol Biol Cell 6(8):1061–1075

Gonzalez-Agosti C, Wiederhold T, Herndon ME, Gusella J, Ramesh V (1999) Interdomain interaction of merlin isoforms and its influence on intermolecular binding to NHE-RF. J Biol Chem 274(48):34438–34442

Goutebroze L, Brault E, Muchardt C, Camonis J, Thomas G (2000) Cloning and characterization of SCHIP-1, a novel protein interacting specifically with spliced isoforms and naturally occurring mutant NF2 proteins. Mol Cell Biol 20(5):1699–1712

Grand RJ, Owen D (1991) The biochemistry of ras p21. Biochem J 279 (Pt 3):609–631

Gronholm M, Vossebein L, Carlson CR, Kuja-Panula J, Teesalu T, Alfthan K, Vaheri A, Rauvala H, Herberg FW, Tasken K, Carpen O (2003) Merlin links to the cAMP neuronal signaling pathway by anchoring the RIbeta subunit of protein kinase A. J Biol Chem 278(42):41167–41172

Grossman SA, Osman M, Hruban R, Piantadosi S (1999) Central nervous system cancers in first-degree relatives and spouses. Cancer Invest 17(5):299–308

Guo HF, The I, Hannan F, Bernards A, Zhong Y (1997) Requirement of Drosophila NF1 for activation of adenylyl cyclase by PACAP38-like neuropeptides. Science 276(5313):795–798

Guo HF, Tong J, Hannan F, Luo L, Zhong Y (2000) A neurofibromatosis-1-regulated pathway is required for learning in Drosophila. Nature 403(6772): 895–898

Gutman DH, Andersen LB, Cole JL, Swaroop M, Collins FS (1993) An alternatively-spliced mRNA in the carboxy terminus of the neurofibromatosis type 1 (NF1) gene is expressed in muscle. Hum Mol Genet 2(7):989–992

Gutmann DH, Donahoe J, Brown T, James CD, Perry A (2000) Loss of neurofibromatosis 1 (NF1) gene expression in NF1-associated pilocytic astrocytomas. Neuropathol Appl Neurobiol 26(4):361–367

Gutmann DH, Wood DL, Collins FS (1991) Identification of the neurofibromatosis type 1 gene product. Proc Natl Acad Sci USA 88(21): 9658–9662

Habib AA, Gulcher JR, Hognason T, Zheng L, Stefansson K (1998) The OMgp gene, a second growth suppressor within the NF1 gene. Oncogene 16(12):1525–1531

Hamilton SR, Liu B, Parsons RE, Papadopoulos N, Jen J, Powell SM, Krush AJ, Berk T, Cohen Z, Tetu B, et al. (1995) The molecular basis of Turcot's syndrome. N Engl J Med 332(13):839–847

Han S, Santos TM, Puga A, Roy J, Thiele EA, McCollin M, Stemmer-Rachamimov A, Ramesh V (2004) Phosphorylation of tuberin as a novel mechanism for somatic inactivation of the tuberous sclerosis complex proteins in brain lesions. Cancer Res 64(3):812–816

Hannan F, Ho I, Tong JJ, Zhu Y, Nurnberg P, Zhong Y (2006) Effect of neurofibromatosis type I mutations on a novel pathway for adenylyl cyclase activation requiring neurofibromin and Ras. Hum Mol Genet 15(7):1087–1098

Huson SM, Hughes RAC (1994) The Neurofibromatoses: a pathogenetic and clinical overview. Chapman & Hall Medical, London/New York

Inoki K, Li Y, Xu T, Guan KL (2003a) Rheb GTPase is a direct target of TSC2 GAP activity and regulates mTOR signaling. Genes Dev 17(15): 1829–1834

Inoki K, Zhu T, Guan KL (2003b) TSC2 mediates cellular energy response to control cell growth and survival. Cell 115(5):577–590

Jacks T, Shih TS, Schmitt EM, Bronson RT, Bernards A, Weinberg RA (1994) Tumour predisposition in mice heterozygous for a targeted mutation in Nf1. Nat Genet 7(3):353–361

James MF, Manchanda N, Gonzalez-Agosti C, Hartwig JH, Ramesh V (2001) The neurofibromatosis 2 protein product merlin selectively binds F-actin but not G-actin, and stabilizes the filaments through a lateral association. Biochem J 356(Pt 2):377–386

Jannatipour M, Dion P, Khan S, Jindal H, Fan X, Laganiere J, Chishti AH, Rouleau GA (2001) Schwannomin isoform-1 interacts with syntenin via PDZ domains. J Biol Chem 276(35): 33093–33100

Johannessen CM, Reczek EE, James MF, Brems H, Legius E, Cichowski K (2005) The NF1 tumor suppressor critically regulates TSC2 and mTOR. Proc Natl Acad Sci USA 102(24):8573–8578

Kamb A, Gruis NA, Weaver-Feldhaus J, Liu Q, Harshman K, Tavtigian SV, Stockert E, Day RS, 3rd, Johnson BE, Skolnick MH (1994a) A cell cycle regulator potentially involved in genesis of many tumor types. Science 264(5157): 436–440

Kamb A, Shattuck-Eidens D, Eeles R, Liu Q, Gruis NA, Ding W, Hussey C, Tran T, Miki Y, Weaver-Feldhaus J, et al. (1994b) Analysis of the p16 gene (CDKN2) as a candidate for the chromosome 9p melanoma susceptibility locus. Nat Genet 8(1):23–26

Kaufman DK, Kimmel DW, Parisi JE, Michels VV (1993) A familial syndrome with cutaneous malignant melanoma and cerebral astrocytoma. Neurology 43(9):1728–1731

Kaufmann D, Muller R, Kenner O, Leistner W, Hein C, Vogel W, Bartelt B (2002) The N-terminal splice product NF1–10a-2 of the NF1 gene codes for a transmembrane segment. Biochem Biophys Res Commun 294(2):496–503

Kim H, Lim JY, Kim YH, Park SH, Lee KH, Han H, Jeun SS, Lee JH, Rha HK (2002) Inhibition of ras-mediated activator protein 1 activity and cell growth by merlin. Mol Cells 14(1):108–114

Kim HA, Ratner N, Roberts TM, Stiles CD (2001) Schwann cell proliferative responses to cAMP and Nf1 are mediated by cyclin D1. J Neurosci 21(4):1110–1116

Kissil JL, Wilker EW, Johnson KC, Eckman MS, Yaffe MB, Jacks T (2003) Merlin, the product of the Nf2 tumor suppressor gene, is an inhibitor of the p21-activated kinase. Pak1. Mol Cell 12(4):841–849

Kleihues P, Schauble B, zur Hausen A, Esteve J, Ohgaki H (1997) Tumors associated with p53 germline mutations: a synopsis of 91 families. Am J Pathol 150(1):1–13

Kluwe L, Hagel C, Tatagiba M, Thomas S, Stavrou D, Ostertag H, von Deimling A, Mautner VF (2001) Loss of NF1 alleles distinguish sporadic from NF1-associated pilocytic astrocytomas. J Neuropathol Exp Neurol 60(9):917–920

Kwiatkowski DJ, Short MP (1994) Tuberous sclerosis. Arch Dermatol 130(3):348–354

Lau N, Feldkamp MM, Roncari L, Loehr AH, Shannon P, Gutmann DH, Guha A (2000) Loss of neurofibromin is associated with activation of RAS/MAPK and PI3-K/AKT signaling in a neurofibromatosis 1 astrocytoma. J Neuropathol Exp Neurol 59(9):759–767

Lim JY, Kim H, Jeun SS, Kang SG, Lee KJ (2006) Merlin inhibits growth hormone-regulated Raf-ERKs pathways by binding to Grb2 protein. Biochem Biophys Res Commun 340(4):1151–1157

Lim JY, Kim H, Kim YH, Kim SW, Huh PW, Lee KH, Jeun SS, Rha HK, Kang JK (2003) Merlin suppresses the SRE-dependent transcription by inhibiting the activation of Ras-ERK pathway. Biochem Biophys Res Commun 302(2):238–245

Lopez-Correa C, Zucman-Rossi J, Brems H, Thomas G, Legius E (2000) NF2 gene deletion in a family with a mild phenotype. J Med Genet 37(1):75–77

Lucci-Cordisco E, Zito I, Gensini F, Genuardi M (2003) Hereditary nonpolyposis colorectal cancer and related conditions. Am J Med Genet A 122(4):325–334

Lynch HT, McComb RD, Osborn NK, Wolpert PA, Lynch JF, Wszolek ZK, Sidransky D, Steg RE (2000) Predominance of brain tumors in an extended Li-Fraumeni (SBLA) kindred, including a case of Sturge-Weber syndrome. Cancer 88(2):433–439

Ma L, Chen Z, Erdjument-Bromage H, Tempst P, Pandolfi PP (2005) Phosphorylation and functional inactivation of TSC2 by Erk implications for tuberous sclerosis and cancer pathogenesis. Cell 121(2):179–193

Macara IG, Lounsbury KM, Richards SA, McKiernan C, Bar-Sagi D (1996) The Ras superfamily of GTPases. Faseb J 10(5):625–630

Maeda M, Matsui T, Imamura M, Tsukita S (1999) Expression level, subcellular distribution and rho-GDI binding affinity of merlin in comparison with Ezrin/Radixin/Moesin proteins. Oncogene 18(34):4788–4797

Malmer B, Iselius L, Holmberg E, Collins A, Henriksson R, Gronberg H (2001) Genetic epidemiology of glioma. Br J Cancer 84(3):429–434

Manning BD, Cantley LC (2003) United at last: the tuberous sclerosis complex gene products connect the phosphoinositide 3-kinase/Akt pathway to mammalian target of rapamycin (mTOR) signalling. Biochem Soc Trans 31(Pt 3):573–578

Marshall CJ (1996) Ras effectors. Curr Opin Cell Biol 8(2):197–204

Matsui T, Maeda M, Doi Y, Yonemura S, Amano M, Kaibuchi K, Tsukita S, Tsukita S (1998) Rho-kinase phosphorylates COOH-terminal threonines of ezrin/radixin/moesin (ERM) proteins and regulates their head-to-tail association. J Cell Biol 140(3):647–657

McClatchey AI, Saotome I, Ramesh V, Gusella JF, Jacks T (1997) The Nf2 tumor suppressor gene product is essential for extraembryonic development immediately prior to gastrulation. Genes Dev 11(10):1253–1265

McLaughlin MR, Gollin SM, Lese CM, Albright AL (1998) Medulloblastoma and glioblastoma multiforme in a patient with Turcot syndrome: a case report. Surg Neurol 49(3):295–301

Morrison H, Sherman LS, Legg J, Banine F, Isacke C, Haipek CA, Gutmann DH, Ponta H, Herrlich P (2001) The NF2 tumor suppressor gene product, merlin, mediates contact inhibition of growth through interactions with CD44. Genes Dev 15(8):968–980

Morrison H, Sperka T, Manent J, Giovannini M, Ponta H, Herrlich P (2007) Merlin/neurofibromatosis type 2 suppresses growth by inhibiting the activation of Ras and Rac. Cancer Res 67(2):520–527

Murthy A, Gonzalez-Agosti C, Cordero E, Pinney D, Candia C, Solomon F, Gusella J, Ramesh V (1998) NHE-RF, a regulatory cofactor for Na(+)-H + exchange, is a common interactor for merlin and

ERM (MERM) proteins. J Biol Chem 273(3): 1273–1276

Neill GW, Crompton MR (2001) Binding of the merlin-I product of the neurofibromatosis type 2 tumour suppressor gene to a novel site in beta-fodrin is regulated by association between merlin domains. Biochem J 358(Pt 3):727–735

Nishi T, Lee PS, Oka K, Levin VA, Tanase S, Morino Y, Saya H (1991) Differential expression of two types of the neurofibromatosis type 1 (NF1) gene transcripts related to neuronal differentiation. Oncogene 6(9):1555–1559

Obremski VJ, Hall AM, Fernandez-Valle C (1998) Merlin, the neurofibromatosis type 2 gene product, and beta1 integrin associate in isolated and differentiating Schwann cells. J Neurobiol 37(4):487–501

Oliner JD, Kinzler KW, Meltzer PS, George DL, Vogelstein B (1992) Amplification of a gene encoding a p53-associated protein in human sarcomas. Nature 358(6381):80–83

Pan D, Dong J, Zhang Y, Gao X (2004) Tuberous sclerosis complex: from Drosophila to human disease. Trends Cell Biol 14(2):78–85

Parry DM, MacCollin MM, Kaiser-Kupfer MI, Pulaski K, Nicholson HS, Bolesta M, Eldridge R, Gusella JF (1996) Germ-line mutations in the neurofibromatosis 2 gene: correlations with disease severity and retinal abnormalities. Am J Hum Genet 59(3):529–539

Paunu N, Syrjakoski K, Sankila R, Simola KO, Helen P, Niemela M, Matikainen M, Isola J, Haapasalo H (2001) Analysis of p53 tumor suppressor gene in families with multiple glioma patients. J Neurooncol 55(3):159–165

Petronzelli F, Sollima D, Coppola G, Martini-Neri ME, Neri G, Genuardi M (2001) CDKN2A germline splicing mutation affecting both p16(ink4) and p14(arf) RNA processing in a melanoma/neurofibroma kindred. Genes Chromosomes Cancer 31(4):398–401

Platten M, Giordano MJ, Dirven CM, Gutmann DH, Louis DN (1996) Up-regulation of specific NF 1 gene transcripts in sporadic pilocytic astrocytomas. Am J Pathol 149(2):621–627

Portwine C, Lees J, Verselis S, Li FP, Malkin D (2000) Absence of germline p16(INK4a) alterations in p53 wild type Li-Fraumeni syndrome families. J Med Genet 37(8):E13

Prowse AH, Schultz DC, Guo S, Vanderveer L, Dangel J, Bove B, Cairns P, Daly M, Godwin AK (2003) Identification of a splice acceptor site mutation in p16INK4A/p14ARF within a breast cancer, melanoma, neurofibroma prone kindred. J Med Genet 40(8):e102

Randerson-Moor JA, Harland M, Williams S, Cuthbert-Heavens D, Sheridan E, Aveyard J, Sibley K, Whitaker L, Knowles M, Bishop JN, Bishop DT (2001) A germline deletion of p14(ARF) but not CDKN2A in a melanoma-neural system tumour syndrome family. Hum Mol Genet 10(1):55–62

Rasmussen SA, Yang Q, Friedman JM (2001) Mortality in neurofibromatosis 1: an analysis using U.S. death certificates. Am J Hum Genet 68(5):1110–1118

Raught B, Peiretti F, Gingras AC, Livingstone M, Shahbazian D, Mayeur GL, Polakiewicz RD, Sonenberg N, Hershey JW (2004) Phosphorylation of eucaryotic translation initiation factor 4B Ser422 is modulated by S6 kinases. Embo J 23(8):1761–1769

Richardson CJ, Broenstrup M, Fingar DC, Julich K, Ballif BA, Gygi S, Blenis J (2004) SKAR is a specific target of S6 kinase 1 in cell growth control. Curr Biol 14(17):1540–1549

Roach ES, Gomez MR, Northrup H (1998) Tuberous sclerosis complex consensus conference: revised clinical diagnostic criteria. J Child Neurol 13(12):624–628

Rong R, Tang X, Gutmann DH, Ye K (2004) Neurofibromatosis 2 (NF2) tumor suppressor merlin inhibits phosphatidylinositol 3-kinase through binding to PIKE-L. Proc Natl Acad Sci USA 101(52):18200–18205

Rouleau GA, Merel P, Lutchman M, Sanson M, Zucman J, Marineau C, Hoang-Xuan K, Demczuk S, Desmaze C, Plougastel B, et al. (1993) Alteration in a new gene encoding a putative membrane-organizing protein causes neuro-fibromatosis type 2. Nature 363(6429):515–521

Roussel MF (1999) The INK4 family of cell cycle inhibitors in cancer. Oncogene 18(38): 5311–5317

Roux PP, Ballif BA, Anjum R, Gygi SP, Blenis J (2004) Tumor-promoting phorbol esters and activated Ras inactivate the tuberous sclerosis tumor suppressor complex via p90 ribosomal S6 kinase. Proc Natl Acad Sci USA 101(37): 13489–13494

Ruttledge MH, Andermann AA, Phelan CM, Claudio JO, Han FY, Chretien N, Rangaratnam S, MacCollin M, Short P, Parry D, Michels V, Riccardi VM, Weksberg R, Kitamura K, Bradburn JM, Hall BD, Propping P, Rouleau GA (1996) Type of mutation in the neurofibromatosis type 2 gene (NF2) frequently determines severity of disease. Am J Hum Genet 59(2):331–342

Ryu CH, Kim SW, Lee KH, Lee JY, Kim H, Lee WK, Choi BH, Lim Y, Kim YH, Hwang TK, Jun TY, Rha HK (2005) The merlin tumor suppressor interacts with Ral guanine nucleotide dissociation stimulator and inhibits its activity. Oncogene 24(34):5355–5364

Sainio M, Zhao F, Heiska L, Turunen O, den Bakker M, Zwarthoff E, Lutchman M, Rouleau GA, Jaas-kelainen J, Vaheri A, Carpen O (1997) Neuro-fibromatosis 2 tumor suppressor protein colocalizes with ezrin and CD44 and associates with actin-containing cytoskeleton. J Cell Sci 110 (Pt 18):2249–2260

Sarbassov DD, Guertin DA, Ali SM, Sabatini DM (2005) Phosphorylation and regulation of Akt/PKB by the rictor-mTOR complex. Science 307(5712):1098–1101

Scoles DR, Huynh DP, Chen MS, Burke SP, Gutmann DH, Pulst SM (2000) The neurofibromatosis 2 tumor suppressor protein interacts with hepatocyte growth factor-regulated tyrosine kinase substrate. Hum Mol Genet 9(11):1567–1574

Scoles DR, Huynh DP, Morcos PA, Coulsell ER, Robinson NG, Tamanoi F, Pulst SM (1998) Neurofibromatosis 2 tumour suppressor schwannomin interacts with betaII-spectrin. Nat Genet 18(4):354–359

Scoles DR, Yong WH, Qin Y, Wawrowsky K, Pulst SM (2006) Schwannomin inhibits tumorigenesis through direct interaction with the eukaryotic initiation factor subunit c (eIF3c). Hum Mol Genet 15(7):1059–1070

Sharma MK, Mansur DB, Reifenberger G, Perry A, Leonard JR, Aldape KD, Albin MG, Emnett RJ, Loeser S, Watson MA, Nagarajan R, Gutmann DH (2007) Distinct genetic signatures among pilocytic astrocytomas relate to their brain region origin. Cancer Res 67(3):890–900

Sharma MK, Zehnbauer BA, Watson MA, Gutmann DH (2005) RAS pathway activation and an oncogenic RAS mutation in sporadic pilocytic astrocytoma. Neurology 65(8):1335–1336

Shaw RJ, Bardeesy N, Manning BD, Lopez L, Kosmatka M, DePinho RA, Cantley LC (2004) The LKB1 tumor suppressor negatively regulates mTOR signaling. Cancer Cell 6(1):91–99

Shen MH, Harper PS, Upadhyaya M (1996) Molecular genetics of neurofibromatosis type 1 (NF1). J Med Genet 33(1):2–17

Sherman L, Xu HM, Geist RT, Saporito-Irwin S, Howells N, Ponta H, Herrlich P, Gutmann DH (1997) Interdomain binding mediates tumor growth suppression by the NF2 gene product. Oncogene 15(20):2505–2509

Sigal A, Rotter V (2000) Oncogenic mutations of the p53 tumor suppressor: the demons of the guardian of the genome. Cancer Res 60(24):6788–6793

Stone JG, Eeles RA, Sodha N, Murday V, Sheriden E, Houlston RS (1999) Analysis of Li-Fraumeni syndrome and Li-Fraumeni-like families for germline mutations in Bcl10. Cancer Lett 147(1–2):181–185

Stone S, Jiang P, Dayananth P, Tavtigian SV, Katcher H, Parry D, Peters G, Kamb A (1995) Complex structure and regulation of the P16 (MTS1) locus. Cancer Res 55(14):2988–2994

Tachibana I, Smith JS, Sato K, Hosek SM, Kimmel DW, Jenkins RB (2000) Investigation of germline PTEN, p53, p16(INK4A)/p14(ARF), and CDK4 alterations in familial glioma. Am J Med Genet 92(2):136–141

Tang X, Jang SW, Wang X, Liu Z, Bahr SM, Sun SY, Brat D, Gutmann DH, Ye K (2007) Akt phosphorylation regulates the tumour-suppressor merlin through ubiquitination and degradation. Nat Cell Biol 9(10):1199–1207

The I, Hannigan GE, Cowley GS, Reginald S, Zhong Y, Gusella JF, Hariharan IK, Bernards A (1997) Rescue of a Drosophila NF1 mutant phenotype by protein kinase A. Science 276(5313):791–794

Tikoo A, Varga M, Ramesh V, Gusella J, Maruta H (1994) An anti-Ras function of neurofibromatosis type 2 gene product (NF2/Merlin). J Biol Chem 269(38):23387–23390

Tong J, Hannan F, Zhu Y, Bernards A, Zhong Y (2002) Neurofibromin regulates G protein-stimulated adenylyl cyclase activity. Nat Neurosci 5(2):95–96

Trofatter JA, MacCollin MM, Rutter JL, Murrell JR, Duyao MP, Parry DM, Eldridge R, Kley N, Menon AG, Pulaski K, et al. (1993) A novel moesin-, ezrin-, radixin-like gene is a candidate for the neurofibromatosis 2 tumor suppressor. Cell 72(5):791–800

Upadhyaya M, Huson SM, Davies M, Thomas N, Chuzhanova N, Giovannini S, Evans DG, Howard E, Kerr B, Griffiths S, Consoli C, Side L, Adams D, Pierpont M, Hachen R, Barnicoat A, Li H, Wallace P, Van Biervliet JP, Stevenson D, Viskochil D, Baralle D, Haan E, Riccardi V, Turnpenny P, Lazaro C, Messiaen L (2007) An absence of cutaneous neurofibromas associated with a 3-bp inframe deletion in exon 17 of the NF1 gene (c.2970–2972 delAAT): evidence of a clinically significant NF1 genotype-phenotype correlation. Am J Hum Genet 80(1):140–151

van Slegtenhorst M, de Hoogt R, Hermans C, Nellist M, Janssen B, Verhoef S, Lindhout D, van den Ouweland A, Halley D, Young J, Burley M, Jeremiah S, Woodward K, Nahmias J, Fox M, Ekong R, Osborne J, Wolfe J, Povey S, Snell RG, Cheadle JP, Jones AC, Tachataki M, Ravine D, Sampson JR, Reeve MP, Richardson P, Wilmer F, Munro C, Hawkins TL, Sepp T, Ali JB, Ward S, Green AJ, Yates JR, Kwiatkowska J, Henske EP, Short MP, Haines JH, Jozwiak S, Kwiatkowski DJ (1997) Identification of the tuberous sclerosis gene TSC1 on chromosome 9q34. Science 277(5327):805–808

Vandenbroucke I, Van Oostveldt P, Coene E, De Paepe A, Messiaen L (2004) Neurofibromin is actively transported to the nucleus. FEBS Lett 560(1–3):98–102

Vanhaesebroeck B, Alessi DR (2000) The PI3K-PDK1 connection: more than just a road to PKB. Biochem J 346 Pt 3:561–576

Varley J (2003) TP53, hChk2, and the Li-Fraumeni syndrome. Methods Mol Biol 222:117–129

Vikhanskaya F, Lee MK, Mazzoletti M, Broggini M, Sabapathy K (2007) Cancer-derived p53 mutants suppress p53-target gene expression–potential mechanism for gain of function of mutant p53. Nucleic Acids Res 35(6):2093–2104

Viskochil D, Buchberg AM, Xu G, Cawthon RM, Stevens J, Wolff RK, Culver M, Carey JC, Copeland NG, Jenkins NA, et al. (1990) Deletions and a translocation interrupt a cloned gene at the neurofibromatosis type 1 locus. Cell 62(1):187–192

Viskochil D, Cawthon R, O'Connell P, Xu GF, Stevens J, Culver M, Carey J, White R (1991) The gene encoding the oligodendrocyte-myelin glycoprotein is embedded within the neurofibromatosis type 1 gene. Mol Cell Biol 11(2):906–912

von Deimling A, Louis DN, Menon AG, von Ammon K, Petersen I, Ellison D, Wiestler OD, Seizinger BR (1993) Deletions on the long arm of chromosome 17 in pilocytic astrocytoma. Acta Neuropathol (Berl) 86(1):81–85

Vousden KH, Lu X (2002) Live or let die: the cell's response to p53. Nat Rev Cancer 2(8):594–604

Weber JD, Taylor LJ, Roussel MF, Sherr CJ, Bar-Sagi D (1999) Nucleolar Arf sequesters Mdm2 and activates p53. Nat Cell Biol 1(1):20–26

Welti S, Fraterman S, D'Angelo I, Wilm M, Scheffzek K (2007) The sec14 homology module of neurofibromin binds cellular glycerophospholipids: mass spectrometry and structure of a lipid complex. J Mol Biol 366(2):551–562

Wiederhold T, Lee MF, James M, Neujahr R, Smith N, Murthy A, Hartwig J, Gusella JF, Ramesh V (2004) Magicin, a novel cytoskeletal protein associates with the NF2 tumor suppressor merlin and Grb2. Oncogene 23(54):8815–8825

Wimmer K, Eckart M, Meyer-Puttlitz B, Fonatsch C, Pietsch T (2002) Mutational and expression analysis of the NF1 gene argues against a role as tumor suppressor in sporadic pilocytic astrocytomas. J Neuropathol Exp Neurol 61(10):896–902

Winston LA, Hunter T (1995) JAK2, Ras, and Raf are required for activation of extracellular signal-regulated kinase/mitogen-activated protein kinase by growth hormone. J Biol Chem 270(52):30837–30840

Xiao ZX, Chen J, Levine AJ, Modjtahedi N, Xing J, Sellers WR, Livingston DM (1995) Interaction between the retinoblastoma protein and the oncoprotein MDM2. Nature 375(6533):694–698

Xu HM, Gutmann DH (1998) Merlin differentially associates with the microtubule and actin cytoskeleton. J Neurosci Res 51(3):403–415

Zhang Y, Gao X, Saucedo LJ, Ru B, Edgar BA, Pan D (2003) Rheb is a direct target of the tuberous sclerosis tumour suppressor proteins. Nat Cell Biol 5(6):578–581

Zhu Y, Guignard F, Zhao D, Liu L, Burns DK, Mason RP, Messing A, Parada LF (2005a) Early inactivation of p53 tumor suppressor gene cooperating with NF1 loss induces malignant astrocytoma. Cancer Cell 8(2):119–130

Zhu Y, Harada T, Liu L, Lush ME, Guignard F, Harada C, Burns DK, Bajenaru ML, Gutmann DH, Parada LF (2005b) Inactivation of NF1 in CNS causes increased glial progenitor proliferation and optic glioma formation. Development 132(24):5577–5588

Part II
Management of Gliomas

Surgical Management of Intracranial Gliomas

6

Matthias Simon and Johannes Schramm

Abstract Surgery is indicated in almost all glioma patients at some point during the course of their disease. The surgical intervention aims at obtaining a tissue diagnosis, providing symptom relief, improving patient survival by reducing the tumor burden, and in rare cases even effecting a cure.

A resection will reduce symptoms related to the mass effect of the tumor, and offers a good chance for seizure control. An increasing body of data suggests that glioma patients will benefit from a maximal safe surgical cytoreduction. However, the size of the effect may vary for the different glioma entities. Modern adjuvant neuro-oncological treatment strategies rely heavily on the histological diagnosis. A (stereotactic) biopsy should therefore be offered to patients with nonresectable gliomas to allow for histology-guided adjuvant therapy. Some gliomas can be managed successfully with stereotactic interstitial radiosurgery (brachytherapy). Intra- and extraoperative electrophysiological mapping and/or monitoring, functional MRI, intraoperative imaging, and neuronavigation are increasingly used in many neurosurgical centers in order to reduce surgical morbidity.

Matthias Simon (✉)
Neurochirurgische Klinik
Universitätskliniken Bonn Sigmund-Freud-Straße 25
53105 Bonn Germany
E-mail: Matthias.Simon@ukb.uni-bonn.de

A definite effect on long-term outcome needs yet to be proven.

Advances in computers, imaging, and other technologies will continue to play a large role in the evolution of neurosurgical treatment for gliomas. This may well lead to further centralization of care. There will be an increasing pressure on neurosurgeons to justify the costs involved by showing that patients will actually benefit from complex treatments in highly specialized centers.

6.1
Surgical Management: Overview

Surgical intervention is indicated in almost all glioma patients at least at some point during the course of their disease. Surgical intervention has three principal goals, i.e., (1) obtaining a histological diagnosis, (2) providing symptom relief, and (3) improving patient survival by reducing the tumor burden. In some cases, surgery will even result in a cure.

Arguably, much of the progress made in neuro-oncology in the last one to two decades relates to the consequent implementation of histology-guided adjuvant therapy (see Chapters 7 and 8) rather than the introduction of truly new therapeutic strategies. The need of providing appropriate tissue for a histological diagnosis with ever-increasing therapeutic consequences has strengthened the role of the neurosurgeon in the management of glioma patients. The concept of individualized treatment based on histological, i.e., intrinsic features of gliomas is currently extended to the molecular level (see Chapters 1–4).

An increasing body of data suggests that patients will benefit from glioma resections with respect to overall survival as well as quality of life. Various mapping techniques for the identification of eloquent brain areas, intraoperative neurophysiological monitoring, intraoperative imaging, and neuronavigation are increasingly used in many centers. The value of these techniques lies primarily in the reduction of surgical morbidity. A significant influence on long-term patient survival has not been proven so far.

6.2
Surgical Therapy for Gliomas: Indications and Results

6.2.1
Low-Grade Gliomas

The role for a tumor resection in diffuse supratentorial low-grade gliomas is controversial. The literature contains a number of large series evaluating the extent of resection as a prognostic parameter, some of which are inconclusive and some in favor of extensive resections. However, the more recent literature seems to favor gross total tumor resections over a more conservative approach for low-grade gliomas. Five-year survival rates of 50–70% have been reported following tumor resection, approaching 80% in some of the more recent series. Prognosis after surgery may vary considerably with age, histology, and tumor size. Young patients with smaller tumors and oligodendroglial gliomas fare best (Keles et al. 2001, Pignatti et al. 2002, Schramm et al. 2006). Results of surgical treatment for low-grade gliomas seem to have improved in recent years. Some authors have reasoned that tumors are diagnosed and treated earlier during the course of the disease. Since survival is generally measured as postoperative survival, improvements of this measure may not necessarily indicate more efficacious therapy (Schramm et al. 2006).

Unfortunately, the quality of the available data on the role of surgery for low-grade gliomas is limited. No randomized study has been published, and only four investigations were conducted prospectively (Keles et al. 2001, Karim et al. 2002, Shaw et al. 2002, Pignatti et al. 2002). None of the large studies reported in the literature has utilized a standardized magnetic resonance imaging (MRI) protocol or a centralized review of the radiographic data for the assessment of the degree of the tumor resection and the diagnosis of tumor recurrence. Oligodendroglial tumors, pilocytic astrocytomas, and pediatric low-grade gliomas are often analyzed together with diffuse astrocytomas under the heading of low-grade gliomas despite their much better prognosis.

Another way of looking at the importance of a tumor resection might be to investigate recurrence rates and malignant progression in relation to postoperative tumor volumes. Malignant progression may occur in well over 50% of patients with low-grade gliomas, and very often limits the patient's prognosis (Keles et al. 2001, Schmidt et al. 2003). In a series of 53 low-grade gliomas, Berger et al. observed no tumor recurrence after a complete resection of 13 gliomas after a mean of 54 months, while a 46% recurrence/malignant progression rate was seen among patients with residual tumor greater than 10 ml. The postoperative radiographic tumor volumes were assessed by a computerized volumetry of the hypodense areas on CAT scans and the T2 signal hyperintensity on MR images (Berger et al. 1994). This widely accepted study seems to show at least some beneficial effects for extensive tumor resections with respect to disease-free survival and the risk for malignant progression.

However, there are data to suggest that this may not necessarily translate into an overall survival benefit. Recht and associates compared 20 patients undergoing surgery directly after imaging diagnosis of a low-grade glioma with 26 patients who were initially just followed up with serials MRI. Of the patients, 58% eventually required surgery for clinically relevant symptoms or suspected malignant transformation. However, neither overall survival nor quality of life as measured from the time of initial diagnosis was statistically different between the two groups (Recht et al. 1992). These results are often used to justify a wait-and-see policy for low-grade glioma patients. Of note, in one study almost a third of the patients with non-enhancing tumors thought to represent low-grade gliomas proved to harbor anaplastic tumors (Bernstein and Guha 1994, Fig. 6.1).

Low-grade glioma patients often present with seizures and sometimes with medically intractable epilepsy. A radical tumor resection (lesionectomy) offers a good chance for seizure control in many patients. Patients with medically intractable seizures may require a different surgical approach

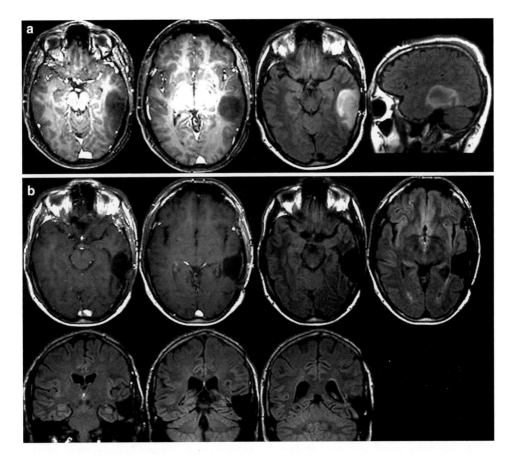

Fig. 6.1 Complete resection of an anaplastic astrocytoma WHO grade III involving the dorsal aspects of the middle and the inferior temporal gyrus. The patient made an uneventful recovery after surgery. Note that the lack of contrast enhancement had led an outside institution to tentatively diagnose a low-grade glioma. Relying on the MRI diagnosis would have clearly resulted in substantial undertreatment. **(a)** Preoperative MR images (*from left to right*: two consecutive axial contrast-enhanced T1-weighted images, an axial and a sagittal FLAIR image). **(b)** Postoperative MRI 3 months after surgery (*upper panel, from left to right*: consecutive axial contrast-enhanced T1-weighted and FLAIR images, *lower panel, from left to right*: three consecutive coronal FLAIR images)

including preoperative and/or intraoperative mapping of extratumoral epileptic foci. Following this approach, we achieved a 71% seizure-free rate in a series of 146 patients with low-grade gliomas (Zentner et al. 1997) and 82% in a later series of 203 cases (Luyken et al. 2003). Patients with tumor-related epilepsy may sometimes even benefit from incomplete tumor resections. In a series of 55 patients from our institution with (para)limbic gliomas (WHO grade I/II: $n=28$, WHO grade III: $n=24$, WHO grade IV: $n=3$) involving the insula, presenting with epilepsy (including 12 cases with medically intractable epilepsy) and with epileptological follow-up, a gross total resection was possible in 28 (51%) cases. Of these patients, 76% remained seizure-free (with or without medication) or had only occasional non-debilitating seizures (Engel's class I status) 1 year after surgery (Simon et al. 2008).

In the absence of prospective randomized data, the authors would suggest the following approach for low-grade glioma patients: There may be no conclusive data supporting a tumor resection, but there is considerable evidence in favor of this (in particular of a complete tumor removal). Hence a complete resection of a suspected low-grade glioma should be offered, whenever the surgical risk is acceptable. The definition of an acceptable risk has to take into account the usually beneficial effects of surgery on tumor-related symptoms such as epilepsy. Symptomatic patients with non-eloquent lobar gliomas are therefore prime surgical candidates, but the presumed oncological benefit will justify surgery also in asymptomatic cases, in which the surgical risk is low. If only a subtotal or a partial resection is possible due to extension of the tumor into eloquent areas, surgery might still provide symptomatic relief, e.g., for tumor-related epilepsy, and the possibility of an oncological benefit should be discussed. All other patients should probably at least have a biopsy to minimize the risk of withholding proper treatment for a non-tumorous lesion or a non-contrast-enhancing high-grade glioma.

6.2.2
Malignant Gliomas

Resecting a high-grade glioma is the fastest way to relieve the mass effect exerted by the tumor. Occasionally, glioma surgery can therefore even be a life-saving procedure. In a recent multicenter study including 408 patients with malignant gliomas, 53% improved neurologically after surgery, while permanent new deficits were seen in only 8% (Chang et al. 2003). No comparable potential for symptomatic improvement exists after tumor biopsy, radiotherapy, or chemotherapy (Fig. 6.2). However, the symptomatic benefits of a surgical resection come at a price. In the above-mentioned study, perioperative complications occurred in 24% of patients and the perioperative mortality rate was 1.5% (Chang et al. 2003).

Many studies have demonstrated that patients with malignant gliomas will survive longer after a complete vs. a partial resection, or a biopsy (Simpson et al. 1993, Albert et al. 1994). In a series of 213 glioblastoma patients operated on in our department, median survival after a complete resection, subtotal or partial resection, or a biopsy was 11, 9.3, and 2.5 months, respectively. The degree of resection correlated significantly with survival during univariate but not multivariate analysis (Simon et al. 2006). A gross total resection proved to be a significant independent positive prognostic parameter in our own series of 24 anaplastic astrocytomas and 24 anaplastic oligodendroglial tumors treated with postoperative radiotherapy and PCV chemotherapy (Kristof et al. 2002). Lacroix and co-workers performed volumetric postoperative MRI in a series of 416 glioblastomas (Lacroix et al. 2001). Their results indicate a modest benefit for more extensive resections. Anecdotal evidence suggests a higher complication rate following a partial rather than a gross total resection. There is some evidence to support the view that less tumor (and therefore maximum surgical cytoreduction) may allow for more efficacious chemotherapy (Keles et al. 2004a).

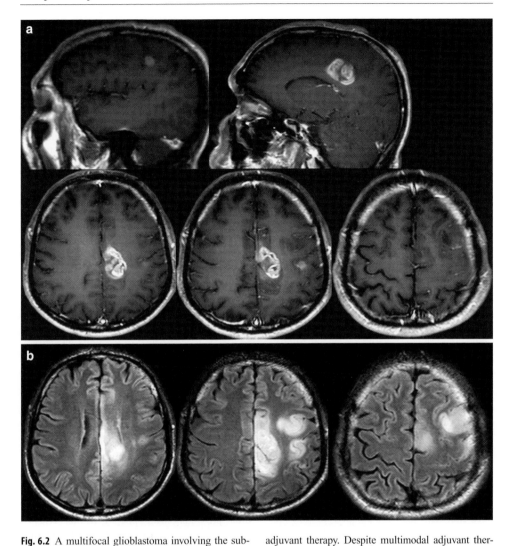

Fig. 6.2 A multifocal glioblastoma involving the subcentral cingulum and the frontocentral white matter and cortex. The patient presented with a moderate right hemiparesis. The extension and growth pattern of the tumor precluded a meaningful resection. The cingular lesion was biopsied in order to obtain a histological diagnosis and allow for the institution of adjuvant therapy. Despite multimodal adjuvant therapy, the patient continued to suffer from moderate hemiparesis. (a) T1-weighted MR images after administration of gadolinium (*upper panel*: two consecutive sagittal scans, *lower panel*: consecutive axial images). (b) Axial FLAIR images show a far more extensive tumor infiltration than the T1-weighted scans

However, there are also some retrospective data to suggest that surgical debulking plays no major role with respect to survival for at least some patients with glioblastoma. Kreth and co-workers found no significant survival difference in a series of patients with glioblastomas undergoing surgical debulking vs. biopsy only, followed by radiotherapy (Kreth et al. 1993).

Vuorinen and coworkers conducted a prospective randomized trial of biopsy vs. surgery for high-grade gliomas (mostly glioblastomas) in patients over 65 years of age. Their data seem to suggest a survival benefit for a tumor resection over a biopsy. However, this trial included only 30 patients (Vuorinen et al. 2003). The recently published prospective study by Stummer and associates attempted to assess the role of fluorescence-guided surgery with 5-aminolevulinic acid for resection control of malignant gliomas. This trial included 270 patients with resectable malignant gliomas (88% glioblastomas) who could be analyzed for postoperative residual tumor using early (< 72 h) standardized postoperative MRI. Median survival after a complete tumor removal was 17.9 months, while median survival for patients who still displayed residual contrast-enhancing tumor on the postoperative MRI was only 12.9 months ($P < 0.0001$) (Stummer et al. 2006).

In conclusion, patients with a resectable malignant glioma should probably undergo tumor removal that is as complete as possible. Surgical cytoreduction will often provide fast symptom relief and the literature supports the concept of an oncological benefit derived from extensive tumor resections. Partial resections may still achieve some of the goals of a complete tumor removal, although to a lesser degree.

6.2.3
Rare Gliomas

A surgical resection may provide a cure for some circumscribed gliomas. In a series of 44 adult patients with pilocytic astrocytomas (mean follow-up of 76±59 months) from our institution, the only recurrences after a gross total resection of the primary tumor were observed in a patient with an atypical tumor of the brainstem, in another patient with an anaplastic tumor, and a third patient with malignant progression (3/26=12%). In contrast, ten (56%) patients experienced further tumor growth after an incomplete resection or biopsy. Overall, anaplastic/malignant tumors were seen in 14% of the patients either at presentation or at tumor recurrence (Stüer et al. 2007). Together these data suggest that pilocytic astrocytomas in adults should be completely resected whenever possible.

Subependymal giant cell astrocytomas (SEGA) complicate the clinical course of 5–10% of patients with tuberous sclerosis. Patients may present with acute obstruction of the foramen of Monroi. Early tumor resections may reduce the substantial morbidity and mortality associated with acute hydrocephalus. SEGA are slow-growing tumors, and symptomatic regrowth even after a subtotal resection is rare (Clarke et al. 2006).

A rare variant of supratentorial astrocytomas termed isomorphic astrocytoma also apparently follows an extremely benign course after a gross total resection (Schramm et al. 2004).

Pleomorphic xanthoastrocytomas (PXA) should be resected as completely as possible. The degree of resection proved to be the most important prognostic factor in the largest case series available (Giannini et al. 1999).

The role of surgery in gliomatosis cerebri is limited. A biopsy may be indicated to conclusively ascertain the diagnosis, and a frontal or temporal lobectomy may be necessary for seizure control or treatment of increased intracranial pressure (Taillibert et al. 2006).

Gangliogliomas are mixed glioneural tumors often presenting with epilepsy. In our series of 184 cases a recurrence rate of only 1% (2/146) was observed following a complete resection, whereas tumor recurrence was seen in 3/38 (8%) of cases with residual tumor (Luyken et al. 2004). Of note, much of the data suggesting a particular benign nature for these neoplasms stem from epilepsy surgery series, i.e., may be biased towards patients with a particularly good prognosis. Some series in the literature have reported a much worse outcome after (subtotal) surgery for gangliogliomas (Rumana et al. 1999). Somewhat similar to our experience with gangliogliomas, we saw no tumor recurrence after resection of 29 dysembryoplastic neuroepithelial tumors (DNTs, Luyken et al. 2003). The relatively benign clinical course of gangliogliomas and DNTs may allow one to defer surgical treatment in some cases. However, this has to be balanced carefully against the often very substantial benefits of surgery in terms of symptom relief (i.e., cure or amelioration of the seizure disorder) and the very low surgical risks (0% mortality, 1% permanent morbidity; $n=207$, Luyken et al. 2003).

6.2.4
Cytoreductive Surgery for Gliomas in Difficult and Eloquent Locations

Patients with lobar gliomas without extension into eloquent areas are prime surgical candidates. Operations for gliomas located in or close to eloquent neurovascular structures, however, carry an increased risk for neurological deterioration. A reduced postoperative functional status, e.g., measured as KPI (Karnofsky performance index), has been correlated with reduced survival for both patients with low-grade and malignant gliomas (Weir 1973, Bauman et al. 1999). Nevertheless, it is clearly possible to extend the benefit of surgical cytoreduction to gliomas in eloquent or near-eloquent locations, while at the same time preserving neurological function. In a series of 235 *temporomesiobasal* gliomas we have seen only a 1.7% rate of permanent deficits with 15.7% transient neurological deficits, apart from 5.4% new hemianopias (Schramm and Aliashkevich 2007).

Gliomas extending into the *dorsal superior frontal gyrus* can be successfully resected with very acceptable risks. The patient frequently has to expect only a transient hemiparesis or hemiparesis and aphasia (if the tumor extends into the middle frontal gyrus of the dominant hemisphere). This has been termed the supplementary motor area (SMA) syndrome. In a series from our institution, a complete SMA syndrome was seen in 9/12 patients (75%) after total resection of the SMA region and an incomplete deficit in the remaining three patients. Subtotal SMA resections resulted in an 81% rate (13/16) of new (but incomplete) deficits. All patients with deficits recovered almost to normal after 3–42 days (mean 11 days) (Zentner et al. 1996b). Similar results have also been reported by other groups (Peraud et al. 2002, Russell and Kelly 2003).

Insular (paralimbic) gliomas are not rare. In the past decade, several centers have begun to publish their experience with operations for intra-axial *tumors of the insula* (Yasargil et al. 1992, Zentner et al. 1996a, Vanaclocha et al. 1997). Even complete tumor resections are possible. However, the surgical risks are not negligible. In our series of 101 operations performed 1995–2005 for insular gliomas, a gross total resection was achieved in 42%. Persistent dysphasia was seen after 13% of 39 operations for left-sided tumors (Simon et al. 2008). Among 84 cases undergoing MEP monitoring, a new or worsened hemiparesis occurred in 30%. A *permanent* paresis was seen in 11%, which remained *severely* disabling in 4% (Neuloh et al. 2007).

Indications for the resection of certain brainstem and thalamic tumors will be discussed in Sect 6.2.6.

6.2.5
Recurrent Gliomas

Operations for recurrent gliomas have been evaluated only in very few prospective studies. No randomized trial has been published. The oncological benefit of a repeat resection is probably smaller than that of the first surgery, particularly if a complete tumor removal is not possible (Fig. 6.3). Repeat surgery for malignant gliomas may prolong time to tumor progression, which implies better quality of life, but the effect on overall survival is questionable (Stromblad et al. 1993, Barker et al. 1998). Of note, in one series of 46 patients with recurrent glioblastomas undergoing surgery for recurrent tumor

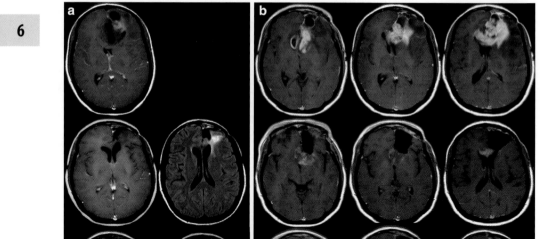

Fig. 6.3 Recurrence and malignant progression of a left frontal anaplastic oligoastrocytoma. The patient underwent surgery in December 1999. (**a**) *Upper panel*: preoperative MRI (T1-weighted axial contrast-enhanced scan). *Middle panel*: postoperative MR imaging (March 2000, axial T1-weighted contrast-enhanced and FLAIR images) reveals possible residual tumor at the laterodorsal aspect of the resection cavity. The patient had completed a course of radiotherapy, and one cycle of PCV chemotherapy. Chemotherapy was continued. *Lower panel*: no tumor growth was seen until June 2005. (**b**) T1-weighted contrast-enhanced axial MR images. *Upper panel*: recurrent contrast-enhancing tumor crossing the midline via the corpus callosum (March 2006). A subtotal resection was performed. The histological diagnosis was glioblastoma. Chemotherapy with temozolomide was instituted. *Middle panel*: residual tumor and even regression of the callosal parts of the tumor (May 2006). *Lower panel*: diffuse tumor progression (July 2006). The patient died in September 2006

(selected from a total of 301 glioblastoma patients), only 28% of the patients had improved KPI scores after undergoing reoperation, 49% were stable, but 23% had declined in KPI scores by 10–30 points (Barker et al. 1998).

Obtaining tumor tissue at repeat surgery will allow one to reliably diagnose the malignant progression of a low-grade glioma (50% in one series, Schmidt et al. 2003) and can guide adjuvant therapy. Current radiotherapy protocols for low-grade vs. high-grade gliomas differ (see Chap. 7), and it is probably safe to defer radiotherapy for a low-grade glioma in many cases until malignant progression (Karim et al. 2002). Chemotherapeutic options for recurrent low-grade tumor are limited with the possible exception of oligodendroglial regrowths, while chemotherapy for malignant gliomas is an effective treatment at least for some patients (see Chap. 8).

Therefore, repeat resections should probably be offered to most patients with recurring low-grade gliomas, many with anaplastic tumors, but only a few with glioblastomas. Factors that may argue against surgery for recurrent gliomas include a KPI < 70, an elderly or multimorbid patient, a relatively short time interval between the initial surgery and tumor recurrence (i.e., < 6–9 months), and a growth pattern that allows only for a partial resection leaving a large part of the recurrent tumor behind.

6.2.6
Pediatric Gliomas

Gliomas account for approximately 50% of pediatric brain tumors. In comparison to adult patients, diffuse hemispheric astrocytomas (including glioblastomas) and oligodendrogliomas are relatively uncommon. While the prognostic impact of a surgical cytoreduction continues to be debated for diffuse gliomas of adulthood (see Sects. 6.2.1 and 6.2.2), a striking correlation between resection extent and survival has been consistently seen for low- and high-grade pediatric tumors alike (Pollack et al. 1995, Wisoff et al. 1998). Surgery plays an important role in the management of pediatric glioneural tumors as outlined previously (see Sect 6.2.3). High-quality neuroimaging may obviate the need to obtain a biopsy in selected cases, i.e., most optic pathway gliomas (see below) and diffuse pontine gliomas.

Roughly two thirds of childhood brain tumors grow in the infratentorial compartment. Management of the associated hydrocephalus poses specific problems. Timely tumor removal may be all that is needed. In some cases, temporary insertion of a ventricular drain may be necessary. An endoscopic ventriculostomy provides definitive treatment of the hydrocephalus and can be performed before the actual tumor surgery. Insertion of a permanent ventricular shunt has been relegated from an up-front treatment for obstructive hydrocephalus to a second-line therapy for malresorptive hydrocephalus developing after excision of the tumor (Sainte-Rose et al. 2001).

Cerebellar astrocytomas are typical and frequent infratentorial gliomas of childhood. The histological examination will most often reveal a low-grade pilocytic or fibrillary astrocytoma. The prognostic impact of this latter histological distinction is controversial. Cerebellar astrocytomas are often ideal surgical candidates. A complete excision of the tumors is possible in more than 80% of the cases, and 10-year recurrence-free survival rates after a complete resection of cerebellar astrocytomas in children approach 100% (Campbell and Pollack 1996, Pencalet et al. 1999). Extension of the tumors into the brainstem or cerebellar peduncles may preclude a total resection. A recurrence rate of 50% was seen after a median of 8 years in one series of incompletely resected cerebellar astrocytomas. Arrested growth and spontaneous tumor regression may account, in part, for the relatively good prognosis even after an incomplete tumor excision (Palma et al. 2004).

Another characteristic childhood tumor is the optic pathway glioma. Optic pathway gliomas commonly occur in neurofibromatosis type 1 (NF1) patients. The histological diagnosis is usually pilocytic astrocytoma. A particularly aggressive variant of pilocytic astrocytomas termed pilomyxoid astrocytoma has been recently described. Prognosis may vary considerably with tumors extending into the hypothalamus and young children having a worse outcome. There is no consensus on whether NF1 patients do better or worse. Tumors confined to one optic nerve may be amenable to a complete resection if there is no functional vision left. The course of some nerve fibers in the base of the contralateral optic nerve (Wilbrand's knee) has to be taken into account when operating close to the chiasm. Surgery for more posteriorly located tumors may be indicated for mass effect or hydrocephalus (O'Kelly and Rutka 2005).

Intrinsic tumors of the thalamus and brainstem play a much larger role in pediatric than adult patients. Focal as opposed to diffuse or bilateral thalamic gliomas may be amenable to aggressive resection strategies. A recent review quotes mortality and persistent morbidity rates of 0–6% and less than 10%, respectively (Souweidane 2005).

Some subsets of brainstem gliomas, i.e., dorsally exophytic gliomas and cervicomedullary gliomas are amenable to microneurosurgical treatment (Epstein and McCleary 1986). However, a subtotal or partial removal is often all that is feasible. Nevertheless, the prognosis is generally good and seems to primarily reflect the tumor histology (Young Poussaint et al. 1999).

6.2.7
Stereotactic Biopsy and Interstitial Radiosurgery (Brachytherapy)

A stereotactic biopsy will allow for a histological diagnosis in cases for which an open tumor resection is not a reasonable option such as multifocal gliomas and most tumors of the basal ganglia. A stereotactic biopsy carries a lower risk than craniotomy and tumor resection (Hall 1998). In a retrospective series of 5,000 consecutive stereotactic brain biopsies (including 3,260 gliomas, 1988 through 1999), a diagnosis could neither be made intraoperatively nor postoperatively in only 4.6% (Tilgner et al. 2005). However, underestimating the tumor grade is not altogether infrequent. In the study by Jackson and co-workers, 38% of diagnoses differed between stereotactic biopsies and resection, in 26% this had therapeutic and in 38% prognostic implications (Jackson et al. 2001). Some centers will therefore perform an open biopsy with larger sample volumes (sometimes using frameless stereotaxy) for superficial lesions, and reserve frame-based stereotactic techniques for deep midline lesions.

Stereotactic techniques can also be used to treat selected gliomas by interstitial radiosurgery (IRS, brachytherapy). After the histological diagnosis is ascertained through a serial biopsy, radioactive sources (usually iodine 125 or iridium 192) are implanted, producing a well-defined small necrosis over time. Implants can be permanent or temporary. IRS is particularly effective for non-lobar low-grade gliomas that are circumscribed and located in the hypothalamus, thalamus, basal ganglia, optic tracts and chiasm, and upper brainstem. Previous radiotherapy is not a contraindication against additional interstitial radiosurgery. Results for interstitial radiosurgery for circumscribed WHO grade I and II gliomas of the hypothalamus, basal ganglia, optic pathways, and upper brainstem compare favorably with the results of microsurgical series (Kreth et al. 1995).

6.3
Technical Aspects of Glioma Surgery

6.3.1
Electrophysiological Mapping and Monitoring of Eloquent Brain Areas

Operating close to eloquent brain and neurovascular structures supplying them requires their precise identification and spatial delineation ("mapping"). Intraoperative monitoring of the corresponding functions may conceptually lead to a lower rate of postoperative neurological deficits. Consequently, mapping and monitoring of the perisylvian cortical language areas and the primary sensorimotor cortex play a major role in glioma surgery. More recently, some experience has also been gained with the mapping and monitoring of subcortical structures subserving motor and language function (Duffau et al. 2003, Keles et al. 2004b).

Direct cortical stimulation for the identification of the primary motor, the somatosensory, and the language cortices has been used for many decades. With the exception of the identification of the rolandic cortex, cortical mapping relies on a functional block rather than elicitation of function. Hence, general anesthesia is not possible ("awake craniotomy"). Awake craniotomies with direct electrical stimulation for the identification and monitoring of language and motor function have gained considerable popularity in recent years (Taylor and Bernstein 1999). There are limitations in pediatric patients (Ojemann et al. 2003), and there is a risk for intraoperatively induced seizures (Sartorius and Berger 1998).

The rolandic fissure can also be localized very reliably using a strip electrode and somatosensory evoked potentials (SEP) phase reversal (Cedzich et al. 1996, Romstöck et al. 2002), when the electrophysiological information is combined with anatomical data. General anesthesia can be used with this technique. SEP phase reversal for the identification of the perirolandic cortices can be combined with SEP and/or MEP monitoring (see below). Ease of use and reliability render it the method of choice in our institution for all glioma surgeries close to the primary motor cortex (or the pyramidal tract; Neuloh et al. 2004).

Evoked potentials have been used since the 1980s for monitoring purposes. Initial work focused on surgery for spinal cord and posterior fossa lesions. SEP monitoring during aneurysm surgery has become somewhat accepted, and has been employed for surgery of perirolandic tumors (Cedzich et al. 1996, Romstöck et al. 2002). However, SEP monitoring does not directly evaluate the functional integrity of the motor pathways. More recently, cortical and transcranial stimulation and monitoring of motor evoked potentials during brain tumor surgery was introduced allowing for a more direct and continuous intraoperative assessment of motor function (Fig. 6.4). Several groups have since reported their results (Kombos et al. 2001, Zhou and Kelly 2001, Neuloh et al. 2004). Using MEP monitoring during 182 operations for brain tumors in the immediate vicinity of the primary motor cortex and/or the pyramidal tract, we observed permanent neurological deficits in only 4.9% of the patients (Neuloh et al. 2004). Wiedemayer and coworkers estimated that neuromonitoring lowered the rate of neurological deficits by 5.2% in a series of 423 patients (including 174 patients with brain tumors; Wiedemayer et al. 2002).

Extraoperative mapping of both motor and language areas is possible with subdural grid electrodes. We and others primarily use this technique in patients with chronic epilepsy in order to define the epileptogenic focus as well as eloquent areas (Kutsy et al. 1999). It may also be used for eloquent tumors as an alternative to awake craniotomy. After recovery from implantation surgery, direct cortical mapping is performed on the awake patient. The tumor is resected a few days later (Fig. 6.5). In a series of 16 such cases a gross total resection (90–100%) as assessed on postoperative MRI scans was possible in nine patients. Only biopsies were taken as a result of the mapping information in two cases (Kral et al. 2006). We have seen patients with subdural bleeds or tumor swelling making emergency explantation of the grid necessary. Mapping results may be less than optimal in the presence of neurological deficits.

6.3.2
Imaging of Functional Brain Areas for Glioma Surgery

Several imaging modalities have been employed for the extraoperative localization of functional brain areas ("functional imaging"). Functional MRI (fMRI) works well to localize motor and to some degree language functions to cortical structures (Yetkin et al. 1997). fMRI has also been employed for the identification of the visual cortex (Fried et al. 1995). Similarly to fMRI, PET can be used for the identification of motor, language, and visual areas (Fried et al. 1995, Bookheimer et al. 1997). Magnetencephalography is the third imaging modality that has been employed for functional imaging (Alberstone et al. 2000). The use of diffusion tensor imaging (DTI) for the visualization of the subcortical fiber tracts, e.g., the pyramidal tract during glioma surgery, has been reported (Nimsky et al. 2005).

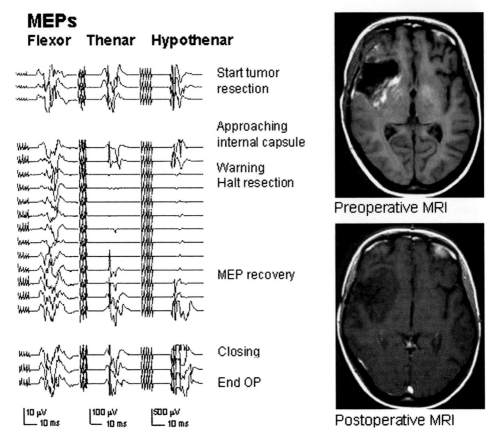

Fig. 6.4 Upper extremity motor evoked potentials (MEPs) were recorded during resection of a right insular astrocytoma WHO grade II in order to monitor motor tract function. Resection at the dorsal aspect of the tumor was halted after MEP deterioration occurred. Clinical outcome was uneventful, and postoperative imaging showed a > 90% resection with some minor residual tumor at the dorsal aspect of the resection cavity. (From Neuloh and Schramm 2002. With permission)

Several important shortcomings of all imaging modalities need to be mentioned: Little is known about their reliability to delineate the complete extent and the borders of the eloquent structure in question, and the intraoperative shift of brain structures during debulking surgery may invalidate the preoperative images.

6.3.3 Image-Guided Surgery: Neuronavigation

Removal of a glial tumor necessitates a concept of the spatial relationships between the tumor and the surrounding brain as delineated from MRI data and an understanding of the principles of glioma growth. Applying this concept to

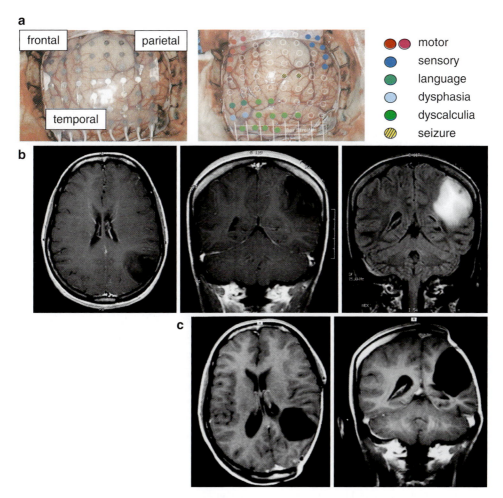

Fig. 6.5 Implantation of a subdural grid electrode for extraoperative functional mapping of the left (dominant) temporoparietal cortex. (**a**) *Left*: A 64-contact subdural grid electrode was placed to cover the tumor and presumed eloquent cortex. *Right*: Extraoperative mapping in the awake patient during the following 3 days showed that no relevant function localized to the tumor-infiltrated cortex. Functional test results are depicted on digitized photos of the brain surface after electrode removal before tumor surgery. The tumor has apparently displaced the motor cortex anteriorly and the sensory cortex posteriorly. Mapping also identified the language-relevant cortex and the eloquent parts of the inferior parietal lobule in the immediate vicinity of the tumor. (**b**) Preoperative coronal and axial contrast-enhanced T1-weighted and coronal FLAIR images. (**c**) Postoperative axial and coronal T1-weighted images obtained 1 year after the operation show that a complete resection had been accomplished. The patient did not incur a neurological deficit. However, an epidural abscess necessitated removal of the bone flap. Histology showed an anaplastic mixed glioma of WHO grade III

the intraoperative scenario is often hampered by the lack of anatomical landmarks in particular within the subcortical white matter. Also, there will be a continuous shift of the surgical target due to CSF loss and resection of parts of the tumor.

Frame-based stereotactic techniques have been employed for tumor resections (Kelly 1988). However, the use of a stereotactic frame restricts surgical maneuvers and there is limited capability of intraoperative updating, i.e., the problem of brain shift outlined above cannot really be accounted for.

Frameless stereotaxy or neuronavigation has been made possible primarily by the development of computers able to generate and manipulate 3D images. The patient's head and surgical instruments are referenced via infrared LEDs to the computer ("registration"). This set-up enables the surgeon to navigate within the (artificial) space defined by the patient's preoperative MRI data. Neuronavigational techniques allow for minimally invasive tailored craniotomies and a comparatively atraumatic approach to small subcortical lesions.

Neuronavigation-assisted biopsies have gained considerable popularity. While they may lack the accuracy of stereotactic biopsies necessary for deep-seated small lesions, they allow for more representative tissue sampling of subcortical lesions not visible on the cortical surface. Neuronavigation-guided biopsies have all but replaced stereotactic and open free-hand biopsies for this indication in our institution.

Resection control can be facilitated by neuronavigational techniques. It may be possible to account for the problem of brain shift to some extent by adjusting one's techniques of tumor resection or by intraoperative updating of the system by using markers placed on the brain just before the actual resection (Barnett 2004). However, the accuracy of such maneuvers at this point does not surpass the accuracy of a trained surgeon's eye. A recent prospective randomized study involving 45 patients with contrast-enhancing intracerebral tumors failed to show a significant benefit for the use of a neuronavigation system when neuronavigation was only used for resection control (Willems et al. 2006). Ultrasound and MRI (Nimsky et al. 2004, Unsgaard et al. 2005) have been used to update neuronavigation systems during resective surgery. Finally, neuronavigation computers can integrate the information obtained by a variety of imaging and mapping techniques such as MRI (including DTI and fMRI), CT, PET, and MEG (Nimsky et al. 2004, Mahvash et al. 2006).

6.3.4
Intraoperative Imaging

A different approach to the problem of intraoperative localization and delineation of the surgical target is obtaining a real-time image during surgery. CT has been used for that purpose. Ultrasonography (US) has also been used to localize and delineate intra-axial tumors. Employing intraoperative US to update a neuronavigation system has gained some popularity. A larger or separate craniotomy may be required to place the US transducer (Unsgaard et al. 2005).

Intraoperative MRI has been investigated by several groups (Black et al. 1997, Tronnier et al. 1997, Steinmeier et al. 1998, Albayrak et al. 2004). There is one commercially available system which allows for the simultaneous completion of the intracranial operation and MRI. An entirely different approach has resulted in the development of a mobile MRI unit. The majority of systems, however, involve transfer of the patient to the MRI unit located at a variable distance from the operating table. This may increase the risks for infections, but gives good access to the patient, while a fixed set-up of the magnet allows for higher field strengths. High magnetic field strengths give much better imaging quality and allow for the simultaneous implementation of accessory MRI modalities. Non-magnetic surgical instruments are usually required for MRI-guided surgery (Albayrak et al. 2004).

Will intraoperative MRI become the intraoperative imaging modality of choice? The central question is whether the rather substantial costs of the set-up can be justified by improved surgical results. Use of intraoperative MRI could allow for improved resection control when compared to conventional navigation techniques, but this may not necessarily translate into better survival. Preliminary experience is promising. Claus and coworkers reported their experience with intraoperative MRI in 156 patients with low-grade gliomas. Overall survival at 1, 2, and 5 years in this series appeared significantly better than that of age- and histology-adjusted controls from a large nationwide American brain tumor registry (Surveillance, Epidemiology, and End Results Registry, SEER) (Claus et al. 2005).

6.4
Perspectives

6.4.1
Technological Progress and Neurosurgery

Technological advances have played an enormous role in the evolution of neurosurgical therapies for brain tumors. This is quite likely to continue. In the near future, the neurosurgeon will have an astonishing array of neuronavigational tools, intraoperative multimodality imaging, and sophisticated monitoring tools at his or her disposal on a routine basis (Nimsky et al. 2004).

New imaging modalities (e.g., multiphoton-excited fluorescence of endogenous fluorophores) allow for a spatial resolution at the cellular or even subcellular level and may provide further help with tumor delineation (Leppert et al. 2006).

Much of the technological progress outlined relates to the ever enlarging computational capabilities. Computer models of glioma growth have been made possible by the emergence of new high-performance computers. Future preoperative planning may well include a simulation of surgery and multimodal therapy (Hatzikirou et al. 2005). Advances in the molecular sciences and biomedical engineering may at some point change our focus from deficit avoidance to reconstruction or restorative neurosurgery (Apuzzo and Liu 2001).

Finally, the full impact of molecular genetics has yet to be felt. Glioma is a loco-regional disease. New targeted therapies for brain tumors are being developed and may require new techniques for local delivery (i.e., convection-enhanced delivery, Dunn and Black 2003).

6.4.2
Clinical Research and Socioeconomic Issues

However, one has to beware of the excitement generated by this proliferation of technologies. Some simple issues deserve just as much attention. We are lacking prospective high-quality studies proving basic surgical tenets, such as the correlation between extent of resection and survival. Quality of life issues have been largely neglected so far (Taphoorn et al. 2005).

Society will increasingly require neurosurgeons to justify the socioeconomic burden of medical care by providing appropriate data. Studies on provider volume and complication rates have already been conducted with predictable results, i.e., high-volume surgeons or hospitals seem to have lesser complications than low-volume providers (Cowan et al. 2003). However, these studies uniformly have methodological flaws, and many important questions remain unanswered. What are the critical numbers necessary to realize the beneficial effect of high-volume neurosurgery? What is the influence of the general neurosurgical experience, i.e., is there something useful to be learned for a surgical neuro-oncologist from nonneuro-oncological cases? Of note, a recent paper by Latif et al. failed to show a benefit for surgical treatment delivered by a specialized neuro-oncological surgeon when compared to a general neurosurgeon (Latif et al. 1998).

References

Albayrak B, Samdani AF, Black PM (2004) Intraoperative magnetic resonance imaging in neurosurgery. Acta Neurochir 146:543–556

Alberstone CD, Skirboll SL, Benzel EC, Sanders JA, Hart BL, Baldwin NG, Tessman CL, Davis JT, Lee RR (2000). Magnetic source imaging and brain surgery: presurgical and intraoperative planning in 26 patients. J Neurosurg 92:79–90

Albert FK, Forsting M, Sartor K, Adams HP, Kunze S (1994) Early postoperative magnetic resonance imaging after resection of malignant glioma: objective evaluation of residual tumor and its influence on regrowth and prognosis. Neurosurgery 34:45–60

Apuzzo ML, Liu CY (2001) Things to come. Neurosurgery 49:765–778

Barker FG 2nd, Chang SM, Gutin PH, Malec MK, McDermott MW, Prados MD, Wilson CB (1998) Survival and functional status after resection of recurrent glioblastoma multiforme. Neurosurgery 42:709–720

Barnett GH (2004) Surgical navigation for brain tumors. In: Winn HR (ed) Youmansh neurological surgery. WB Saunders, Philadelphia, pp 941–949

Bauman G, Lote K, Larson D, Stalpers L, Leighton C, Fisher B, Wara W, MacDonald D, Stitt L, Cairncross JG (1999) Pretreatment factors predict overall survival for patients with low-grade glioma: a recursive partitioning analysis. Int J Radiat Oncol Biol Phys 45:923–299

Berger MS, Deliganis AV, Dobbins J, Keles GE (1994) The effect of extent of resection on recurrence in patients with low grade cerebral hemisphere gliomas. Cancer 74:1784–1791

Bernstein M, Guha A (1994) Biopsy of low-grade astrocytomas. J Neurosurg. 80:776–777

Bookheimer SY, Zeffiro TA, Blaxton T, Malow BA, Gaillard WD, Sato S, Kufta C, Fedio P, Theodore WH (1997) A direct comparison of PET activation and electrocortical stimulation mapping for language localization. Neurology 48:1056–1065

Black PM, Moriarty T, Alexander E 3rd, Stieg P, Woodard EJ, Gleason PL, Martin CH, Kikinis R, Schwartz RB, Jolesz FA (1997) Development and implementation of intraoperative magnetic resonance imaging and its neurosurgical applications. Neurosurgery 41:831–842

Campbell JW, Pollack IF.(1996) Cerebellar astrocytomas in children. J Neurooncol 28:223–231

Cedzich C, Taniguchi M, Schafer S, Schramm J (1996) Somatosensory evoked potential phase reversal and direct motor cortex stimulation during surgery in and around the central region. Neurosurgery 38:962–970

Claus EB, Horlacher A, Hsu L, Schwartz RB, Dello-Iacono D, Talos F, Jolesz FA, Black PM (2005) Survival rates in patients with low-grade glioma after intraoperative magnetic resonance image guidance. Cancer 103:1227–1233

Chang SM, Parney IF, McDermott M, Barker FG 2nd, Schmidt MH, Huang W, Laws ER Jr, Lillehei KO, Bernstein M, Brem H, Sloan AE, Berger M; Glioma Outcomes Investigators (2003) Glioma Outcomes Investigators. Perioperative complications and neurological outcomes of first and second craniotomies among patients enrolled in the Glioma Outcome Project. J Neurosurg 98: 1175–1181

Clarke MJ, Foy AB, Wetjen N, Raffel C (2006) Imaging characteristics and growth of subependymal giant cell astrocytomas. Neurosurg Focus 20:E5

Cowan JA Jr, Dimick JB, Leveque JC, Thompson BG, Upchurch GR Jr, Hoff JT (2003) The impact of provider volume on mortality after intracranial tumor resection. Neurosurgery 52:48–53

Duffau H, Capelle L, Denvil D, Sichez N, Gatignol P, Taillandier L, Lopes M, Mitchell MC, Roche S, Muller JC, Bitar A, Sichez JP, van Effenterre R (2003) Usefulness of intraoperative electrical subcortical mapping during surgery for low-grade gliomas located within eloquent brain regions: functional results in a consecutive series of 103 patients. J Neurosurg 98:764–778

Dunn IF, Black PM (2003) The neurosurgeon as local oncologist: cellular and molecular neurosurgery in malignant glioma therapy. Neurosurgery 52:1411–1422

Epstein F, McCleary EL (1986) Intrinsic brain-stem tumors of childhood: surgical indications. J Neurosurg 64:11–15

Fried I, Nenov VI, Ojemann SG, Woods RP (1995). Functional MR and PET imaging of rolandic and visual cortices for neurosurgical planning. J Neurosurg 83:854–861

Giannini C, Scheithauer BW, Burger PC, Brat DJ, Wollan PC, Lach B, O'Neill BP (1999) Pleomorphic xanthoastrocytoma: what do we really know about it? Cancer 85:2033–2045

Hall WA (1998) The safety and efficacy of stereotactic biopsy for intracranial lesions. Cancer 82:1749–1755

Hatzikirou B, Deutsch A, Schaller C, Simon M, Swanson KR (2005) Mathematical modelling of glioblastoma tumour development: a review. Math Models Meth Appl Sci 15:1779–1794

Jackson RJ, Fuller GN, Abi-Said D, Lang FF, Gokaslan ZL, Shi WM, Wildrick DM, Sawaya R (2001) Limitations of stereotactic biopsy in the initial management of gliomas. Neurooncol 3:193–200

Karim AB, Afra D, Cornu P, Bleehan N, Schraub S, De Witte O, Darcel F, Stenning S, Pierart M, van Glabbeke M (2002) Randomized trial on the efficacy of radiotherapy for cerebral low-grade glioma in the adult: European Organization for research and treatment of Cancer Study 22845 with the Medical Research Council study BRO4: an interim analysis. Int J Radiat Oncol Biol Phys 52:316–324

Keles GE, Lamborn KR, Berger MS (2001) Low-grade hemispheric gliomas in adults: a critical review of extent of resection as a factor influencing outcome. J Neurosurg 95:735–745

Keles GE, Lamborn KR, Chang SM, Prados MD, Berger MS (2004a) Volume of residual disease as a predictor of outcome in adult patients with recurrent supratentorial glioblastomas multiforme who are undergoing chemotherapy. Volume of residual disease as a predictor of outcome in adult patients with recurrent supratentorial glioblastomas multiforme who are undergoing chemotherapy. J Neurosurg 100:41–46

Keles GE, Lundin DA, Lamborn KR, Chang EF, Ojemann G, Berger MS (2004b) Intraoperative subcortical stimulation mapping for hemispherical perirolandic gliomas located within or adjacent to the descending motor pathways: evaluation of morbidity and assessment of functional outcome in 294 patients. J Neurosurg 100:369–375

Kelly PJ (1988) Volumetric stereotactic surgical resection of intra-axial brain mass lesions. Mayo Clin Proc 63:1186–1198

Kombos T, Suess O, Ciklatekerlio O, Brock M (2001) Monitoring of intraoperative motor evoked potentials to increase the safety of surgery in and around the motor cortex. J Neurosurg 95:608–614

Kral T, Kurthen M, Schramm J, Urbach H, Meyer B (2006) Stimulation mapping via implanted grid electrodes prior to surgery for gliomas in highly eloquent cortex. Neurosurgery 58(Suppl):ONS36–43

Kreth FW, Warnke PC, Scheremet R, Ostertag CB (1993) Surgical resection and radiation therapy versus biopsy and radiation therapy in the treatment of glioblastoma multiforme. J Neurosurg 78:762–766

Kreth FW, Faist M, Warnke PC, Rossner R, Volk B, Ostertag CB (1995) Interstitial radiosurgery of low-grade gliomas. J Neurosurg 82:418–429

Kristof RA, Neuloh G, Hans V, Deckert M, Urbach H, Schlegel U, Simon M, Schramm J (2002) Combined surgery, radiation, and PCV chemotherapy for astrocytomas compared to oligodendrogliomas and oligoastrocytomas WHO grade III. J Neurooncol 59:231–237

Kutsy RL, Farrell DF, Ojemann GA (1999) Ictal patterns of neocortical seizures monitored with intracranial electrodes: correlation with surgical outcome. Epilepsia 40:257–266

Lacroix M, Abi-Said D, Fourney DR, Gokaslan ZL, Shi W, DeMonte F, Lang FF, McCutcheon IE, Hassenbusch SJ, Holland E, Hess K, Michael C, Miller D, Sawaya R (2001) A multivariate analysis of 416 patients with glioblastoma multiforme: prognosis, extent of resection, and survival. J Neurosurg 95:190–198

Latif AZ, Signorini D, Gregor A, Whittle IR (1998) The costs of managing patients with malignant glioma at a neuro-oncology clinic. Br J Neurosurg 12:118–122

Leppert J, Krajewski J, Kantelhardt SR, Schlaffer S, Petkus N, Reusche E, Huttmann G, Giese A (2006) Multiphoton excitation of autofluorescence for microscopy of glioma tissue. Neurosurgery 58:759–767

Luyken C, Blumcke I, Fimmers R, Urbach H, Elger CE, Wiestler OD, Schramm J (2003) The spectrum of long-term epilepsy-associated tumors: long-term seizure and tumor outcome and neurosurgical aspects. Epilepsia 44:822–830

Luyken C, Blumcke I, Fimmers R, Urbach H, Wiestler OD, Schramm J (2004) Supratentorial gangliogliomas: histopathologic grading and tumor recurrence in 184 patients with a median follow-up of 8 years. Cancer 101:146–155

Mahvash M, Konig R, Urbach H, von Ortzen J, Meyer B, Schramm J, Schaller C (2006) FLAIR-/T1-/T2-co-registration for image-guided diagnostic and resective epilepsy surgery. Neurosurgery 58 (Suppl):ONS69–75

Neuloh G, Schramm J (2002) Intraoperative neurophysiological mapping and monitoring. In: Deletis V, Shils JL (eds) Neurophysiology in neurosurgery. Academic Press, Amsterdam, The Netherlands, pp 339–401

Neuloh G, Pechstein U, Cedzich C, Schramm J (2004) Motor evoked potential monitoring with supratentorial surgery. Neurosurgery 54:1061–1070

Neuloh G, Pechstein U, Schramm J (2007) Motor tract monitoring during insular glioma surgery. J Neurosurg 106:582–592

Nimsky C, Ganslandt O, Fahlbusch R (2004) Functional neuronavigation and intraoperative MRI. Adv Tech Stand Neurosurg 29:229–263

Nimsky C, Grummich P, Sorensen AG, Fahlbusch R, Ganslandt O (2005) Visualization of the pyramidal tract in glioma surgery by integrating diffusion tensor imaging in functional neuronavigation. Zentralbl Neurochir 66:133–141

Ojemann SG, Berger MS, Lettich E, Ojemann GA. Localization of language function in children: results of electrical stimulation mapping (2003) J Neurosurg 98:465–470

O'Kelly, Rutka JT (2005) Optic pathway gliomas. In: Berger MS, Prados MD (eds) Textbook of neuro-oncology. WB Saunders, Philadelphia, pp 579–586

Palma L, Celli P, Mariottini A (2004) Long-term follow-up of childhood cerebellar astrocytomas after incomplete resection with particular reference to arrested growth or spontaneous tumour regression. Acta Neurochir 146:581–588

Pencalet P, Maixner W, Sainte-Rose C, Lellouch-Tubiana A, Cinalli G, Zerah M, Pierre-Kahn A, Hoppe-Hirsch E, Bourgeois M, Renier D (1999) Benign cerebellar astrocytomas in children. J Neurosurg 90:265–273

Peraud A, Meschede M, Eisner W, Ilmberger J, Reulen HJ (2002) Surgical resection of grade II astrocytomas in the superior frontal gyrus. Neurosurgery 50:966–975

Pignatti F, van den Bent M, Curran D, Debruyne C, Sylvester R, Therasse P, Afra D, Cornu P, Bolla M, Vecht C, Karim AB; European Organization for Research and Treatment of Cancer Brain Tumor Cooperative Group; European Organization for Research and Treatment of Cancer Radiotherapy Cooperative Group (2002) Prognostic factors for survival in adult patients with cerebral low-grade glioma. J Clin Oncol 20:2076–2084

Pollack IF, Claassen D, al-Shboul Q, Janosky JE, Deutsch M (1995) Low-grade gliomas of the cerebral hemispheres in children: an analysis of 71 cases. J Neurosurg 82:536–547

Recht LD, Lew R, Smith TW (1992) Suspected low-grade glioma: is deferring treatment safe? Ann Neurol 31:431–436

Romstöck J, Fahlbusch R, Ganslandt O, Nimsky C, Strauss C (2002) Localisation of the sensorimotor cortex during surgery for brain tumours: feasibility and waveform patterns of somatosensory evoked potentials. J Neurol Neurosurg Psychiatry 72:221–229

Rumana CS, Valadka AB, Contant CF (1999) Prognostic factors in supratentorial ganglioglioma. Acta Neurochir 141:63–68

Russell SM, Kelly PJ (2003) Incidence and clinical evolution of postoperative deficits after volumetric stereotactic resection of glial neoplasms involving the supplementary motor area. Neurosurgery 52:506–516

Sainte-Rose C, Cinalli G, Roux FE, Maixner R, Chumas PD, Mansour M, Carpentier A, Bourgeois M, Zerah M, Pierre-Kahn A, Renier D (2001) Management of hydrocephalus in pediatric patients with posterior fossa tumors: the role of endoscopic third ventriculostomy. J Neurosurg 95:791–797

Sartorius CJ, Berger MS (1998) Rapid termination of intraoperative stimulation-evoked seizures with application of cold Ringer's lactate to the cortex. Technical note. J Neurosurg 88:349–351

Schmidt MH, Berger MS, Lamborn KR, Aldape K, McDermott MW, Prados MD, Chang SM (2003) Repeated operations for infiltrative low-grade gliomas without intervening therapy. J Neurosurg 98:1165–1169

Schramm J, Luyken C, Urbach H, Fimmers R, Blumcke I (2004) Evidence for a clinically distinct new subtype of grade II astrocytomas in patients with long-term epilepsy. Neurosurgery 55:340–347

Schramm J, Blümcke I, Ostertag CB, Schlegel U, Simon M, Lutterbach J (2006) Low-grade gliomas - current concepts. Zentralbl Neurochir 67:55–66

Schramm J, Aliashkevich AF (2007) Surgery for temporal mediobasal tumors: Experience based on a series of 235 cases. Neurosurgery 60:285–294

Shaw E, Arusell R, Scheithauer B, O'Fallon J, O'Neill B, Dinapoli R, Nelson D, Earle J, Jones C, Cascino T, Nichols D, Ivnik R, Hellman R, Curran W, Abrams R (2002). Prospective randomized trial of low- versus high-dose radiation therapy in adults with supratentorial low-grade glioma: initial report of a North Central Cancer Treatment Group/Radiation Therapy Oncology Group/Eastern Cooperative Oncology Group study. J Clin Oncol 20:2267–2276

Simon M, Ludwig M, Fimmers R, Mahlberg R, Müller-Erkwoh A, Köster G, Schramm J (2006) A variant of the *CHEK2* gene as a prognostic marker in glioblastoma multiforme Neurosurgery 59:1078–1085

Simon M, Neuloh G, von Lehe M, Meyer B, Schramm J (2008) Insular gliomas: the case for surgical management. J Neurosurg (in press)

Simpson JR, Horton J, Scott C, Curran WJ, Rubin P, Fischbach J, Isaacson S, Rotman M, Asbell SO, Nelson JS, et al (1993) Influence of location and extent of surgical resection on survival of patients with glioblastoma multiforme: results of three consecutive Radiation Therapy Oncology Group (RTOG) clinical trials. Int J Radiat Oncol Biol Phys 26:239–244

Souweidane MM (2005) Thalamic gliomas. In: Berger MS, Prados MD (eds) Textbook of neuro-oncology. WB Saunders, Philadelphia, pp 587–598

Steinmeier R, Fahlbusch R, Ganslandt O, Nimsky C, Buchfelder M, Kaus M, Heigl T, Lenz G, Kuth R, Huk W (1998) Intraoperative magnetic resonance imaging with the magnetom open scanner: concepts, neurosurgical indications, and procedures: a preliminary report. Neurosurgery 43:739–747

Stromblad LG, Anderson H, Malmstrom P, Salford LG (1993) Reoperation for malignant astrocytomas: personal experience and a review of the literature. Br J Neurosurg 7:623–633

Stüer C, Vilz B, Majores M, Becker A, Schramm J, Simon M (2007) Frequent recurrence and progression in pilocytic astrocytoma in adults. Cancer 110:2799–2808

Stummer W, Pichlmeier U, Meinel T, Wiestler OD, Zanella F, Reulen HJ; ALA-Glioma Study Group (2006) Fluorescence-guided surgery with 5-aminolevulinic acid for resection of malignant glioma: a randomised controlled multicentre phase III trial. Lancet Oncol 7:392–401

Taillibert S, Chodkiewicz C, Laigle-Donadey F, Napolitano M, Cartalat-Carel S, Sanson M (2006) Gliomatosis cerebri: a review of 296 cases from the ANOCEF database and the literature. J Neurooncol 76:201–205

Taphoorn MJ, Stupp R, Coens C, Osoba D, Kortmann R, van den Bent MJ, Mason W, Mirimanoff RO, Baumert BG, Eisenhauer E, Forsyth P, Bottomley A; European Organisation for Research and Treatment of Cancer Brain Tumour Group; EORTC Radiotherapy Group; National Cancer Institute of Canada Clinical Trials Group (2005) Health-related quality of life in patients with glioblastoma: a randomised controlled trial. Lancet Oncol 6:937–944

Taylor MD, Bernstein M (1999) Awake craniotomy with brain mapping as the routine surgical approach to treating patients with supratentorial intraaxial tumors: a prospective trial of 200 cases. J Neurosurg 90:35–41

Tilgner J, Herr M, Ostertag CB, Volk B (2005) Validation of intraoperative diagnoses using smear preparations from stereotactic brain biopsies: intraoperative versus final diagnosis; relevance of tumor location, age and gender patients. Neurosurgery 56:257–265

Tronnier VM, Wirtz CR, Knauth M, Lenz G, Pastyr O, Bonsanto MM, Albert FK, Kuth R, Staubert A, Schlegel W, Sartor K, Kunze S (1997) Intraoperative diagnostic and interventional magnetic resonance imaging in neurosurgery. Neurosurgery 40: 891–900

Unsgaard G, Rygh OM, Selbekk T, Muller TB, Kolstad F, Lindseth F, Hernes TA (2005) Intraoperative 3D ultrasound in neurosurgery. Acta Neurochir 148:235–253

Vanaclocha V, Saiz-Sapena N, Garcia-Casasola C (1997) Surgical treatment of insular gliomas. Acta Neurochir 139:1126–1134

Vuorinen V, Hinkka S, Farkkila M, Jaaskelainen J (2003) Debulking or biopsy of malignant glioma in elderly people - a randomised study. Acta Neurochir 145:5–10

Weir B (1973) The relative significance of factors affecting postoperative survival in astrocytomas, grades 3 and 4. J Neurosurg 38:448–452

Wiedemayer H, Fauser B, Sandalcioglu IE, Schafer H, Stolke D (2002) The impact of neurophysiological intraoperative monitoring on surgical decisions: a critical analysis of 423 cases. J Neurosurg 96:255–262

Willems PW, Taphoorn MJ, Burger H, Berkelbach van der Sprenkel JW, Tulleken CA (2006) Effectiveness of neuronavigation in resecting solitary intracerebral contrast-enhancing tumors: a randomized controlled trial. J Neurosurg 104:360–368

Wisoff JH, Boyett JM, Berger MS, Brant C, Li H, Yates AJ, McGuire-Cullen P, Turski PA, Sutton LN, Allen JC, Packer RJ, Finlay JL (1998) Current neurosurgical management and the impact of the extent of resection in the treatment of malignant gliomas of childhood: a report of the Children's Cancer Group trial no. CCG-945. J Neurosurg 89:52–59

Yasargil MG, von Ammon K, Cavazos E, Doczi T, Reeves JD, Roth P (1992) Tumours of the limbic and paralimbic systems. Acta Neurochir 118:40–52

Yetkin FZ, Mueller WM, Morris GL, McAuliffe TL, Ulmer JL, Cox RW, Daniels DL, Haughton VM (1997) Functional MR activation correlated with intraoperative cortical mapping. AJNR Am J Neuroradiol 18:1311–1315

Young Poussaint T, Yousuf N, Barnes PD, Anthony DC, Zurakowski D, Scott RM, Tarbell NJ (1999) Cervicomedullary astrocytomas of childhood: clinical and imaging follow-up. Pediatr Radiol 29:662–668

Zhou HH, Kelly PJ (2001) Transcranial electrical motor evoked potential monitoring for brain tumor resection. Neurosurgery 48:1075–1080

Zentner J, Meyer B, Stangl A, Schramm J (1996a) Intrinsic tumors of the insula: a prospective surgical study of 30 patients. J Neurosurg 85:263–71

Zentner J, Hufnagel A, Pechstein U, Wolf HK, Schramm J (1996b) Functional results after resective procedures involving the supplementary motor area. J Neurosurg 85:542–549

Zentner J, Hufnagel A, Wolf HK, Ostertun B, Behrens E, Campos MG, Elger CE, Wiestler OD, Schramm J (1997) Surgical treatment of neoplasms associated with medically intractable epilepsy. Neurosurgery 41:378–386

Radiation Therapy

Stephanie E. Combs

Abstract Radiation therapy is a main pillar in the multimodal treatment of gliomas. However, application of radiation has to be adapted to the distinct characteristics of the various glioma subtypes, with respect to dosing, time-point of irradiation, choice of treatment technique, and more recently, of radiation quality.

Treatment of low-grade gliomas has been characterized by much controversy, which is still ongoing. For anaplastic gliomas, addition of chemotherapy to radiation alone is currently being discussed and is evaluated in prospective trials. For glioblastomas, a change in treatment paradigm has taken place with the alkylating agent temozolomide, which could increase survival significantly for the first time in many centuries. Moreover, the first steps toward pretreatment stratification have been established by defining the role of MGMT-promotor methy-lation for treatment response and outcome.

Over the last few years, particle therapy with protons and carbon ions has become available. These new radiation qualities now offer promising treatment alternatives that will be evaluated within clinical studies in the near future and have the potential to further improve outcome in patients with gliomas.

7.1 Low-Grade Gliomas

There is ongoing controversy about the radiotherapeutic management of low-grade gliomas. Since low-grade gliomas are commonly slow-growing tumors, immediate treatment after initial diagnosis may not always be necessary. Thus, main issues of discussion were not only the identification of the optimal time-point for radiation therapy (RT), but also dose-finding for an optimal dose–response relationship.

The natural course of low-grade gliomas depends mainly on the histologic subtype. Patients with WHO grade I tumors, also termed pilocytic astrocytomas, present with overall survival rates of up to 80% at 10 years, whereas WHO grade II astrocytomas, oligoastrocytomas, or oligodendrogliomas lead to 10-year survival rates of around 17%, 33%, and 49%, respectively (Daumas-Duport et al. 1987; Kelly et al. 1987; Shaw et al. 1997). Due to the favorable history, especially compared with higher-grade gliomas, a number of physicians have favored a

Stephanie E. Combs, MD (✉)
Department of Radiation Oncology
University Hospital of Heidelberg
Im Neuenheimer Feld 400
69120 Heidelberg , Germany
E-mail: Stephanie.Combs@med.uni-heidelberg.de

delay of RT particularly with respect to long-term morbidity and the lack of a convincing benefit of RT for overall survival (Westergaard et al. 1993; Janny et al. 1994; Philippon et al. 1993; Piepmeier 1987, 1996; Nicolato et al. 1995; Bahary et al. 1996; Leighton et al. 1997). On the other hand, some studies have shown a benefit of early RT, with a significant increase in survival with early versus delayed radiation treatment (Shaw et al. 1989; Shibamoto et al. 1993). Additionally, some studies not only recommended early RT, but also suggested a dose–response relationship with an improved outcome after radiation doses of more than 53 Gy (Shaw et al. 1989).

To clarify the two open questions on time-point and dose, large prospective multicenter trials were conducted in patients with low-grade gliomas.

7.1.1
Dose Prescription: High Versus Low

For a number of tumor entities, a clear dose–response relationship has been shown. Therefore, this issue was of main concern also in the treatment of low-grade gliomas. This question was addressed mainly by two large prospective randomized trials.

The North Central Cancer Treatment Group (NCCTG) in conjunction with the Radiation Therapy Oncology Group (RTOG) and the Eastern Cooperative Oncology Group (ECOG) randomized 203 adult patients with low-grade gliomas aged 18 and older between 1986 and 1995 to either 50.4 Gy delivered in 28 fractions or 64.8 Gy in 36 fractions to localized treatment fields including the tumor plus 1–2-cm safety margins. The histological types included were WHO grade II astrocytoma, oligoastrocytoma, as well as oligodendroglioma. Overall survival as well as progression-free survival were not statistically significant between the two treatment arms (Shaw et al. 2002). The high-dose arm demonstrated a slightly lower overall survival, while the incidence of severe radiation-induced toxicity was increased in the high-dose treatment arm.

A second randomized trial conducted by the European Organization of Research and Treatment of Cancer (EORTC), which is also called the *believer trial* favoring adjuvant RT for patients with low-grade gliomas, randomized 379 adults with low-grade gliomas to receive postoperative or post-biopsy irradiation with either 45 Gy in 5 weeks or 59.4 Gy in 6.6 weeks (EORTC 22844; Karim et al. 1996). With survival rates of 58% and 59% for the low- and high-dose treatment arms, no statistically significant difference could be observed between the two dosing schedules. Moreover, progression-free survival was comparable, with 47% and 50% between the two treatment arms. Although survival differences were not significant, the study did find that age and extent of resection were prognostically important, with younger patients and those undergoing more extensive resection having superior outcomes. In principle, long-term side effects were equally distributed between both treatment arms: A quality of life (QoL) questionnaire consisting of 47 items assessing a range of physical, psychological, social, and symptom domains was included in the trial to measure the impact of treatment over time. Patients who received high-dose RT tended to report lower levels of functioning and more symptom burden following completion of RT. These group differences were statistically significant for fatigue/malaise and insomnia immediately after RT and in leisure time and emotional functioning at 7–15 months after randomization. These findings suggest that in conventional RT for low-grade cerebral glioma, a schedule of 45 Gy in 5 weeks not only saves valuable resources, but also spares patients a prolonged treatment at no loss of clinical efficacy (Kiebert et al. 1998).

7.1.2
Timing of Radiation Therapy: Early Versus Delayed

To evaluate the optimal timing of RT in patients with low-grade gliomas, EORTC Trial 22845 randomized 311 patients to 54 Gy of RT directly after biopsy or neurosurgical resection, versus following a wait-and-see strategy (Van den Bent et al. 2005). This trial is also known as the *non-believer trial*. Included were patients with histologically proven supratentorial astrocytoma, oligoastrocytoma, and oligodendroglioma classified as WHO grade II, and treatment was performed within 24 centers worldwide. After a median follow-up time of 7.8 years, 70% of the patients showed tumor progression, and 50% of the patients had died, of which 91% died of tumor progression. Both overall survival and progression-free survival were the primary endpoints of the analysis.

Between both treatment groups, no difference in overall survival could be demonstrated. However, progression-free survival could be increased significantly by early RT from a median of 3.4 years to 5.3 years at $P < 0.0001$.

One main argument against early RT are the potential neurocognitive deficits that might result from RT. From studies on patients with brain metastases treated with whole-brain RT (WBRT), it is known that the incidence of dementia increases with increased fraction sizes. Patients treated with single doses of less than 3 Gy commonly do not develop radiation-induced neurocognitive deficits (DeAngelis et al. 1989). Other studies have confirmed that over time there might be only limited effects of neurocognition after RT (Taylor et al. 1998). However, there still remains a lack of long-term follow-up data. A study published by Brown et al. in 2003 evaluated 203 patients with supratentorial low-grade gliomas treated with radiation doses of 50.4 Gy or higher. Neurocognitive evaluation revealed a stable function during follow-up; moreover, patients with abnormal mini-mental state examination (MMSE) showed even an improvement in function after treatment. Only a small percentage of patients developed deterioration, with 5.3% at 5 years after treatment (Brown et al. 2003).

From the radiation oncologist point of view, sparing of normal brain tissue, besides fraction size, helps reduce the risk of treatment-related side effects. Modern high-precision photon techniques, such as fractionated stereotactic radiotherapy (FSRT), allow millimeter-precise delivery of radiation with a steep dose gradient around the target volume. This technique was evaluated in a group of 143 patients with low-grade gliomas; the outcome was comparable to other conventional photon techniques, especially with no increased rate of field-border recurrences (Plathow et al. 2003). This was also confirmed in a smaller group of patients with oligodendroglial tumors (Combs et al. 2005). Newer radiation qualities, such as proton RT, offering distinct physical characteristics leading to optimal sparing of normal tissue, might offer further benefit.

Besides the known effectiveness of RT for controlling low-grade gliomas, a number of study groups have provided some evidence that temozolomide (TMZ) may represent an interesting alternative option as primary treatment after surgery (Hoang-Xuan et al. 2004; Levin et al. 2006; Kaloshi et al. 2007). In particular, tumors with 1p/19q loss have been shown to profit most from up-front chemotherapy. A study performed by the EORTC is currently comparing progression-free survival in patients with low-grade gliomas after stratification for genetic 1p loss after treatment with primary TMZ versus RT in a phase III trial (EORTC 22033).

However, based on the above-mentioned three major trials, RT to date remains the standard treatment after surgery in patients with low-grade gliomas. No clear survival advantage for early versus delayed RT could be shown, and additionally no benefit of high-dose RT in the 59.4–64.8 Gy range compared to 45 Gy or 50.4 Gy for adults with low-grade supratentorial gliomas could be observed. Survival in this patient group is clearly more dependent on patient age, histologic subtype, as well as the extent of neurosurgical resection. Patients aged 40 years and older undergoing incomplete removal of the tumor appear to have the worst outcome.

Therefore, within the group of low-grade gliomas, certain risk factors should be considered when opting for early RT, such as gemistocytic histology, age over 40 years, progressive clinical symptoms, as well as contrast enhan-cement on computed tomography (CT) and magnetic resonance imaging (MRI). A clear indication for RT can be seen for progressive tumors after wait-and-see or after neurosurgical resection, as well as tumors after only minimal surgical removal. In general, this indication is found in the interdisciplinary setting of modern neurooncology considering individual risk factors (Fig. 7.1).

7.2 Anaplastic Gliomas

Anaplastic gliomas are moderately growing primary brain tumors; they are considered to be WHO grade III tumors, and are subclassified as pure astrocytomas, anaplastic oligoastrocytomas, or anaplastic oligodendrogliomas.

In spite of numerous clinical investigations on the treatment of anaplastic gliomas, microsurgical resection is generally still recommended as the first treatment of choice after diagnosis, especially for large lesions. In general, it is recommended that neurosurgical resection should be as radical as possible; however, a complete resection is rarely possible due to the infiltrative

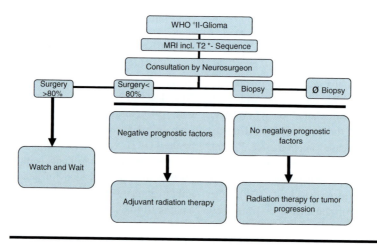

Fig. 7.1 Flow diagram developed at the interdisciplinary neuro-oncology team at the University of Heidelberg, Germany, considering the treatment of patients with low-grade gliomas with respect to individual risk factors

growth pattern of gliomas. In anaplastic gliomas, the role of the extent of tumor resection remains controversial: As opposed to glioblastoma multiforme (GBM), a number of analyses have shown that the extent of surgery is not of prognostic value (Curran et al. 1992; Nitta and Sato 1995). Superiority of a subtotal or complete resection to a biopsy only has been shown for elderly patients with grade III and IV gliomas (Vuorinen et al. 2003); however, a number of studies could not support this idea in the general population (Nitta and Sato 1995; Curran et al. 1992).

Current management strategies for anaplastic gliomas include neurosurgical resection followed by postoperative RT.

Over 2 decades ago, Walker et al. demonstrated that postoperative RT significantly increases overall survival in patients with malignant gliomas, including glioblastomas as well as anaplastic gliomas (Walker et al. 1979, 1980). In spite of extensive research, this treatment approach still remains the standard-of-care in patients with WHO grade III gliomas. In the literature, few reports focus on anaplastic gliomas alone; in general, they are analyzed together with glioblastomas.

Since Walker et al. published a significant increase in overall survival of patients with malignant gliomas treated with RT. Postoperative RT remains the treatment standard for patients with anaplastic gliomas. The Brain Tumor Study Group (BTCG) published a median survival time of 14 months with surgery only and 36 months after surgery and postoperative RT (Walker et al. 1978, 1980). Laperriere et al. performed a meta-analysis on six randomized studies comparing surgery alone with surgery followed by postoperative RT; the risk ratio was lowered by postoperative RT to 0.81 ($P < 0.00001$), underlying the significant prognostic value of postoperative RT (Laperriere et al. 2002).

In a multivariate analysis of a study performed by Do et al., the variables significantly associated with worse survival in patients with anaplastic gliomas were older age, reduced dose, and prolonged waiting time on RT calculated from presentation. The risk of death increased by 2% for each day of waiting for RT (Do et al. 2000).

The value of postoperative RT was re-evaluated in a recent study on elderly patients. In an interim analysis, addition of RT showed significantly improved outcome than in patients treated with best supportive care only; study recruitment was therefore stopped based on these results (Keime-Guibert et al. 2007).

In the past, considerable discussion was focused on dose–volume concepts as well as fractionation schemes in postoperative RT. As early as 1989, Shapiro et al. demonstrated that whole-brain RT did not show significant benefit over RT of the tumor volume adding a sufficient safety margin (Shapiro et al. 1989). The implementation of accelerated fractionation schemes, e.g., 2×1.6 Gy/die as well as hyperfractionated protocols, e.g., 2×1.2 Gy/die, could not show any difference in outcome. For patients in RPA class III and IV, hypofractionated RT with single doses of 2.5Gy, 3Gy, or 3.4Gy were proven to be equieffective to conventional fractionation, while overall treatment time was substantially shortened (Brada et al. 1999; Laperriere et al. 2002).

In patients with glioblastoma, postoperative RT was replaced by radiochemotherapy with TMZ (Stupp et al. 2005; Combs et al. 2005). In a study performed by Stupp and colleagues, a dosing of 75 mg/m^2 of TMZ was prescribed on a daily basis during RCHT (Stupp et al. 2005). Comparable results have been obtained by the Heidelberg Temozolomide Dosing Regimen of 50 mg/m^2: Outcome is most likely to be equivalent with both dosing regimens, while the toxicity profile is more beneficial in the 50 mg/m^2 group (Combs et al. 2008); (Combs et al. 2005). A retrospective analysis on patients with anaplastic gliomas treated with this combined radiochemotherapy regimen compared to patients treated with postoperative irradiation alone, however, did not show a statistically significant advantage of combination treatment (Combs et al. 2008).

The NOA-01 protocol also demonstrated excellent results for RCHT, using concomitant

ACNU and VM26 or cytarabine (AraC); however, a standard treatment arm with RT only was not included into this study. Moreover, only 61 patients with anaplastic gliomas were included. However, median overall survival was 93 months for ACNU + VM26 and 72 months for ACNU + AraC, with 5-year overall survival rates of 88% and 92%, respectively (Weller et al. 2003).

In general, chemotherapy has been widely used for patients with primary anaplastic gliomas, and meta-analyses have shown significant benefit (Stewart 2002). Especially patients with pure oligodendrogliomas or mixed oligoastrocytomas profit from chemotherapy; for fist-line therapy after surgical resection, RT and chemotherapy with TMZ or PCV (procarbazine, lomustine, vincristine) are considered to be equieffective. This concept was evaluated in the NOA-04-Study conducted by the German Society of Neuro-Oncology. Results from this study were first presented at the ASCO meeting in 2008 (Wick and Weller 2008): Wick and colleagues could show that there is no difference in progression-free survival with RT compared to chemotherapy with PCV or TMZ. MGMT-promotor methylation was significantly associated with better outcomes, irrespective of treatment arm; toxicity was higher in the PCV-treated patients compared to TMZ.

Oligodendroglial tumors are the first neoplasms of the central nervous system presenting with distinct genetic signatures such as 1p/19q deletions that significantly correlate with outcome in phase III trials. Two large randomized studies, RTOG 9402 and EORTC 26951, evaluated addition of PCV chemotherapy to postoperative RT in patients with oligodendroglioma (EORTC 26951) and the role of neoadjuvant intensive PCV administered before RT (RTOG 9402) (Cairncross et al. 2004a, b; van den Bent et al. 2007; Jaeckle et al. 2006). The findings of these two phase III studies suggest that there is no improvement in survival by adding PCV chemotherapy to RT, and that timing of chemotherapy (adjuvant vs. neoadjuvant) seems to be irrelevant to outcome. 1p/19q loss could be identified as favorable prognostic factors in both groups; however, data have not yet reached sufficient levels of evidence to serve as a basis for therapeutic decision making.

TMZ has been used with increasing frequency in the treatment of anaplastic oligodendrogliomas and oliogoastrocytomas, and results seem to be comparable to those obtained with PCV (Jaeckle et al. 2006). RTOG 0131 analyzed the outcome of patients with anaplastic gliomas with an oligodendroglial component after 6 months of TMZ prior to RT. In all, 33% of the evaluable patients responded well to TMZ with complete or partial remissions, and only 10% of all patients progressed during adjuvant TMZ, which is favorable compared to 20% of patients progressing during PCV in RTOG 9402 (Cairncross et al. 2004a, b; Vogelbaum et al. 2005).

To date, no large randomized trials have been conducted evaluating the potential benefit of TMZ concomitant to RT versus RT alone after primary diagnosis. Currently, a four-armed prospective randomized study on RT and RCHT using TMZ in patients with anaplastic gliomas without 1p/19q loss is being performed (EORTC 26053, phase III trial on concurrent and adjuvant TMZ chemotherapy in non-1p/19q deleted anaplastic glioma; the CATNON intergroup trial).

For elderly patients, it has been discussed whether TMZ as first-line treatment is equieffective to postoperative RT. A large randomized phase III trial conducted by the German Society for Neuro-Oncology is currently evaluating postoperative RT versus TMZ in a 1-week on–1-week off schedule in patients with anaplastic gliomas and glioblastomas over 65 years of age (NOA-08 – Methusalem).

Outside of studies, however, postoperative RT is still considered the standard of care. For patients with oligodendroglial tumors, up-front chemotherapy might be considered as an alternative, favoring TMZ over the combined PCV regimen.

7.3
Glioblastoma

WHO Grade IV astrocytomas are characterized by a aggressive, rapid, and infiltrating growth pattern, leading to fast and often uncontrollable neurologic deterioration. Early studies have shown that only palliative treatment leads to an overall survival of 2–3 months. A great value has been attributed to neurosurgical resection, which should be as radical as possible; however, when performed alone without adjuvant treatment, it increases overall survival to only 4–5 months (Ammirati et al. 1987; Hess 1999). In the late 1970s, Walker et al. demonstrated a significant increase in outcome by adding postoperative RT (Walker et al. 1978, 1979, 1980). This was supported by a number of other early reports (Andersen 1978). However, with a median survival time of 10–12 months, outcome was still unsatisfactory. Early on, chemotherapy was added to postoperative irradiation, and in most cases a combination of procarbazine, vincristine, and lomustine (PCV) was included in the protocols. However, a statistically significant benefit for postoperative radiation compared with supportive care alone or compared with single- or multi-agent chemotherapy without radiation was shown (Walker et al. 1978, 1979, 1980; Shapiro and Young 1976; Andersen 1978; Kristiansen et al. 1981; Sandberg-Wollheim et al. 1991). Therefore, over a long period of time, postoperative irradiation alone was considered to be the standard of care in patients with glioblastomas.

Radiation oncologist focused on optimizing the application of RT by improving the target volume, as well as identifying superior dosing regimens. Prior to the CT and MRI era, most studies applied whole-brain radiotherapy (WBRT). Over the years it could be shown that regional fields around the enhancing tumor lesions including adequate safety margins in order to account for the infiltrative nature of the disease were adequate. This concept improved with newer imaging possibilities associated with superior tumor localization with CT and MRI, and the fact that most recurrences are within the original tumor site, treated with high-dose irradiation, in over 90% of all cases. On the other hand, larger irradiation fields, as used for WBRT, are associated with high morbidity and risk for side effects (Hochberg and Pruitt 1980; Wallner et al. 1989). Initially, lateral opposing radiation fields were applied. However, with the advent of 3D conformal irradiation techniques, more conformal treatment plans using multiple non-coplanar fields are used today.

The impact of field size was evaluated in two randomized studies by Shapiro and colleagues and Kita et al. (Shapiro et al. 1989; Kita et al. 1989). In both studies, WBRT plus a boost to the tumor site were compared with local RT. In both studies, there was no statistically significant difference in outcome. In the study by Shapiro et al., three treatment arms were designed, also evaluating the use of three different chemotherapy regimens, of which none showed any impact on outcome. Thus, local RT became the treatment of choice in this patient collective.

In order to improve outcome, different radiation techniques and dosing schemes were evaluated in a number of randomized and non-randomized studies.

Hyperfractionated RT as well as accelerated treatment schemes, however, did not show any increase in treatment response, and did not convert into prolonged overall survival in most studies. In hyperfractionation, an increased amount of smaller treatment fractions are used up to a total dose that is commonly higher than with conventionally fractionated irradiation over the same treatment time. The only study demonstrating an advantage for the hyperfractionated arm was by Shin et al., evaluating a small number of patients per arm (Shin et al. 1985). Additionally, outcome in the conventionally fractionated group is significantly worse than in most other published analyses on conventionally fractionated RT. The largest report by Scott et al.

could demonstrate no benefit for hypofractionated irradiation in malignant gliomas (Scott et al. 1998). The studies' experimental arm was in accordance with a report by Nelson et al., who analyzed four different hyperfractionated schemes up to total doses of 64.8 Gy, 72.0 Gy, 76.8 Gy, and 81.6 Gy (Nelson et al. 1988).

Besides hyperfractionation, accelerated treatment schemes were implemented for patients with gliomas. While in hyperfractionation the idea is that normal tissue shows a pronounced ability to repair sublethal damage at lower sized fractions thus resulting in a lower risk for side effects, the aim of accelerated RT is to reduce overall treatment time aiming at reducing the possibility of tumor repopulation during treatment. Commonly this is done by delivering two or three fractions per day with normal sized fractions. This concept was studied by the European Organization for Research and Treatment of Cancer (EORTC) within protocol 22803 (Horiot et al. 1988); however, the study did not show any increase in treatment response, and did not convert into prolonged overall survival. In this study, patients were randomized to conventional RT versus accelerated fractionation with or without misonidazole. In the accelerated group, three fractions were applied per day at 2 Gy, with a 4-h time span between fractions; therefore, 30 Gy could be delivered in 1 week. After a 2-week break, this dosing scheme was repeated, up to a total dose of 60 Gy. Survival was not different in both groups, and toxicity was not increased by accelerated RT. The RTOG evaluated dose escalation in 305 patients delivering 1.6 Gy twice daily up to 48 Gy or 54.4 Gy; however, while toxicity was low in the accelerated group, outcome was not significantly different (Werner-Wasik et al. 1996).

Local dose escalation has also been studied using the placement of radioactive seeds as brachytherapy. Using this technique, a rapid decrease in dose outside the high-dose treatment volume can be achieved, resulting in local dose escalation and sparing of normal tissue. However, interstitial radiation did not convert into an improved in patients with gliomas. The group led by Laperrierre randomized 140 patients to external RT with 50 Gy in 25 fractions, or external RT plus temporary stereotactic iodine-125 implants delivering a minimum peripheral tumor dose of 60 Gy (Laperriere et al. 1998). Median survival for patients randomized to the brachytherapy arm was 13.8 months versus 13.2 months without brachytherapy at a P-level of 0.49, showing no significant benefit of the interstitial implants. A second study performed by the Brain Tumor Cooperative Group (BTCG) evaluated RT plus carmustine with and without an interstitial boost delivered to a total dose of 60 Gy (Selker et al. 2002). The authors concluded that there is no long-term survival advantage of increased radiation dose with (125)I seeds in newly diagnosed glioma patients.

Taking together the RT data to date, 60 Gy in conventional fractionation is considered the standard of care, and is applied in most treatment regiments initiated thereafter.

Keeping in mind the relatively low survival rates, however, novel treatment concepts were followed up. Combination of RT and chemotherapy became a central point of interest, and ultimately could offer significant benefit.

The triple-combination PCV scheme could manage a slight increase in overall survival; however, it is associated with substantial rates of side effects, such as neuropathies (Schmidt et al. 2006; Postma et al. 1998). For a long time, nitrosoureas were evaluated as salvage-chemotherapy in recurrent gliomas; additionally, several other chemotherapy regimens have shown moderate efficacy in recurrent malignant gliomas (Wong et al. 1999; Yung et al. 1999). The role of chemotherapy in addition to RT as first-line treatment was less well defined in the past: Only scarce data supported the idea that carmustine (BCNU) or any other systemic chemotherapeutic agent could in combination with RT significantly increase outcome compared to RT alone (Walker et al. 1980; Green et al. 1983). In different protocols, first-line chemotherapy as radiochemotherapy was evaluated or re-evaluated using carmustine (BCNU) or nimustine (ACNU), in combination with other agents. A trial by the German Austrian Glioma (GAG) group recruited 501 patients with malignant glioma between 1983 and 1988, comparing WBRT plus BCNU and teniposide versus BCNU alone. Progression-free survival was significantly increased by the combination arm; however, overall survival was unchanged. A high rate of pulmonary toxicity was reported within this trial, leading to a replacement of BCNU by nimustine (ACNU) in a subsequent trial.

In a large randomized study performed by the Neuro-oncology Society of the German Cancer Society (NOA), the combination of ACNU and VP16 versus ACNU and cytarabine was analyzed compared with RT alone (Weller et al. 2003).

A major breakthrough and a change in treatment recommendation have been achieved by the oral applicable alkylating substance TMZ. A large randomized trial performed by the EORTC evaluated postoperative RT alone versus postoperative radiochemotherapy using TMZ in patients with primary glioblastoma (Stupp et al. 2005). The combination treatment could increase overall survival from 12.1 to 14.6 months. TMZ was applied daily, 7 days per week, at a dose of 75 mg/m^2. Radiochemotherapy was followed by six cycles of adjuvant TMZ. At about the same time, a phase I/II study on radiochemotherapy with TMZ at daily doses of 50 mg/m^2 on each day of irradiation (5 days/week) without adjuvant TMZ was performed at the University Hospital of Heidelberg. The outcome in this study was comparable; however, treatment-related toxicity was lower compared to the EORTC trial, in which 7% of the patients developed grade 3 and 4 toxicities (Combs et al. 2005). Long-term evaluation of the two dosing schemes confirmed that outcome seems to be equieffective, but with somewhat lower rates of side effects (Combs et al. 2008).

This issue might be of great importance for future treatment initiatives, since outcome in patients with glioblastoma still remains unsatisfactory, and combination of standard treatment with further approaches is being considered. Modern systemic treatments targeting distinct molecular pathways, such as by ways of antibodies or small molecules selectively inhibiting tyrosine kinases, promise improvement in outcome. However, a number of studies to date have shown only modest benefit, for primary as well as for recurrent gliomas, alone or in combination with RT.

For example, it is known that glioblastoma cells show high expression of the epidermal growth factor receptor (EGFR); thus, combination of postoperative radiochemotherapy with TMZ and EGFR inhibition by a monoclonal antibody seems to be a promising treatment alternative (Combs et al. 2007). This trimodal concept is currently being investigated in a phase I/II study (Combs et al. 2006).

For optimal implementation of targeted therapies, effective stratification and selection of patients may be very important for outcome. The first molecular characteristic promising to be a stratification marker for treatment of patients with primary glioblastoma is the methylation status of the repair enzyme O6-methylguanine-DNA methyltransferase status (MGMT). From the EORTC 22981 study, we have learned that patients without MGMT-promoter methylation are characterized by a significantly worse prognosis than patients with MGMT-promoter methylation, irrespective of treatment arm. Sub-group analyses from this study have shown that benefit from the addition of TMZ to radiation is only limited in patients without MGMT-promoter methylation (Stupp et al. 2005; Hegi et al. 2005; Mirimanoff et al. 2006; Gorlia et al. 2008). Therefore, MGMT-promoter methylation status could be used for stratification in subse-quent studies.

Regarding the treatment of elderly patients with glioblastoma, the subgroup of the EORTC 22981 study revealed only a modest benefit of radiochemotherapy with increasing age (Mirimanoff et al. 2006). On the other hand, other groups report safety and efficacy of combined chemoradiation in elderly patients with glioblastoma, perhaps by implementing alternative dosing regimens to prevent TMZ-associated side effects (Combs et al. 2008). Postoperative treatment of elderly patients with TMZ only as compared to postoperative radiation alone is currently evaluated in a large multicenter randomized trial performed by the German Neuro-Oncology Working Group (NOA 08 Trial; Methusalem).

Facing the high rates of tumor recurrences, novel radiation qualities offer a promising alternative for patients with glioblastoma. Particle therapy offers distinct physical and biological characteristics that have proven to be beneficial in certain tumor entities (Schulz-Ertner et al. 2007a, b. RT with charged particles is characterized by an inverted dose profile, with low doses in the entry channel of the beam and a high local dose-deposition termed the Bragg peak, with a sharp dose fall-off thereafter. Moreover, carbon ion RT is characterized by an increased relative biological effectiveness (RBE).

Preclinical studies have shown an increased relative biological effectiveness of carbon ion RT in glioblastoma cell lines (Iwadate et al. 2001).

A first clinical study published by Mizoe et al. treated patients with primary glioblastoma with photon RT up to a total dose of 50 Gy, followed by a carbon ion RT boost in a dose-escalation study (Mizoe et al. 2007). Concomitantly, chemotherapy with ACNU was applied. The study could show the safety and feasibility of the carbon ion boost to the macroscopic tumor, and median overall survival was 17 months. Moreover, the study could show that patients treated with higher doses of carbon ion RT demonstrated a significantly better outcome than patients treated with lower doses. However, these results are based only on a small patient collective, and standard chemotherapy with TMZ was not applied. Therefore, further analysis is needed to evaluate the role of carbon ion RT for glioblastomas.

7.4
Re-irradiation

In the past, a second course or RT was only applied reluctantly in patients with gliomas due to the high risk of treatment-related side effects using conventional RT. Different radiotherapeutic treatment alternatives were evaluated, commonly with only modest palliative effect and substantial toxicity (Combs et al. 2007). Interstitial brachytherapy as well as intraoperative RT were analyzed in several small studies; however, clinical results were never convincing. Modern radiation techniques, such as fractionated stereotactic radiotherapy (FSRT) or stereotactic radiosurgery (SRS), offer the possibility to deliver high local doses, while sparing of normal tissue is possible due to the steep dose gradient around the target volume. The largest series on re-irradiation using FSRT was published by the Department of Radiation Oncology at the University Hospital of Heidelberg, Germany (Combs et al. 2005). Between 1990 and 2004, 172 patients with recurrent gliomas were treated with re-irradiation with a median dose of 36 Gy in single fractions of 2 Gy (Fig. 7.2). Included were 71 patients with recurrent

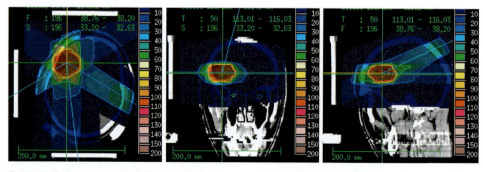

Fig. 7.2. Typical treatment plan of Fractionated Stereotactic Radiotherapy (FSRT) for a patient with a recurrent glioma. A total dose of 36 Gy was applied in daily single fractions of 2 Gy. Axial, coronal and sagittal view

or progressive low-grade gliomas showing signs of malignization, 42 patients with WHO grade III gliomas, and 59 patients with glioblas-toma. Overall survival was 21 months, 50 months, and 111 months for glioblastomas, anaplastic tumors, and low-grade gliomas, respectively. Median survival after re-irradiation was 8, 16, and 22 months, respectively. Toxicity was very low, and treatment was well tolerated.

Stereotactic radiosurgery (SRS) offers the main benefit of a dose application in one single fraction resulting in a significant lower treatment time. However, it is known that severe treatment-related side effects increase with the size of the treatment volume. Therefore, SRS should be considered from smaller lesions only. For a subgroup of patients, however, this treatment alternative is safe and effective and treatment results are convincing (Combs et al. 2005).

To further improve outcome after re-irradiation, concomitant application of chemotherapy was evaluated. A number of different substances have been added to re-irradiation, with often high rates of side effects and only modest benefit. Addition of TMZ in analogy to the standard-of-care chemoradiation regimen for primary glioblastoma was reported to be a safe and effective combination treatment for re-irradiation with FSRT (Combs et al. 2008). Median overall survival was 59 months, and median survival from re-irradiation was 8 months. Actuarial survival rates at 6 and 12 months were 81% and 25%. No severe treatment-related side effects could be documented.

Particle therapy, such as proton and carbon ion RT, might also open new horizons for the treatment of recurrent gliomas.

7.5
Conclusion

Over the past decades, radiation oncology has progressed significantly, and the results of various clinical studies have had significant impact on patient outcome. In the future, the role of RT alone or in combination with different systemic substances warrants evaluation. The new potential associated with particle therapy, such as protons and carbon ions, should be widely exploited and is most likely to improve treatment itself and clinical results.

References

Daumas-Duport C, Scheithauer BW, Kelly PJ (1987) A histologic and cytologic method for the spatial definition of gliomas. Mayo Clin Proc 62:435–49

Kelly PJ, Daumas-Duport C, Scheithauer BW, Kall BA, Kispert DB (1987) Stereotactic histologic correlations of computed tomography- and magnetic resonance imaging-defined abnormalities in patients with glial neoplasms. Mayo Clin Proc 62:450–459

Shaw EG, Scheithauer BW, O'Fallon JR (1997) Supratentorial gliomas: a comparative study by grade and histologic type. J Neurooncol 31:273–278

Westergaard L, Gjerris F, Klinken L (1993) Prognostic parameters in benign astrocytomas. Acta Neurochir (Wien.) 123:1–7

Janny P, Cure H, Mohr M, Heldt N, Kwiatkowski F, Lemaire JJ et al. (1994) Low grade supratentorial astrocytomas. Management and prognostic factors. Cancer 73:1937–1945

Philippon JH, Clemenceau SH, Fauchon FH, Foncin JF (1993) Supratentorial low-grade astrocytomas in adults. Neurosurgery 1993;32:554–559.

Piepmeier JM (1987) Observations on the current treatment of low-grade astrocytic tumors of the cerebral hemispheres. J Neurosurg 67:177–181.

Leighton C, Fisher B, Bauman G, Depiero S, Stitt L, Macdonald D et al. (1997) Supratentorial low-grade glioma in adults: an analysis of prognostic factors and timing of radiation. J Clin Oncol 15: 1294–301 Nicolato A, Gerosa MA, Fina P, Iuzzolino P, Giorgiutti F, Bricolo A (1995) Prognostic factors in low-grade supratentorial astrocytomas: a uni-multivariate statistical analysis in 76 surgically treated adult patients. Surg Neurol 44:208–221

Piepmeier J, Christopher S, Spencer D, Byrne T, Kim J, Knisel JP et al. (1996) Variations in the natural history and survival of patients with supra-tentorial low-grade astrocytomas. Neurosurgery 38:872–878

Bahary JP, Villemure JG, Choi S, Leblanc R, Olivier A, Bertrand G et al. (1996) Low-grade pure and mixed cerebral astrocytomas treated in the CT scan era. J Neurooncol 27:173–177

Shaw EG, Daumas-Duport C, Scheithauer BW, Gilbertson DT, O'Fallon JR, Earle JD et al. (1989) Radiation therapy in the management of low-grade supratentorial astrocytomas. J Neurosurg 70:853–861

Shibamoto Y, Kitakabu Y, Takahashi M, Yamashita J, Oda Y, Kikuchi H et al. (1993) Supratentorial low-grade astrocytoma. Correlation of computed tomography findings with effect of radiation therapy and prognostic variables. Cancer 72:190–195

Shaw E, Arusell R, Scheithauer B, O'Fallon J, O'Neill B, Dinapoli R et al. (2002) Prospective randomized trial of low- versus high-dose radiation therapy in adults with supratentorial low-grade glioma: initial report of a North Central Cancer Treatment Group/Radiation Therapy Oncology Group/Eastern Cooperative Oncology Group study. J Clin Oncol 20:2267–2276

Karim AB, Maat B, Hatlevoll R, Menten J, Rutten EH, Thomas DG et al. (1996) A randomized trial on dose-response in radiation therapy of low-grade cerebral glioma: European Organization for Research and Treatment of Cancer (EORTC) Study 22844. Int.J Radiat.Oncol Biol.Phys 36:549–556

Kiebert GM, Curran D, Aaronson NK, Bolla M, Menten J, Rutten EH et al. (1998) Quality of life after radiation therapy of cerebral low-grade gliomas of the adult: results of a randomised phase III trial on dose response (EORTC trial 22844). EORTC Radiotherapy Co-operative Group. Eur.J Cancer 34:1902–1909

Van den Bent MJ, Afra D, de Witte O, Ben Hassel M, Schraub S, Hoang-Xuan K et al. (2005) Long-term efficacy of early versus delayed radiotherapy for low-grade astrocytoma and oligodendroglioma in adults: the EORTC 22845 randomised trial. Lancet 366:985–990

DeAngelis LM, Delattre JY, Posner JB (1989) Radiation-induced dementia in patients cured of brain metastases. Neurology 39:789–796

Taylor BV, Buckner JC, Cascino TL, O'Fallon JR, Schaefer PL, Dinapoli RP et al. (1998) Effects of radiation and chemotherapy on cognitive function in patients with high-grade glioma. J Clin Oncol 16:2195–2201

Brown PD, Buckner JC, O'Fallon JR, Iturria NL, Brown CA, O'Neill BP et al. (2003) Effects of radiotherapy on cognitive function in patients with low-grade glioma measured by the folstein mini-mental state examination. J Clin Oncol 21:2519–2524

Plathow C, Schulz-Ertner D, Thilman C, Zuna I, Lichy M, Weber MA et al. (2003) Fractionated stereotactic radiotherapy in low-grade astrocytomas: long-term outcome and prognostic factors. Int J Radiat Oncol Biol Phys 57:996–1003

Combs SE, Schulz-Ertner D, Thilmann C, Edler L, Debus J (2005) Fractionated stereotactic radiation therapy in the management of primary oligodendroglioma and oligoastrocytoma. Int J Radiat Oncol Biol Phys 62:797–802

Levin N, Lavon I, Zelikovitsh B, Fuchs D, Bokstein F, Fellig Y et al. (2006) Progressive low-grade oligodendrogliomas: response to temozolomide and correlation between genetic profile and O6-methylguanine DNA methyltransferase protein expression. Cancer 106:1759–1765

Hoang-Xuan K, Capelle L, Kujas M, Taillibert S, Duffau H, Lejeune J et al. (2004) Temozolomide as initial treatment for adults with low-grade oligodendrogliomas or oligoastrocytomas and correlation with chromosome 1p deletions. J Clin Oncol 22:3133–3138

Kaloshi G, Benouaich-Amiel A, Diakite F, Taillibert S, Lejeune J, Laigle-Donadey F et al. (2007) Temozolomide for low-grade gliomas: predictive impact of 1p/19q loss on response and outcome. Neurology 68:1831–1836

Curran WJ, Jr., Scott CB, Horton J, Nelson JS, Weinstein AS, Nelson DF et al. (1992) Does extent of surgery influence outcome for astrocytoma with atypical or anaplastic foci (AAF)? A report from three Radiation Therapy Onco-logy Group (RTOG) trials. J Neurooncol 12:219–227

Nitta T, Sato K (1995) Prognostic implications of the extent of surgical resection in patients with intracranial malignant gliomas. Cancer 75:2727–2731

Vuorinen V, Hinkka S, Farkkila M, Jaaskelainen J (2003) Debulking or biopsy of malignant glioma in elderly people - a randomised study. Acta Neurochir (Wien) 145:5–10

Nitta T, Sato K (1995) Prognostic implications of the extent of surgical resection in patients with intracranial malignant gliomas. Cancer 75: 2727–2731

Curran WJ, Jr., Scott CB, Horton J, Nelson JS, Weinstein AS, Nelson DF et al. (1992) Does extent of surgery influence outcome for astrocytoma with atypical or anaplastic foci (AAF)? A report from three Radiation Therapy Oncology Group (RTOG) trials. J Neurooncol 12:219–227

Walker MD, Strike TA, Sheline GE (1979) An analysis of dose-effect relationship in the radiotherapy of malignant gliomas. Int J Radiat Oncol Biol Phys 5:1725–1731

Walker MD, Green SB, Byar DP, Alexander E Jr, Batzdorf U, Brooks WH et al. (1980) Randomized comparisons of radiotherapy and nitrosoureas for the treatment of malignant glioma after surgery. N Engl J Med 303:1323–1329

Walker MD, Alexander E Jr, Hunt WE, MacCarty CS, Mahaley MS Jr, Mealey J Jr. et al. (1978) Evaluation of BCNU and/or radiotherapy in the treatment of anaplastic gliomas. A cooperative clinical trial. J Neurosurg 49:333–343

Walker MD, Green SB, Byar DP, Alexander E Jr, Batzdorf U, Brooks WH et al. (1980) Randomized comparisons of radiotherapy and nitrosoureas for the treatment of malignant glioma after surgery. N Engl J Med 303:1323–1329

Laperriere N, Zuraw L, Cairncross G (2002) Radiotherapy for newly diagnosed malignant glioma in adults: a systematic review. Radiother Oncol 64:259–273

Do V, Gebski V, Barton MB (2000) The effect of waiting for radiotherapy for grade III/IV gliomas. Radiother.Oncol 57:131–136

Keime-Guibert F, Chinot O, Taillandier L, Cartalat-Carel S, Frenay M, Kantor G et al. (2007) Radiotherapy for glioblastoma in the elderly. N Engl J Med 356:1527–1535

Shapiro WR, Green SB, Burger PC, Mahaley MS, Jr., Selker RG, VanGilder JC et al. (1989) Randomized trial of three chemotherapy regimens and two radiotherapy regimens and two radiotherapy regimens in postoperative treatment of malignant glioma. Brain Tumor Cooperative Group Trial 8001. J Neurosurg 71:1–9

Brada M, Sharpe G, Rajan B, Britton J, Wilkins PR, Guerrero D et al. (1999) Modifying radical radiotherapy in high grade gliomas; shortening the treatment time through acceleration. Int J Radiat Oncol Biol Phys 43:287–292

Laperriere N, Zuraw L, Cairncross G (2002) Radiotherapy for newly diagnosed malignant glioma in adults: a systematic review. Radiother Oncol 64:259–273

Stupp R, Mason WP, Van den Bent MJ, Weller M, Fisher B, Taphoorn MJ et al. (2005) Radiotherapy plus concomitant and adjuvant temozolomide for glioblastoma. N Engl J Med 352:987–996

Combs SE, Gutwein S, Schulz-Ertner D, van Kampen M, Thilmann C, Edler L et al. (2005) Temozolomide combined with irradiation as postoperative treatment of primary glioblastoma multiforme. Phase I/II study. Strahlenther Onkol 181: 372–377

Stupp R, Mason WP, Van den Bent MJ, Weller M, Fisher B, Taphoorn MJ et al. (2005) Radiotherapy plus concomitant and adjuvant temozolomide for glioblastoma. N Engl J Med 352:987–996

Combs SE, Wagner J, Bischof M, Welzel T, Edler L, Rausch R et al. (2008a) Radiochemotherapy in patients with primary glioblastoma comparing two temozolomide dose regimens. Int J Radiat Oncol Biol Phys 70:67–74

Combs SE, Gutwein S, Schulz-Ertner D, van Kampen M, Thilmann C, Edler L et al. (2005) Temozolomide combined with irradiation as postoperative treatment of primary glioblastoma multiforme. Phase I/II study. Strahlenther Onkol 181:372–377

Combs SE, Nagy M, Edler L, Rausch R, Bischof M, Welzel T et al. (2008b) Comparative evaluation of radiochemotherapy with temozolomide versus standard-of-care radiation alone in patients with WHO grade III astrocytic tumors. Radiother Oncol 88(2):177–182

Weller M, Muller B, Koch R, Bamberg M, Krauseneck P (2003) Neuro-Oncology Working Group 01 trial of nimustine plus teniposide versus nimustine plus cytarabine chemotherapy in addition to involved-field radiotherapy in the first-line treatment of malignant glioma. J Clin Oncol 21:3276–3284

Stewart LA (2002) Chemotherapy in adult high-grade glioma: a systematic review and meta-analysis of individual patient data from 12 randomised trials. Lancet 359:1011–1018

Wick W, Weller M, and on behalf of the German Neurooncology Working Group (NOA) (2008) Randomized phase III study of sequential radiochemotherapy of oligoastrocytic tumors of WHO-grade III with PCV or temozolomide: NOA-04. J Clin Oncol 26:(May 20 suppl; abstr LBA2007)

Cairncross G, Seiferheld W, Shaw E, et al. (2004a) An intergroup randomized controlled clinical trial (RCT) of chemotherapy plus radiation (RT) versus RT alone for pure and mixed anaplastic oligodendrogliomas. Initial report of RTOG 9402. J Clin Oncol 22, 107s

Cairncross G, Seiferheld W, Shaw E, et al. (2004b) Intergroup randomized controlled clinical trial (RCT) of chemotherapy plus radiotherapy (RT) versus RT alone for pure and mixed anaplastic oligodendroglioma: Initial report of RTOG 9402. Presented at the Society for Neuro-Oncology 9th Annual Scientific Meeting, Toronto, Canada. November 18–21, 2004

van den Bent MJ, Delattre JY, Brandes AA, et al. (2007) First analysis of EORTC trial 26951, a randomized phase III study of adjuvant PCV chemotherapy in patients with highly anaplastic oligodendroglioma. Presented at the American Society of Clinical Oncology 41st Annual Meeting, Orlando, FL, May 13–17, 2005

Jaeckle KA, Ballman KV, Rao RD, Jenkins RB, Buckner JC (2006) Current strategies in treatment of oligodendroglioma: evolution of molecular signatures of response. J Clin Oncol 24: 1246–1252

Jaeckle KA, Ballman KV, Rao RD, Jenkins RB, Buckner JC (2006) Current strategies in treatment of oligodendroglioma: evolution of molecular signatures of response. J Clin Oncol 24: 1246–1252

Vogelbaum M, Berkey B, Peerenboom D, et al. (2005) Phase II trial of pre-irradiation and concurrent temozolomide in patients with newly diagnosed anaplastic oligodendrogliomas and mixed anaplastic oligodendrogliomas. J Clin Oncol 23:119s, 2005 (abstr 1520)

Ammirati M, Vick N, Liao YL, Ciric I, Mikhael M (1987) Effect of the extent of surgical resection on survival and quality of life in patients with supratentorial glioblastomas and anaplastic astrocytomas. Neurosurgery 21:201–206

Hess KR (1999) Extent of resection as a prognostic variable in the treatment of gliomas. J Neurooncol 42:227–231

Walker MD, Alexander E Jr, Hunt WE, MacCarty CS, Mahaley MS Jr, Mealey J Jr, et al. (1978) Evaluation of BCNU and/or radiotherapy in the treatment of anaplastic gliomas. A cooperative clinical trial. J Neurosurg 49:333–343

Walker MD, Strike TA, Sheline GE (1979) An analysis of dose-effect relationship in the radiotherapy of malignant gliomas. Int J Radiat Oncol Biol Phys 5:1725–1731

Walker MD, Green SB, Byar DP, Alexander E Jr, Batzdorf U, Brooks WH et al. (1980) Randomized comparisons of radiotherapy and nitrosoureas for the treatment of malignant glioma after surgery. N Engl J Med 303:1323–1329

Andersen AP (1978) Postoperative irradiation of glioblastomas. Results in a randomized series. Acta Radiol Oncol Radiat Phys Biol 17:475–484

Shapiro WR, Young DF (1976) Treatment of malignant glioma. A controlled study of chemotherapy and irradiation. Arch Neurol 33:494–450

Kristiansen K, Hagen S, Kollevold T, Torvik A, Holme I, Nesbakken R et al. (1981) Combined modality therapy of operated astrocytomas grade III and IV. Confirmation of the value of postoperative irradiation and lack of potentiation of bleomycin on survival time: a prospective multicenter trial of the Scandinavian Glioblastoma Study Group. Cancer 47:649–652

Sandberg-Wollheim M, Malmstrom P, Stromblad LG, Anderson H, Borgstrom S, Brun A et al. (1991) A randomized study of chemotherapy with procarbazine, vincristine, and lomustine with and without radiation therapy for astrocytoma grades 3 and/or 4. Cancer 68:22–29

Hochberg FH, Pruitt A (1980) Assumptions in the radiotherapy of glioblastoma. Neurology 30:907–911

Wallner KE, Galicich JH, Krol G, Arbit E, Malkin MG (1989) Patterns of failure following treatment for glioblastoma multiforme and anaplastic astrocytoma. Int J Radiat Oncol Biol Phys 16: 1405–1409

Shapiro WR, Green SB, Burger PC, Mahaley MS Jr, Selker RG, VanGilder JC et al. (1989) Randomized trial of three chemotherapy regimens and two radiotherapy regimens and two radiotherapy regimens in postoperative treatment of malignant glioma. Brain Tumor Cooperative Group Trial 8001. J Neurosurg 71:1–9

Kita M, Okawa T, Tanaka M, Ikeda M (1989) [Radiotherapy of malignant glioma–prospective randomized clinical study of whole brain vs local irradiation]. Gan No Rinsho 35:1289–1294

Shin KH, Urtasun RC, Fulton D, Geggie PH, Tanasichuk H, Thomas H et al. (1985) Multiple daily fractionated radiation therapy and misonidazole in the management of malignant astrocytoma. A preliminary report. Cancer 56:758–760

Scott CB, Curran WJ, Yung WKA (1998) Long term results of RTOG 90.06: A randomized study of hyperfractionated radiotherapy (RT) to 72.0Gy & carmustine vs. standard RT & carmustine for malignant glioma patients with emphasis on anaplastic astrocytoma (AA) patients. Proc Am Soc Clin Oncol 17:401aNelson DF, Diener-West M, Horton J, Chang CH, Schoenfeld D, Nelson JS (1988) Combined modality approach to treatment of malignant gliomas–re-evaluation of RTOG 7401/ECOG 1374 with long-term follow-up: a joint study of the Radiation Therapy Oncology Group and the Eastern Cooperative Oncology Group. NCI Monogr 279–284

Horiot JC, van den BW, Ang KK, Van der SE, Bartelink H, Gonzalez D et al. (1988) European Organization for Research on Treatment of Cancer trials using radiotherapy with multiple fractions per day. A 1978–1987 survey. Front Radiat Ther Oncol 22:149–161

Werner-Wasik M, Scott CB, Nelson DF, Gaspar LE, Murray KJ, Fischbach JA et al. (1996) Final report of a phase I/II trial of hyperfractionated and accelerated hyperfractionated radiation therapy with carmustine for adults with supratentorial malignant gliomas. Radiation Therapy Oncology Group Study 8302. Cancer 77:1535–1543

Laperriere NJ, Leung PM, McKenzie S, Milosevic M, Wong S, Glen J et al. (1998) Randomized study of brachytherapy in the initial management of patients with malignant astrocytoma. Int J Radiat Oncol Biol Phys 41:1005–1011

Selker RG, Shapiro WR, Burger P, Blackwood MS, Arena VC, Gilder JC et al. (2002) The Brain Tumor Cooperative Group NIH Trial 87–01: a randomized comparison of surgery, external radiotherapy, and carmustine versus surgery, interstitial radiotherapy boost, external radiation therapy, and carmustine. Neurosurgery 51:343–355

Schmidt F, Fischer J, Herrlinger U, Dietz K, Dichgans J, Weller M (2006) PCV chemotherapy for recurrent glioblastoma. Neurology 66:587–589

Postma TJ, van Groeningen CJ, Witjes RJ, Weerts JG, Kralendonk JH, Heimans JJ (1998) Neurotoxicity of combination chemotherapy with procarbazine, CCNU and vincristine (PCV) for recurrent glioma. J Neurooncol 38:69–75

Wong ET, Hess KR, Gleason MJ, Jaeckle KA, Kyritsis AP, Prados MD et al. (1999) Outcomes and prognostic factors in recurrent glioma patients enrolled onto phase II clinical trials. J Clin Oncol 17:2572–2578

Yung WK, Prados MD, Yaya-Tur R, Rosenfeld SS, Brada M, Friedman HS et al. (1999) Multicenter phase II trial of temozolomide in patients with anaplastic astrocytoma or anaplastic oligoastrocytoma at first relapse. Temodal Brain Tumor Group. J Clin Oncol 17:2762–2771

Green SB, Byar DP, Walker MD, Pistenmaa DA, Alexander E Jr, Batzdorf U et al. (1983) Comparisons of carmustine, procarbazine, and high-dose methylprednisolone as additions to surgery and radiotherapy for the treatment of malignant glioma. Cancer Treat Rep 67:121–132

Weller M, Muller B, Koch R, Bamberg M, Krauseneck P (2003) Neuro-Oncology Working Group 01 trial of nimustine plus teniposide versus nimustine plus cytarabine chemotherapy in addition to involved-field radiotherapy in the first-line treatment of malignant glioma. J Clin Oncol 21:3276–3284

Stupp R, Mason WP, Van den Bent MJ, Weller M, Fisher B, Taphoorn MJ et al. (2005) Radiotherapy plus concomitant and adjuvant temozolomide for glioblastoma. N Engl J Med 352:987–996

Combs SE, Gutwein S, Schulz-Ertner D, van Kampen M, Thilmann C, Edler L et al. (2005) Temozolomide combined with irradiation as postoperative treatment of primary glioblastoma multiforme. Phase I/II study. Strahlenther Onkol 181:372–377

Combs SE, Wagner J, Bischof M, Welzel T, Edler L, Rausch R et al. (2008) Radiochemotherapy in patients with primary glioblastoma comparing two temozolomide dose regimens. Int J Radiat Oncol Biol Phys 71:999–1005

Combs SE, Schulz-Ertner D, Roth W, Herold-Mende C, Debus J, Weber KJ (2007) In vitro responsiveness of glioma cell lines to multimodality treatment with radiotherapy, temozolomide, and epidermal growth factor receptor inhibition with cetuximab. Int J Radiat Oncol Biol Phys 68: 873–882

Combs SE, Heeger S, Haselmann R, Edler L, Debus J, Schulz-Ertner D (2006) Treatment of primary glioblastoma multiforme with cetuximab, radiotherapy and temozolomide (GERT)–phase I/II trial: study protocol. BMC Cancer 6:133

Hegi ME, Diserens AC, Gorlia T, Hamou MF, de Tribolet N, Weller M et al. (2005) MGMT gene silencing and benefit from temozolomide in glioblastoma. N Engl J Med 352:997–1003

Mirimanoff RO, Gorlia T, Mason W, Van den Bent MJ, Kortmann RD, Fisher B et al. (2006) Radiotherapy and temozolomide for newly diagnosed glioblastoma: recursive partitioning analysis of the EORTC 26981/22981-NCIC CE3 phase III randomized trial. J Clin Oncol 24:2563–2569

Gorlia T, Van den Bent MJ, Hegi ME, Mirimanoff RO, Weller M, Cairncross JG et al. (2008) Nomograms for predicting survival of patients with newly diagnosed glioblastoma: prognostic factor analysis of EORTC and NCIC trial 26981–22981/CE.3. Lancet Oncol 9:29–38

Combs SE, Wagner J, Bischof M, Welzel T, Wagner F, Debus J et al. (2008) Postoperative treatment of primary glioblastoma multiforme with radiation and concomitant temozolomide in elderly patients. Int J Radiat Oncol Biol Phys 70:987–992

Schulz-Ertner D, Karger CP, Feuerhake A, Nikoghosyan A, Combs SE, Jakel O et al. (2007a) Effectiveness of carbon ion radiotherapy in the treatment of skull-base chordomas. Int J Radiat Oncol Biol Phys 68(2):449–457

Schulz-Ertner D, Nikoghosyan A, Hof H, Didinger B, Combs SE, Jakel O et al. (2007b) Carbon ion radiotherapy of skull base chondrosarcomas. Int J Radiat Oncol Biol Phys 67:171–177

Iwadate Y, Mizoe J, Osaka Y, Yamaura A, Tsujii H (2001) High linear energy transfer carbon radiation effectively kills cultured glioma cells with either mutant or wild-type p53. Int J Radiat Oncol Biol Phys 50:803–808

Mizoe JE, Tsujii H, Hasegawa A, Yanagi T, Takagi R, Kamada T et al. (2007) Phase I/II clinical trial of carbon ion radiotherapy for malignant gliomas: combined X-ray radiotherapy, chemotherapy,

and carbon ion radiotherapy. Int J Radiat Oncol Biol Phys 69:390–396
Combs SE, Debus J, Schulz-Ertner D (2007) Radiotherapeutic alternatives for previously irradiated recurrent gliomas. BMC Cancer 7:167
Combs SE, Thilmann C, Edler L, Debus J, Schulz-Ertner D (2005) Efficacy of fractionated stereotactic reirradiation in recurrent gliomas: long-term results in 172 patients treated in a single institution. J Clin Oncol 23:8863–8869
Combs SE, Widmer V, Thilmann C, Hof H, Debus J, Schulz-Ertner D (2005) Stereotactic radiosurgery (SRS): treatment option for recurrent glioblastoma multiforme (GBM). Cancer 104:2168–2173
Combs SE, Bischof M, Welzel T, Hof H, Oertel S, Debus J et al. (2008) Radiochemotherapy with temozolomide as re-irradiation using high precision fractionated stereotactic radiotherapy (FSRT) in patients with recurrent gliomas. J Neurooncol 89(2):205–210. Epub 2008 May 7

Adjuvant Therapy

8

Wolfgang Wick and Michael Weller

Abstract This chapter focuses on the therapeutic strategies for patients with gliomas other than surgery (Chap. 6) and radiotherapy (Chap. 7). It deals with gliomas of all WHO grades and details the primary treatment as well as therapeutic options at recurrence. Chemotherapy is used at recurrence after surgery and radiotherapy, in combination with radiotherapy or as the first treatment after the histological diagnosis has been achieved, prior to radiotherapy.

8.1 Introduction

8.1.1 General Principles

In general, the efficacy of chemotherapy depends on the drug levels achieved in the tumor tissue and on the intrinsic resistance mechanisms to the specific mode of action of a drug. Determinants of drug delivery to the tumor via the systemic route include tumor perfusion, the existence of arteriovenous shunts, and the distance that has to be crossed by a

Wolfgang Wick (✉)
Department of Neurooncology,
University Clinic of Heidelberg
Im Neuenheimer Feld 400,
69120 Heidelberg
Germany
E-mail: wolfgang.wick@med.uni-heidelberg.de

substance from the vasculature to the tumor cell, either by diffusion or bulk flow. Moreover, the limited efficacy of chemotherapeutic agents used to treat patients with gliomas results in part from their inability to penetrate the blood–brain barrier in non-contrast-enhanced areas of the tumor and to achieve meaningful tumoricidal concentrations within the tumor tissue.

The blood–brain barrier (BBB) is comprised of brain capillary endothelial cells (BCECs), pericytes, astrocytes, and neuronal cells (Rubin and Staddon 1999). Its primary role is the maintenance of brain homeostasis, that is, to protect the integrity of neuronal function from toxic metabolites and inflammatory cells derived from the peripheral circulation. BCECs, the major functional constituents of the BBB, differ from peripheral endothelial cells in that they possess tight junctions that prevent the paracellular transport of molecules from the peripheral circulation into the brain (Brightman and Reese 1969). Moreover, BCECs are characterized by low vesicular transport and lack of fenestration, limiting transcellular transport. The integrity of the BBB, however, is not only a result of limited extravasation, but is also actively maintained by several transport systems. These transport systems include cationic and anionic transflux systems such P-glycoprotein (PGP) and multidrug-resistance (MDR) proteins, nucleoside transports, receptor-mediated transport systems such as the transferrin receptors and large amino acid transporters. Diseases altering the function of the BBB such as brain tumors disrupt CNS homeostasis and allow toxic mediators to disturb the neuronal integrity of adjacent brain tissue. This may result in neurological impairment and focal seizures. These transport systems that are found on tumor cells proper inhibit the intracellular deposition of multiple structurally unrelated compounds, such as vincristine, doxorubicin, or teniposide.

Other cell and molecular biological factors also determine the sensitivity of tumor cells toward cytotoxic stimuli. In a further attempt to increase drug exposure of tumor cells, disrupting the BBB has been attempted using hypertonic reagents such as mannitol or vasoactive substances such as the bradykinin analog labradimil (RMP-7). However, in clinical trials neither of these approaches combining conventional intravenous or intra-arterial chemotherapy with BBB disruption has shown superiority over chemotherapy alone in patients with malignant gliomas (Prados et al. 2003).

The first molecular marker that became relevant for the prognosis of brain-tumor patients is the combined loss of heterozygosity (LOH) on chromosomes 1p and 19q in oligodendroglial tumors, presumably as a result of an unbalanced translocation. Patients with 1p/19q-deleted tumors show a longer progression-free and overall survival in response to radio- or chemotherapy than patients whose tumors lack these changes (Cairncross et al. 2006; van den Bent et al. 2006). This prognostic value of the 1p/19q status is less well established for low-grade (I/II) tumors and may be negligible for the time to progression if the patients receive no adjuvant radiotherapy or chemotherapy (Weller et al. 2007). Further, analyses of O^6-methylguanine DNA methyltransferase (MGMT) promoter methylation status in glioblastoma showed that patients with a methylated MGMT promoter derived the greatest survival benefit from treatment with radiotherapy plus nitrosoureas or temozolomide (TMZ) (Esteller et al. 2000; Hegi et al. 2005). These studies established the MGMT promoter methylation status as a predictive marker for the progression-free survival in response to alkylating agents both in the primary as well as in the salvage treatment of glioblastoma (Herrlinger et al. 2006; Wick et al. 2007).

Loss of p53 activity, enhanced activity of the epidermal growth factor receptor (EGFR), or enhanced expression of antiapoptotic BCL-2-family proteins or of inhibitor-of-apoptosis-proteins (IAPs) are associated with resistance toward radio- and chemotherapy.

In human cancers, p53 may be the most common target gene for mutational inactivation; p53 mutations are rather common (65%) in secondary glioblastomas thought to be derived through the malignant progression from grade II or III astrocytomas. In these patients, the same p53 mutations are already found in the less malignant precursor lesion in approximately 90%. In contrast, only 10% of primary glioblastomas exhibit p53 mutations. Interestingly, p53 mutations and amplification of the EGFR gene appear to be mutually exclusive. The molecular basis for this phenomenon remains to be identified.

In untransformed cells, the loss of p53 may enhance rather than decrease the vulnerability to apoptosis. This is because p53 senses DNA damage and promotes cell cycle arrest and DNA repair prior to cell cycle reentry unless this damage is overwhelming. However, within the process of neoplastic transformation, the loss of p53 probably allows the cell to accumulate random genetic and chromosomal aberrations without triggering the endogenous p53-controlled cell death pathway. In human malignant glioma cell lines, there is no apparent correlation between the sensitivity to cytotoxic therapy and genetic or functional p53 status or expression of p53 response genes (Weller et al. 1998). Many tumors, including glioblastomas, overexpress members of the IAP family, whereas IAP levels are rather low or absent in non-neoplastic cells (Liston et al. 2003). The principle mechanism underlying the antiapoptotic activity of IAP has been proposed to be by direct caspase inhibition. Several human IAPs directly bind and inhibit members of the caspase family, e.g., XIAP, cIAP1, cIAP2, and survivin directly target caspases 3, 7, and 9 (Salvesen and Duckett 2002).

Accordingly, inhibition of EGFR has become one of the leading strategies of current experimental clinical trials in human glioma patients. In some glioma cell lines, signaling through other receptor tyrosine kinases such as insulin-like growth factor receptor I may compensate for the inhibition of EGFR (Chakravarti et al. 2002). The combination of EGFR inhibitors with inhibitors of other receptor tyrosine kinases may therefore improve the efficacy of this approach. Recent work has offered an explanation for the possible efficacy of co-inhibition: the kinase c-Src downstream of the EGFR phosphorylates and inhibits the tumor suppressor phosphatase and tensin homolog deleted on chromosome 10 (PTEN). Inhibition of EGFR may restore the function of PTEN and thus put a break on PI3K signaling. Human glioma cell lines express a variety of antiapoptotic and proapoptotic BCL-2 family proteins. Enhanced expression of BCL-2 and BCL-X_L protects these cells from apoptosis induced by diverse stimuli. An up-regulation of BCL-2 and BCL-X_L, but a down-regulation of BAX has been described in recurrent glioblastoma independent from treatment, suggesting therapy-independent pressures for the development of an apoptosis-resistant phenotype. In contrast, BCL-2 or BCL-X_L expressions have not consistently been shown to be associated with increasing WHO grade. Enhanced expression of BCL-2 or BCL-X_L induces complex changes of the glioma cell phenotype in that it not only protects glioma cells from various proapoptotic stimuli but also enhances their motility via mechanisms independent of the prevention of apoptosis (Weiler et al. 2006).

The protein kinase C (PKC) family of serine threonine protein kinases has been implicated in the processes that control tumor cell growth, survival, and progression. Early observations that PKC are activated by tumor promoting phorbol esters suggested that PKC activation may be involved in tumor initiation and progression. Tumor-induced angiogenesis also requires the activation of PKC, particularly PKC-β. PKC activation also contributes to tumor cell survival and proliferation and has been implicated in the malignant progression of human cancers, notably B cell lymphomas, malignant gliomas, and colorectal carcinomas (Goekjian and Jirousek 2001).

8.1.2
Current Therapeutic Strategies

A selection of registered, experimental compounds for glioma therapy are summarized in Table 8.1. Chemotherapeutics are given as monotherapy or in combination regimens (Table 8.2). These regimens aim at synergistic effects and at differential sensitivity of subclones in the tumor toward individual compounds. Most commonly, alkylating agents are used in glioma therapy. Proliferating cells are more or less specific targets in the generally nonproliferating brain. More recently, this concept had to be revised since stem cell compartments with proliferating glial and neuronal stem cells were suggested to reside in the adult human brain in the subventricular zone and the hippocampus. Moreover, the low proliferation rates in glioma, as low as 5% and even in glioblastoma rarely more than 25%, and the difficulties achieving relevant drug levels in the tumor bed for prolonged times hamper this paradigm. Therefore, compounds that act independently from the cell cycle and are administered in a long-term metronomic fashion, preferentially via the oral route, are now preferentially being developed for glial tumors.

Importantly, until now there has been no proof of a synergistic effect of any chemotherapy with radiotherapy in the treatment of glioma. This is also true for the combination of radiotherapy and TMZ in the treatment of newly diagnosed glioblastoma (Stupp et al. 2005) where synergy as opposed to additive effects has not been confirmed. More likely, chemotherapeutics with activity in brain tumors act independently from radiotherapy. Theoretically, chemotherapy before radiotherapy should allow higher drug levels because the vasculature is not yet altered by radiotherapy. Furthermore, tolerability could

Table 8.1 Clinically approved and selected experimental agents (Translated and modified from Wick and Weller (therapie und verlauf neurologischer erkrankungen, 5. aufl., kohlhammer verlag, 2007))

Drug	Mechanism	BBB-penetration[a]	Dosages	Tumor	Adverse events[d]	References
ACNU (Nimustine)	Alkylating agent	++	100 mg/m² [b] × 6 weeks	Anaplastic glioma, glioblastoma	Lung fibrosis	Takakura et al. 1986; NOA 2003
BCNU (Carmustine)	Alkylating agent	++	150–200 mg/m² × 6 weeks	Anaplastic glioma, glioblastoma	Lung fibrosis	Walker et al. 1978, 1980
Bevacizumab (within studies)	VEGF inhibitor	–	5–10 mg/2 weeks	Glioblastoma	Thrombosis	Vredenburgh et al. 2007
Carboplatin	DNA-crosslinks	–	Different regimens, e.g., 360 mg/m² × 4 weeks	Oligodendroglioma	Polyneuropathy, renal toxicity	Alberts and Dorr 1998
CCNU (Lomustine)	Alkylating agent	++	130 mg/m² [b] × 6 weeks, 110 mg/m² [c] × 6 weeks	Anaplastic glioma, Glioblastoma, medulloblastoma	Lung fibrosis	Levin et al. 1990; Schmidt et al. 2006
Cilengitide (within studies)	Anti-integrin	?	500 mg/2×/week	Glioblastoma	Rare	Stupp et al. 2007
Cisplatin	DNA crosslinks	–	Different regimens, e.g., 100 mg/m² × 4 weeks	Oligodendroglioma	Polyneuropathy, renal toxicity, ototoxicity	Alberts and Dorr 1998
Cytarabine		+	Different regimens, e.g., 120 mg/m² D1–3 × 6 weeks	Glioblastoma	rare, pulmonary Edema	NOA 2003
Enzastaurin (within studies)	PKC-β inhibition	?	1 × 500 mg, 2 × 250 mg	Glioblastoma	Rare, lymphopenia	Fine et al. 2005
Etoposide (VP16)	Topoisomerase II inhibitor		Different regimens	Anaplastic glioma, glioblastoma	Diarrhea	Balmaceda et al. 1996; Baranzelli et al. 1997
Procarbazine	Alkylating agent		130–150 mg/m² p.o. D1–D28 × 4 weeks	Anaplastic glioma, glioblastoma	Allergy, polyneuropathy	Rodriguez et al. 1989; Brandes et al. 1999a; Yung et al. 2000
Tamoxifen	Anti-estrogen, protein kinase-C inhibition		20–200 mg daily	Anaplastic glioma, glioblastoma	Nausea, liver toxicity	Couldwell et al. 1996; Brandes et al. 1999b

Temozolomide	Alkylating agent	++	150–200 mg/m² D1–D5 × 4 weeks; 100–150 mg/m² 1 week on/1 week off; 75 mg/m²/day concomitant with XRT[e]	Anaplastic glioma, glioblastoma	Diarrhea	Friedman et al. 1998; Yung et al. 1999, 2000; Stupp et al. 2005; Wick 2007
Teniposide (VM26)	Topoisomerase II inhibitor	–	Different regimens, e.g., 60 mg/m² D1– × 6 weeks	Anaplastic glioma, glioblastoma	Rare	Brandes et al. 1998; NOA 2003
Topotecane	Topoisomerase I Inhibitor	++	1.5 mg/m² D1-5 ×3 weeks	Anaplastic glioma, glioblastoma	Rare	Macdonald et al. 1996
Vincristine	Inhibition of mitosis	–	1.4 mg/m² (max.: 2 mg)[f]	Anaplastic glioma, Glioblastoma, medulloblastoma	Polyneuropathy	Cairncross et al. 1994; Packer et al. 1997

[a]Csf level > 30% blood level: ++, > 5% +, < 5% –
[b]Monotherapy
[c]Combination chemotherapy
[d]Apart from myelosuppression
[e]Pcv regimen
[f]Radiotherapy (xrt)

Table 8.2 Protocols of combination chemotherapies (Translated and modified from Therapie und Verlauf Neurologischer Erkrankungen, 5. Aufl., Kohlhammer Verlag, 2007)

Protocol	Design	Tumor	References
PCV	Procarbazine 60 mg/m² p.o. D8-21 CCNU 110 mg/m² p.o. D1 Vincristine 1.4 mg/m² i.v. D8 + 29 × (6-)8 weeks	(Anaplastic) oligodendroglioma anaplastic astrocytoma glioblastoma	Levin et al. 1990 Streffer et al. 2000
ACNU/VM26 (Teniposid)	ACNU 90 mg/m² D1 VM26 60 mg/m² D1-3 ×6 weeks	Anaplastic astrocytoma glioblastoma	NOA (2003)
CCV	CCNU 75 mg/m² p.o. D1 Cisplatin 70 mg/m² i.v. D1 Vincristine 1.4 mg/m² i.v. D1, 8, 15 × 6–7 weeks	Medulloblastoma	Packer et al. 1994 Kortmann et al. 2000
CV	Carboplatin 175 mg/m² vincristine 1.5 mg/m²	Grade I/II -astrocytoma	Packer et al. 1997
CE	Carboplatin 300 mg/m² D1 Etoposide (VP16) 150 mg/m² D2-3 × 4 weeks (and other regimens)	Recurrent oligodendroglioma Germ cell tumor	Balmaceda et al. 1996 Baranzelli et al. 1997 Streffer et al. 2000

be better. However, this strategy, which shows success in primary CNS lymphoma and most likely oligodendroglial tumors, has failed to be effective in other primary brain tumors so far.

High-dose chemotherapy with autologous stem cell transplantation has been studied in children and young adults with newly diagnosed as well as recurrent malignant brain tumors (Wolff and Finlay 2004). Although there have been objective responses in individual patients, high-dose chemotherapy has not assumed a defined role in the standards of care for any glial brain tumor.

8.1.3
Alternative Modes of Application

Intra-arterial chemotherapy mainly using BCNU or cisplatin was neuro- and oculotoxic and intra-arterial placement of the catheter had led to thromboembolic events. There was no promising activity from these approaches in phase II clinical trials. Since the growth of malignant gliomas is not restricted to single arterial territories, even superselective angiography-guided intra-arterial chemotherapy to limit toxicity is unlikely to improve efficacy. There is no role for intrathecal chemotherapy in the treatment of primary brain tumors apart from the treatment of subarachnoid spread with a significant tumor cell load in the cerebrospinal fluid. Interstitial chemotherapy using BCNU wafers (Gliadel®) is a registered treatment for newly diagnosed and recurrent malignant glioma (Westphal et al. 2003, 2006). Yet, concerns regarding the interpretation of the trial results for newly diagnosed glioblastoma include the overrepresentation of grade III tumors in the control arm and the failure to demonstrate an effect of local BCNU administered at first surgery on progression-free survival.

8.1.4
Alternative Therapies

Given the major steps that have been made in the last few years in the understanding of the genetic and cell biologic mechanisms that are involved in the initiation and progression of gliomas, this clearer understanding should be translated into approaches targeting the key molecular effectors of glioma malignancy. These novel therapeutic strategies are based on new pharmaceutical compounds that are designed to interfere with specific targets in glioma signal transduction pathways or focus on gene therapy to modify the tumor microenvironment. Principally, the induction of differentiation should revert the malignant phenotype. However, candidate substances such as interferons, retinoid acid, or phenylacetate have not fulfilled promises. Infiltrative glioma growth leads to progressive neurological morbidity and prevents complete resection. Hence inhibitors of migration, invasion, and angiogenesis are being tested in patients with progressive or recurrent gliomas or are used initially parallel to radiotherapy. These include thalidomide, PTK787, cilengitide, enzastaurin, bevacizumab, temsirolimus, the PDGF inhibitor imatinib (Gleevec, STI571) or EGFR inhibitors such as gefinitib (Iressa, ZD1839) or erlotinib (Tarceva, OSI774). In analogy to other tumor entities, great efforts are being undertaken to define molecular subgroups of gliomas that specifically respond to such strategies, e.g., inhibition of EGFR (Mellinghoff et al. 2005). Death ligands such as CD95L or TRAIL have not been administered to human brain tumor patients yet. Details on these experimental therapies are given in Chap. 9.

8.1.5
Gene Therapy

The first efforts of somatic gene therapy were in fact merely a novel approach to deliver a chemotherapeutic cytotoxic agent to gliomas more efficiently and more selectively. In fact, glioblastoma was the first and so far the only disease entity subjected to a gene therapy approach in a phase III trial. In this classical paradigm of retroviral gene therapy, actively dividing cells were transduced by prodrug gene therapy with the herpes simplex virus thymidine kinase (HSV-TK) gene and subsequently treated with the antiviral drug ganciclovir (Rainov 2000). That this trial was negative may have mainly resulted from limitations of the GCV/TK system itself, since ganciclovir poorly crosses the blood–brain barrier and since the transduction efficacy of tumor cells was very low. Applications of ganciclovir directly into the tumor or different prodrug/suicide gene systems, e.g., cyclophosphamide/cytochrome P450 2B1, in which the prodrug can cross the blood–brain barrier, are being developed.

Oncolytic virotherapy uses viruses such as adenoviruses or herpes simplex viruses with the natural ability to kill their host cells. An infected cell undergoes lysis. Thereby thousands of new virus particles are released and new cells are infected and killed in successive rounds of infection and cytolysis. Using mutant/attenuated viruses that preferentially replicate in tumor cells or through engineered viruses where genes that are essential for replication are placed under tumor-specific promoters, cell death is restricted to tumor cells. Phase I/II clinical trials showed the safety and some signs of efficacy of dl1520, a replication-competent adenoviral oncolytic mutant. A NABTTtrial of injection of dl1520 at 10^7–10^{10} plaque-forming units in 24 patients with recurrent glioblastomas after surgical resection of tumor exhibited no maximum tolerated dose at 10^{10} plaque-forming units, and a median time to tumor progression of 67.5 days, with a median survival time of 176.6 days (Chiocca et al. 2004). Dl1520 was safe, but the time to progression was short and only one patient showed a subjective partial response.

8.2
Astrocytic Tumors

Chemotherapy has so far no role in the treatment of adult pilocytic astrocytoma but is used with some efficacy, resulting in long-term stabilizations but no cures in recurrent childhood grades I and II glioma at recurrence and also prior to radiotherapy (Packer et al. 1997; Gnekow et al.

2004). Chemotherapy is also used in grade II astrocytoma after failure of radiotherapy.

In the primary situation, PCV and TMZ are used and a definite role at least for TMZ is being investigated in the EORTC trial 22033/26033. The RTOG is already running a phase II trial testing this combination in high-risk low-grade astrocytomas. Nitrosourea-based chemotherapy regimens have been by far most widely studied and clinically used in the treatment of gliomas, in particular oligodendroglial tumors where chemotherapy may be as efficacious as radiotherapy. Nitrosoureas share with TMZ good blood–brain barrier penetration and both cause DNA alkylation. Adjuvant nitrosourea-based radiochemotherapy has been shown to increase survival compared to radiation alone in anaplastic astrocytoma and glioblastoma (Glioma Meta-analysis Trialists Group 2002). The outstanding results of the NOA-01 trial does not prove the efficacy of adjuvant alkylating chemotherapy since a control arm was missing. On the other hand, it is unlikely that the good overall survival of 16 months in glioblastoma would have been reached with radiotherapy alone (NOA 2003).

TMZ was approved for recurrent anaplastic glioma (WHO grade III) in the USA and Europe based on a phase II trial that had demonstrated a 35% response rate (Yung et al. 1999). The superiority over procarbazine in a randomized trial for recurrent glioblastoma (WHO grade IV) (Yung et al. 2000) led to its approval in Europe, but not in the United States, chiefly because no effect on overall survival was demonstrated. The limited efficacy at recurrence and promising survival data in a phase II study on TMZ given concomitantly with radiotherapy and as a maintenance treatment thereafter in the first-line treatment of glioblastoma led to a randomized phase III trial conducted as a joint effort of the European Organization for Research and Treatment of Cancer (EORTC) and the National Cancer Institute of Canada (NCIC). This trial compared standard radiotherapy with radiotherapy plus concomitant TMZ at 75 mg/m^2 plus up to six cycles of adjuvant (maintenance) TMZ at 150–200 mg/m^2 at D1–D5 of 28-day cycles. The trial enrolled 573 patients in 85 centers in 15 countries. TMZ as concomitant and adjuvant therapy has also been shown to increase progression-free survival (rate at 6 months, 53.9% vs. 36.4%) and median survival (14.6 vs. 12.1 months) when added to radiation therapy (EORTC trial 26981, Stupp et al. 2005), but still many patients do not respond to therapy.

Nonhematological toxicity was mild. The DNA repair enzyme MGMT mediated resistance to some DNA lesions induced by alkylating agents. Loss of MGMT expression in cancer cells is commonly the result of methylation in the promotor region of the MGMT gene. The analysis of tumor DNA for MGMT gene methylation showed a striking impact on the clinical course. Patients with MGMT gene promoter methylation gained a much larger benefit from alkylating therapy than patients without this methylation. Survival at 2 years approached 50% for patients with a methylated promoter who received TMZ as first-line treatment. Moreover, patients with a methylated promoter who received radiotherapy only as first-line treatment still appeared to benefit from chemotherapy administered at recurrence, be it TMZ or nitrosourea-based, as indicated by the increase in overall, but not progression-free, survival compared with the patients without a promoter methylation (Hegi et al. 2005).

While differences in MGMT gene promoter methylation may determine the clinical course in glioblastoma patients treated with TMZ, it is at present not recommended to use the MGMT gene promoter methylation assay as a clinical guide to decide which glioma patients should receive TMZ and which should not. An independent confirmation of the results of the EORTC NCIC study and the validation of the assay appear necessary. There is some reason to believe that alternative, dose-intensified schedules such as the 1 week on/1 week of schedule (Wick et al. 2007) or the 3-weeks-out-of-4 schedule may produce more benefit for the nonmethylators than the conventional 5-out-of-28-day schedule. This question is addressed in a RTOG EORTC intergroup trial. At present, the only established alternative is pure or combined nitrosourea-based chemotherapy, which may also depend on MGMT gene promoter methylation status for its efficacy (Herrlinger et al. 2006).

Delay of radiotherapy in glioblastoma was generally not successful. Whether this also applies to anaplastic astrocytoma will be shown by the NOA-04 trial that randomized between primary radio- or chemotherapy with PCV or TMZ in anaplastic astrocytoma (www.neuroonkologie.de). The situation may be also different in elderly patients with anaplastic astrocytoma and glioblastoma because of the side effects of radiotherapy in this population. Hence, the NOA-08 trial compares radiotherapy with a dose-intensified TMZ regimen in patients over 65 years of age (www.neuroonkologie.de).

The role of chemotherapy at recurrence is solid. A meta-analysis of single-center single-arm phase-II trials demonstrated a median progression-free survival for patients with glioblastoma at 9 weeks and anaplastic astrocytoma at 13 weeks. Median overall survival was 25 weeks for glioblastoma and 47 weeks for anaplastic astrocytoma (Wong et al. 1998). Progression-free survival rates with PCV or TMZ are between 20% and 40% at 6 months.

A rare differential entity is termed gliomatosis cerebri. This is the diffuse growth of glial cells in more than two lobes of the brain. Regardless of whether the biopsy reveals a histological grade II or III lesion, this entity has the prognostic features of a grade III astrocytic lesion. Clinical presentation i soften by seizures or personality changes. Due to its nature, diagnosis is made by biopsy – an attempt to resect is not advised – and neuroradiology. Median survival is between 1 and 2 years but varies widely. Radiotherapy as well as chemotherapy with PCV or TMZ are possibly effective in slowing the disease progression (Herrlinger et al. 2002; Sanson et al. 2004). There are no randomized trials exploring this entity.

8.3 Oligodendroglial Tumors

Although resection and postoperative radiotherapy are considered standard of care, data on alternative strategies, i.e., biopsy plus radiotherapy or resection without follow-up treatment, have not been generated in a randomized fashion. In a retrospective series, early radio- or chemotherapy in grade II oligodendroglial tumors did not improve progression-free or overall survival. The role of surgery is less important because radio- or chemotherapy frequently lead to minor or major responses.

Patients with a grade II oligodendroglial tumor can be followed if they are asymptomatic and young. Symptomatic, progressing, or grade III oligodendroglial tumors need further therapy. The mainstay is not defined and will be evaluated between radiotherapy and chemotherapy with PC(V) or TMZ. In addition, other chemotherapies might be effective. A subgroup of TMZ-resistant oligodendroglioma from EORTC 26971 showed a response to following PCV chemotherapy in 50% (Triebels et al. 2004). In anaplastic oligodendroglial tumors, PCV and TMZ have been tested head to head in the NOA-04 trial (www.neuroonkologie.de).

Chromosomal deletions on 1p and 19q are predictive for good response to radio- as well as chemotherapy and therefore it is not appropriate to differentially chose between these options.

Both the RTOG study 94-02 and EORTC study 26951 compared adjuvant PCV in combination with radiotherapy to radiotherapy only in anaplastic oligodendroglial and mixed oligoastrocytic tumors, which are considered chemosensitive. Both studies showed that adjuvant PCV increased progression-free survival, but in neither study could a significant effect on overall survival be demonstrated. Most likely this can be explained by the efficacy of chemotherapy at the time of recurrence in this group of patients. Prolonged progression-free survival in both trials was associated with marked hematological toxicity during the PCV therapy. In addition, both trials on oligodendroglial tumors confirmed that LOH 1p/19q is the most important predictor of long progression-free and overall survival in oligodendroglial tumors, regardless of the treatment the patients were allocated to. Without combined 1p/19q, loss median survival was 2–2.8 years, with combined 1p/19q loss survival is more than 6–7 years. This 2- to 2.8-year survival in patients without 1p/19q deletions is similar to the survival of patients with anaplastic astrocytoma in historical studies (Cairncross et al. 2006; van den Bent et al. 2006). Thus, both from the clinical and the molecular point of view it is logical to combine anaplastic astrocytoma with oligoastrocytomas and oligodendrogliomas without combined 1p/19q loss in new studies on newly diagnosed anaplastic glioma. These trials in combination with the positive results of the EORTC 26981 glioblastoma trial (Stupp et al. 2005) lead to the remarkable observation that chemotherapy in combination with radiotherapy increases overall survival in a relatively chemoresistant disease, but not in a much more chemosensitive tumor type. That conclusion seems counterintuitive. A more rational explanation may be found in the different methodologies of the trials: the glioblastoma trial investigated daily TMZ during the entire period of radiotherapy. A concurrent chemoradiation approach has also been successful in other tumor entities. In contrast, both trials on adjuvant PCV chemotherapy on oligodendroglial tumors used classical sequential treatment of radiotherapy and PCV chemotherapy, and neither observed a significant impact on overall survival. This outcome is similar to the outcome of past trials on sequential adjuvant chemotherapy in glioblastoma, which also failed to observe a survival benefit after adjuvant chemotherapy. These observations suggest that in particular the combined part of the treatment in which daily TMZ is given together with daily irradiation increases survival in glioblastoma. However, the design of EORTC 26981 did not allow any conclusions to be drawn concerning which part of the treatment contributes most to the improved outcome. Moreover, it is unclear whether the observations made in GBM can be extrapolated to anaplastic glioma.

Recurrent treatment is dependent on primary treatment. Importantly, so far high-dose regimens are not superior to conventional recurrence treatments (Cairncross et al. 2000; Zander et al. 2002).

References

Alberts DS, Dorr RT (1998) New perspectives on an old friend: optimizing carboplatin for the treatment of solid tumors. The Oncologist 3:15–34

Balmaceda C, Heller G, Rosenblum M, Diez B, Villablanca JG, Kellie S, Maher P, Vlamis V, Walker RW, Leibel S, Finlay JL (1996) Chemotherapy without irradiation – a novel approach for newly diagnosed CNS germ cell tumors: results of an international cooperative trial. The First International Central Nervous System Germ Cell Tumor Study. J Clin Oncol 14:2908–2915

Baranzelli MC, Patte C, Bouffet E, Couanet D, Habrand JL, Portas M, Lejars O, Lutz P, Le Gall E, Kalifa C (1997) Nonmetastatic intracranial germinoma: the experience of the French Society of Pediatric Oncology. Cancer 80:1792–1797

Brandes AA, Rigon A, Zampieri P, Ermani M, Carollo C, Altavilla G, et al. (1998) Carboplatin and teniposide concurrent with radiotherapy in patients with glioblastoma multiforme. A phase II study. Cancer 82: 355–361

Brandes AA, Ermani M, Turazzi S, Scelzi E, Berti F, Amistà P, et al. (1999a) Procarbazine and high-dose tamoxifen as a second-line regimen in recurrent high-grade gliomas: a phase II study. J Clin Oncol 17: 645–650

Brandes AA, Palmisano V, Monfardini S (1999b) Medulloblastoma in adults: clinical characteristics and treatment. Cancer Treat Rev 25:3–12

Brightman MW, Reese TS (1969) Junctions between intimately apposed cell membranes in the vertebrate brain. J Cell Biol 40:648–677

Cairncross G, Macdonald D, Ludwin S, Lee D, Cascino T, Buckner J, Fulton D, Dropcho E, Stewart D, Schold C Jr, et al. (1994) Chemotherapy for anaplastic oligodendroglioma. National Cancer Institute of Canada Clinical Trials Group. J Clin Oncol 12(10):2013–2021

Cairncross G, Swinnen L, Bayer R, Rosenfeld S, Salzman D, Paleologos N, et al. (2000) Myeloablative chemotherapy for recurrent aggressive oligodendroglioma. Neurooncol 2:114–119

Cairncross G, Berkey B, Shaw E, Jenkins R, Scheithauer B, Brachman D, Buckner J, Fink K, Souhami L, Laperierre N, Mehta M, Curran W (2006) Phase III trial of chemotherapy plus radiotherapy compared with radiotherapy alone for pure and mixed anaplastic oligodendroglioma: Intergroup Radiation Therapy Oncology Group Trial 9402. J Clin Oncol 24:2707–2714

Chakravarti A, Loeffler JS, Dyson NJ (2002) Insulin-like growth factor receptor I mediates resistance to anti-epidermal growth factor receptor therapy in primary human glioblastoma cells through continued activation of phosphoinositide 3-kinase signaling. Cancer Res 62:200–207

Chiocca EA, Abbed KM, Tatter S, et al. (2004) A phase I open-label, dose-escalation, multi-institutional trial of injection with an E1B-attenuated adenovirus, ONYX-015, into the peritumoral region of recurrent malignant gliomas, in the adjuvant setting. Mol Ther 10:958–966

Couldwell WT, Hinton DR, Surnock AA, DeGiorgio CM, Weiner LP, Apuzzo ML, et al. (1996) Treatment of recurrent malignant gliomas with chronic oral high-dose tamoxifen. Clin Cancer Res 2:619–622

Esteller M, Garcia-Foncillas J, Andion E, Goodman SN, Hidalgo OF, Vanaclocha V, et al. (2000) Inactivation of the DNA-repair gene MGMT and the clinical response of gliomas to alkylating agents. N Engl J Med 343:1350–1354

Fine HA, Kim L, Royce C, et al. (2005) Results from phase II trial of enzastaurin (LY317615) in patients with recurrent high grade gliomas. Proc. ASCO 1504

Friedman HS, McLendon RE, Kerby T, Dugan M, Bigner SH, Henry AJ, et al. (1998) DNA mismatch repair and O6-alkylguanine-DNA alkyltransferase analysis and response to Temodal in newly diagnosed malignant glioma. J Clin Oncol 16:3851–3857

Glioma Meta-analysis Trialists (GMT) Group (2002) Chemotherapy in adult high-grade glioma: a systematic review and meta-analysis of individual patient data from 12 randomised trials. Lancet 359:1011–1018

Gnekow AK, Kortmann RD, Pietsch T, Emser A (2004) Low grade chiasmatic-hypothalamic glioma-carboplatin and vincristine chemotherapy effectively defers radiotherapy within a comprehensive treatment strategy – report from the multicenter treatment study for children and adolescents with a low grade glioma - HIT-LGG 1996 - of the Society of Pediatric Oncology and Hematology (GPOH). Klin Pädiatr 216:331–342

Goekjian PG, Jirousek MR (2001) Protein kinase C inhibitors as novel anticancer drugs. Expert Opin Investig Drugs 10:2117–2214

Hegi M, Diserens A, Gorlia T, et al. (2005) MGMT gene silencing and benefit from temozolomide in glioblastoma. N Engl J Med 352:997–1003

Herrlinger U, Felsberg J, Küker W, Bornemann A, Plasswilm L, Knobbe CB, et al. (2002) Gliomatosis cerebri. Molecular pathology and clinical course. Ann Neurol 52:390–399

Herrlinger U, Rieger J, Koch D, Loeser S, Blaschke B, Kortmann R-D, Steinbach JP, Hundsberger T, Wick W, Meyermann R, Sommer C, Bamberg M, Reifenberger G, Weller M (2006) UKT-03 phase II trial of CCNU plus temozolomide chemotherapy in addition to radiotherapy in newly diagnosed glioblastoma. J Clin Oncol 24:4412–4417

Levin VA, Silver P, Hannigan J, Wara WM, Gutin PH, Davis RL, Wilson CB (1990) Superiority of post-radiotherapy adjuvant chemotherapy with CCNU, procarbazine, and vincristine (PCV) over BCNU for anaplastic gliomas: NCOG 6G61 final report. Int J Radiat Oncol Biol Phys 18:321–324

Liston P, Fong WG, Korneluk RG (2003) The inhibitors of apoptosis: there is more to life than Bcl-2. Oncogene 22:8568–8580

Macdonald D, Cairncross G, Stewart D, Forsyth P, Sawka C, Wainman N, Eisenhauer E (1996)

Phase II Study of topotecan in patients with recurrent malignant glioma. National Clinical Institute of Canada Clinical Trials Group. Ann Oncol 7(2):205–207

Mellinghoff IK, Wang MY, Vivanco I, Haas-Kogan DA, Zhu S, Dia EQ, et al. (2005) Molecular determinants of the response of glioblastomas to EGFR kinase inhibitors. N Engl J Med 353:2012–2024

Neuro-Oncology Working Group (NOA) of the German Cancer Society (2003) Neuro-Oncology Working Group (NOA)-01 trial of ACNU/VM26 *versus* ACNU/Ara-C chemotherapy in addition to involved-field radiotherapy in the first-line treatment of malignant glioma. J Clin Oncol 21:3276–3284

Packer RJ, Ater J, Allen J, Phillips P, Geyer R, Nicholson HS, et al. (1997) Carboplatin and vincristine chemotherapy for children with newly diagnosed progressive low-grade gliomas. J Neurosurg 86:747–754

Prados MD, Schold SC JR SC, Fine HA, Jaeckle K, Hochberg F, Mechtler L, et al. (2003) A randomized, double-blind, placebo-controlled, phase 2 study of RMP-7 in combination with carboplatin administered intravenously for the treatment of recurrent malignant glioma. Neurooncol 5:96–103

Rainov NG (2000) A phase III clinical evaluation of herpes simplex virus type 1 thymidine kinase and ganciclovir gene therapy as an adjuvant to surgical resection and radiation in adults with previously untreated glioblastoma multiforme. Hum Gene Ther 112389–2401

Rodriguez LA, Prados M, Silver P, Levin VA (1989) Reevaluation of procarbazine for the treatment of recurrent malignant central nervous system tumors. Cancer 64:2420–2423

Rubin LL, Staddon JM (1999) The cell biology of the blood-brain barrier. Annu Rev Neurosci 22:11–28

Salvesen GS, Duckett CS (2002) IAP proteins: blocking the road to death's door. Nat Rev Mol Cell Biol 3:401–410

Sanson M, Cartalat-Carel S, Taillibert S, Napolitano M, Djafari L, Cougnard J, et al. (2004) Initial chemotherapy in gliomatosis cerebri. Neurology 63:270–275

Schmidt F, Fischer J, Herrlinger U, Dietz K, Dichgans J, Weller M (2006) PCV chemotherapy for recurrent glioblastoma. Neurology 66:587–589

Stupp R, Mason WP, van den Bent MJ, Weller M, Fisher B, Taphoorn MJB, et al. (2005) Radiotherapy plus concomitant and adjuvant temozolomide for patients with newly diagnosed glioblastoma. N Engl J Med 352:987–996

Stupp R, Goldbrunner R, Neyns B, Schlegel U, Clement P, Grabenbauer GG, Hegi ME, Nippgen J, Picard M, Weller M (2007) Phase I/IIa Trial of Cilengitide (EMD121974) and Temozolomide With Concomitant Radiotherapy, Followed by Temozolomide and Cilengitide Maintenance Therapy in Patients With Newly Diagnosed Glioblastoma. ASCO 2007

Takakura K, Abe H, Tanaka R, Kitamura K, Miwa T, Takeuchi K, et al. (1986) Effects of ACNU and radiotherapy on malignant glioma. J Neurosurg 64:53–57

Triebels VH, Taphoorn MJ, Brandes AA, Menten J, Frenay M, Tosoni A, et al. (2004) Salvage PCV chemotherapy for temozolomide-resistant oligodendrogliomas. Neurology 63:904–906

van den Bent M, Carpentier AF, Brandes AA, Sanson M, Taphoorn MJ, Bernsen HJ, Frenay M, Tijssen CC, Grisold W, Sipos L, Haaxma-Reiche H, Kros JM, van Kouwenhoven MC, Vecht CJ, Allgeier A, Lacombe D, Gorlia T (2006) Adjuvant procarbazine, lomustine, and vincristine improves progression-free survival but not overall survival in newly diagnosed anaplastic oligodendrogliomas and oligoastrocytomas: a randomized European Organisation for Research and Treatment of Cancer phase III trial. J Clin Oncol 24;2715–2722

Vredenburgh JJ, Desjardins A, Herndon JE 2nd, Dowell JM, Reardon DA, Quinn JA, Rich JN, Sathornsumetee S, Gururangan S, Wagner M, Bigner DD, Friedman AH, Friedman HS. (2007) Phase II trial of bevacizumab and irinotecan in recurrent malignant glioma. Clin Cancer Res 13:1253–1259

Walker MD, Alexander E, Hunt WE, MacCarty CS, Mahaley MS, Mealey J, et al. (1978) Evaluation of BCNU and/or radiotherapy in the treatment of anaplastic gliomas. A cooperative clinical trial. J Neurosurg 49:333–343

Walker MD, Green SB, Byar DP, Alexander E, Batzdorf U, Brooks WH, et al. (1980) Randomized comparisons of radiotherapy and nitrosoureas for the treatment of malignant glioma after surgery. N Engl J Med 303:1323–1329

Weiler M, Bähr O, Hohlweg U, et al. (2006) BCL-x_L: time-dependent dissociation between modulation of apoptosis and invasiveness in human malignant glioma cells. Cell Death and Differ 13:1156–1169

Weller M, Rieger J, Grimmel C, et al. (1998) Predicting chemoresistance in human malignant glioma cells: the role of molecular genetic analyses. Int J Cancer 79:640–644

Weller M, Berger H, Hartmann C, Schramm J, Westphal M, Simon M, Goldbrunner R, Krex D, Steinbach JP, Ostertag CB, Loeffler M, Pietsch T, von Deimling A; German Glioma Network (2007) Combined 1p/19q loss in oligodendroglial tumors: predictive or prognostic biomaker? Clin Cancer Res 13(23):6933–6937

Westphal M, Hilt DC, Bortey E, Delavault P, Olivares R, Warnke PC, et al. (2003) A phase 3 trial of local chemotherapy with biodegradable wafers (Gliadel wafers) in patients with primary malignant glioma. Neurooncol 5:79–88

Westphal M, Ram Z, Riddle V, Hilt D, Bortey E; On behalf of the Executive Committee of the Gliadel Study Group (2006) Gliadel wafer in initial surgery for malignant glioma: long-term follow-up of a multicenter controlled trial. Acta Neurochir (Wien) 148:269–275

Wick A, Felsberg J, Steinbach JP, Herrlinger U, Platten M, Blaschke B, Meyermann R, Reifenberger G, Weller M, Wick.W (2007) Efficacy and tolerability of Temozolomide in an one week on/one week off regimen in patients with recurrent glioma. J Clin Oncol (in press)

Wolff JE, Finlay JL (2004) High-dose chemotherapy in childhood brain tumors. Onkologie 27:239–245

Wong WW, Hirose T, Scheithauer BW, Schild SE, Gunderson LL (1998) Malignant peripheral nerve sheath tumor: analysis of treatment outcome. Int J Radiat Oncol Biol Phys 42:351–360

Yung WKA, Prados MD, Yaga-Tur R, Rosenfeld SS, Brada M, Friedman HS, et al. for the Temodal Brain Tumor Group (1999) Multicenter phase II trial of temozolomide in patients with anaplastic astrocytoma or anaplastic oligoastrocytoma at first relapse. J Clin Oncol 17:2762–2771

Yung WKA, Albright RE, Olson J, Fredericks R, Fink K, Prados MD, et al. (2000) A phase II study of temozolomide vs. procarbazine in patients with glioblastoma multiforme at first relapse. Br J Cancer 83:588–593

Zander T, Nettekoven W, Kraus JA, Pels H, Ko YD, Vetter H, Klockgether T, Schlegel U (2002) Intensified PCV-chemotherapy with optional stem cell support in recurrent malignant oligodendroglioma. J Neurol 249:1055–1057

Other Experimental Therapies for Glioma

9

Manfred Westphal and Katrin Lamszus

Abstract Experimental therapies for glioma are mostly based on the insights into the cell biology of the tumors studied by modern methods including genomics and metabolomics. In surgery, intraoperative visualization of residual tumor by fluorescence has helped with the radicality of resection. Although temozolamide has become an important agent in the combined radiochemotherapy of newly diagnosed glioblastoma, understanding the underlying mechanisms of action and resistance has led to alterations in dosing schemes, which may be more beneficial than the introduction of new agents. Targeted therapies that have been highly promising in other solid tumors have been rather disappointing in gliomas, not for the lack of promising targets but most likely due to inefficacy of the reagents to reach their target. Direct delivery of reagents with interstitial infusion via convection-enhanced delivery has proven to be safe and effective, but the potential of that technology has not been exploited because many technicalities are still to be worked out, and better, more selective reagents are needed. Gene therapy has been reactivated with direct adenoviral application to transfer HSV-Tk into tumor cells by adenoviral vectors, still awaiting final analysis. Oncolytic viruses are also under long-term refinement and await definitive pivotal clinical trials. Immunotherapy is currently focusing on vaccination strategies using either specifically pulsed dendritic cells or immunization with a specific peptide, which is unique to the vIII variant of the epidemal growth factor receptor. An area attracting immense attention for basic research as well as translation into clinical use is the characterization of neural stem cells and their theraputic potential when appropriately manipulated.

In general, there is a wide spectrum of specific neuro-oncological therapy developments, which are not only extrapolated from general oncology but also based on translational research in the field of glioma biology.

9.1 Introduction

Most newly developed therapies are centered around the theme of targeted therapies. In that respect, this chapter is divided into separate sections that cover surgical advances, new developments in chemotherapy, radiotherapy, and new

Manfred Westphal (✉)
Department of Neurosurgery
University Hospital Hamburg Eppendorf
Martinistraβe 52
20251 Hamburg, Germany
E-mail: westphal@plexus.uke.uni-hamburg.de

experimental therapies. Targeting in neuro-oncology has two very different meanings. Firstly, as in general oncology, targeted therapies attempt to interfere with some very specific, select intrinsic tumor pathways that are either reflected on the cell surface or in the intracellular signaling pathways. Secondly, however, therapy for intrinsic brain tumors faces the problem of getting the agents to the tumor cells, which in the postsurgical adjuvant setting are mostly beyond the blood–brain barrier. Therefore, the physical act of targeting, meaning delivery of a therapeutic agent to the required location, is also a major aspect of targeting.

9.2
Surgery

An important development in the surgical management of gliomas is the use of intraoperative guidance. Whereas magnetic resonance imaging, computerized tomography, and ultrasound are purely imaging technologies that compete in importance and impact and all lack evidence of cost-effective efficacy, intraoperative fluorescence has just been shown to be a simple technique by which resections of high-grade gliomas can be guided. In a recent phase III randomized trial, which will most likely lead to marketing the reagent, a fluorescent compound was found to increase the proportion of patients who underwent total gross resection (as assessed by early postoperative MRI) (Stummer et al. 2006). According to protocol, the patient drinks a hematoporphyrin compound 2 h prior to surgery, which is then selectively taken up by tumor cells and metabolized to 5-aminolevuleic acid (5-ALA). Using a specific UV light source in the operating microscope, the fluorescent compound will become visible by lighting up and areas of undetected tumor can be removed. This being the first trial aimed to assess the effect of resection. A meta-analysis confirmed that combining the patients with a complete resection of contrast enhancing tumor from both arms and comparing them to patients with residual tumor from both arms, a significant difference could be objectivated for the more radically resected patients (Stummer et al. 2008). Using this and related compounds as truly photodynamic interstitial cytotoxic therapy, applied to deep seated, nonresectable tumors, is experimental. A laser beam guided by a glass fiber is inserted into the tumor and then excites the compound leading to direct cytotoxic reaction. This treatment is currently under evaluation.

9.3
Chemotherapy

The basic concept for experimental chemotherapy for gliomas is based on extrapolation from general oncology. These are reviewed in Chap. 8. More recently, the developments focus on modifications of existing regimens. Temozolamide which has been found to be beneficial mainly in patients in whom the repair mechanism responsible for part of the drug resistance has been epigenetically silenced by methylation of the MGMT gene (Hegi et al. 2005), will be evaluated in a risk-adapted larger multinational trial where the MGMT status determines the use of the agent (M. van den Bent, personal communication). Also, because MGMT is a suicide enzyme that is trial innitiated used up in action, thought has been given to the use of temozolamide in a chronic, low-dose application scheme called taxonomic chemotherapy, which aims at taking advantage of the exhaustion of MGMT by the chronic presence of its substrate what has led to the dose dense trials currently innitiated.

Intracavitary chemotherapy has been established for newly diagnosed malignant glioma as well as for recurrent disease (Brem et al. 1995; Westphal et al. 2003). Modifying a major resistance mechanism by the application of 0-6 benzylguanine may additionally enhance its efficacy (Friedman et al. 2002; Weingart et al. 2007). In contrast to the combination of chemotherapy with modifiers given systemically, the combination of a systemic modifier with local chemotherapy is much better tolerated and systemically nontoxic.

In a further development of modified ways to administer chemotherapy, direct application of chemotherapeutic agents by interstitial infusion is under investigation. This so-called convection method has been the basis of recent clinical trials aiming at the delivery of large molecules (see below) but may also be used to deliver Taxol, temozolamide, and other agents (Yamashita et al. 2007).

Recognizing the insufficiency of most single agents, approved agents are being combined experimentally. More recently, an antibody against the vascular endothelial growth factor (VEGF), which is approved for colorectal cancer (bevacizumab, Avastin®), has been combined with CPT11 (irinotecan) a topoisomerase inhibitor and has provided promising early results (Pope et al. 2006). Using an anti-VEGF antibody will probably lead to vessel normalization, reducing the neoangiogenesis what clinically correlates with the disappearance of contrast enhancement. It must be assumed that the intratumoral tissue pressure that results in part from the "leaky" angiogenic vessels is thereby reduced, making it easier for substances like irinotecan to enter the tumor. It has been observed by some investigators, that there is a very rapid resolution of edema and contrast enhancement with a marked improvement of the functional status of the patient but in subsequent controls, very diffusely infiltrating progression can be seen and it is the goal for currently designed trials to estimate the relationship between progression free survival and an improvement in overall survival.

9.4 Radiation

Much of the experimental therapy around the field of radiation is concerned with dosing schemes, fractionation, and improvement of precision of delivery to only the targeted area (see Chap. 7). In addition, there is a wealth of experimental studies of radiation sensitizers, all of which so far seem not to have worked; no reagent from that concept has entered clinical use. In that context, temozolamide was also thought to act partially as a radiosensitizing agent, explaining why it has now become standard therapy to combine it at a reduced dose with radiation before giving the full dose (Stupp et al. 2005). Another classical chemotherapeutic agent believed to be radiosensitizing is 5-FU (Roullin et al. 2004). It has to be noted also, that the considerations following the standardized use of temozolamide in the proposed regimen noticed that in the period of radiotherapy, temozolamide is given daily which is emulating the dose dense schedules currently under evaluation and that such taxonomic therapy may have its. In this context, a slow-release biopolymer has been developed that slowly releases 5-FU over time. In a phase II design, these 5-FU containing microspheres were injected into the circumference of the wall of the resection cavity at the end of surgery and then radiation follows 2 weeks later, assuming that by then most of the slowly released local 5-FU is taken up by the tumor cells, rendering them more susceptible to radiation (Menei et al. 2005).

Another method of targeting radiation other than by beam shape and rotating beam sources uses radiolabeled molecules to immobilize radiation at the targeted site. This can be achieved using radiolabeled ligands to receptors that are selectively overexpressed on the surface of tumor cells or by antibodies to cell surface determinants, which can be transmembrane receptors but also other molecules that belong to the realm of adhesion molecules or posttranslational modifications such as gangliosides or other sugar moieties. In general, this type of radiotherapy is summarized as brachytherapy.

The most widely explored form of local carrier-bound radiation therapy is intracavitary brachytherapy, which makes use of a surgically created cavity that is then secondarily filled with the therapeutic agent via an Ommaya reservoir. Prototypically, radiolabeled antibodies have been used, which are directed against epitopes that are carried by the tumor cells in abundance. These have also been modified extensively with different radioactive isotopes, which vary in half-life and delivered energy. For reasons of handling, radiochemistry, manufacturing, and dispensing, I-131 seems to be the most practical agent, but I-125 has also been widely used and astatine and technetium are less widely used (Zalutsky 2005). As for targets, the adhesion molecule called tenascin has been most elaborately explored. Two antibodies have been used in clinical trials over the last few years. The BC-1 antibody (Riva et al. 1997) has been used combined with Y-90, I-125, or I-131 for recurrent completely resectable glioblastoma (Goetz et al. 2003). Depending on the long-term results, a phase III trial might be started. Another antibody with a long track record is the 81C6 antibody against tenascin, which is currently going to phase III trials as an I-131 radiolabeled agent (Reardon et al. 2002).

A highly selective agent has been developed by the in-depth analysis of the EGF/EGF-receptor system, which is also abundantly activated in gliomas. A specific mutation in the EGF-R was found by deletion of a gene segment that shifts the reading frame such that a new amino acid is inserted, creating a unique site of immunogenicity (VIII variant; Kuan et al. 2001). Using that site as an immunogen, a highly selective antibody has been created that can also be used for a highly selective radioimmunotherapy (Shankar et al. 2006).

Other agents that over the years have come into early phase clinical trials are radiolabeled short somatostatin peptide analog binding to the somatostatin receptor and substance P-based radiochemicals, which are both delivered by convection (Kneifel et al. 2007; Schumacher et al. 2002).

9.5
New Developments

9.5.1
Targeted Therapies for Glioma

When describing targeted therapies for any cancer, specific molecules or pathways have usually been identified on the tumor cells and these offer a selective therapeutic window. Apart from extrapolation of therapies from general oncology (Rich and Bigner 2004) and findings from correlative molecular genetics; 1p/19), the gene expression profiling will most likely provide new highly selected targets that will yield effective reagents in the next decade. The most advanced attempt in this direction has come from the "cancer genome sequencing" of a series of glioblastoma specimens in which very interestingly many of the already known molecules like p53 or the EGF-R came up in the display (Nature 2008). Presently, many targets under investigation have been identified by extrapolation, immunohistochemistry, or by general biological insights such as the transferrin receptor, which is overexpressed on dividing cells, and the retroviral vector selectivity for gene therapy, which is also based on cell division (Ram et al. 1997).

9.5.2
Targeting New Targets by Convection

Many candidate molecules such as IL-4, IL-13, the EGF receptor including its variants, and transferrin have been discovered to be overexpressed on the surface of gliomas. All these molecules have become targets for what are called toxin conjugates for convection-enhanced delivery.

Convection encompasses the placement of an intraparenchymal catheter connected to a pump, which over several days continuously delivers very minute amounts (10 µl/min), which eventually will result in large distribution volumes in the parenchyma on the other side of the blood–brain barrier. Using this technique, with new reagents represents a tandem-evaluation of the assumptions of volume distribution in brain parenchyma and the efficacy of a given drug against a target itself. After promising phase I/II data (Kunwar 2003; Kunwar et al. 2007; Laske et al. 1997), two convection trials went to phase III, the pseudomonas toxin conjugated IL-13 (cintredekin-besudotox; the PRECISE trial) and the diphtheria-toxin-coupled transferrin (the TransMID trial). IL-13 was administered intraparenchymally into the brain surrounding a resection cavity of a gross total resection of a case of recurrent glioblastoma. Up to three stereotactically placed catheters were used. Compared to the authorities-prescribed comparator, a carmustine implant (Gliadel® wafer), no statistically superior efficacy could be seen on unstratified analysis. The diphtheria toxin coupled to transferrin was delivered via stereotactically placed catheters intratumorally to patients who were nonsurgical candidates with recurrent glioblastoma. In addition, that study was halted for lack of positive results at an early interim analysis based on unstratified results that still need to be clarified for the technical quality of the delivery mode.

Convection delivery, despite the above-mentioned superficial setbacks of two phase III trials ending inconclusively, seems to be the most promising concept of drug delivery to the brain. The failure of the two trials has reasons which do not affect the promise of CED as such. While the Il-13 trial lacked from the target specificity and possibly a misassumption of target quantity, the TransMid Trial may have targeted a population of patients for whom this therapy is simply inadequate without being inefficient as such when applied in the correct context. With the target organ being the human brain, however, progress will be very slow because drug and delivery technologies must progress simultaneously. As for drug delivery technology there is considerable progress with new catheter systems and catheter placement schedules (Dickinson et al. 2008). More careful evaluation will have to be invested into the characteristics of the reagents. Each reagent will have its own biophysical properties determining distribution by charge-related matrix interaction, the solubility-dependent radius of distribution, its stability in the extracellular space and the size-dependent penetration of extracellular spaces. These parameters come on top of the efficacy of the reagent to the target in the context of tumor biology, which can only very partially be estimated in the cell culture dish.

Reagents targeting the EGF-R are manifold. Apart from tyrosine kinase inhibitors (see Chap. 8), there is a very promising agent that is also a ligand-coupled toxin to be distributed by convection-enhanced delivery, the TGF-alpha-pseudomonas exotoxin conjugate called TP38 (Sampson et al. 2003), which has undergone a yet unpublished but promising phase II trial and awaits further development. In addition, there are unarmed antibodies that have shown efficacy via systemic administration in phase II trials (Sampson et al. 2000) and will go soon into phase III evaluation. One of these, an antibody against the EGF-receptor (nimotuzumab) has been used for pediatric brain stem glioma with some efficacy (Ramos et al. 2006) and is currently half way through a phase III.

9.6
Immunotherapy

The majority of immunotherapies are now focusing on some kind of vaccination. Autologous dendritic cells that have been pulsed with materials from human glioma tissue, be it protein extracts, whole

DNA, or other derivatives (de Vleeschouwer et al. 2006). Although already commercialized, proof of principle has not come from advanced clinical trials (Parajuli et al. 2007).

A more substantiated approach aims at the isolation of tumor-specific antigens that are already bound to an antigen-presenting protein: HSP96. After isolating and purifying this complex from the patient's tumor, it will be given back to the patient, and after being processed in dendritic cells, it will initiate an immune response (A. Parsa, personal communication).

Other strategies use specific immunogens such as the fusion peptide of the vIII variant of the EGF-R, which is present in 40–60% of patients with glioblastoma. Early trials have shown safety and anecdotal evidence of efficacy, so there are now plans for a phase III trial to follow in which the peptide will be administered in three biweekly injections starting 2 weeks after surgery followed by monthly injections thereafter until progression.

stepwise process has led to a series of early-phase clinical trials (Markert et al. 2006) but no definitive phase III trial to date.

Many other viruses are being developed to be intracranially selectively oncolytic vehicles, but the necessary proofs of principle and safety tests are time-consuming. The best example may be the poliovirus, which can be modified to lose all its neurotoxicity and be selectively intracerebrally oncolytic (Gromeier et al. 2000). With a wide spectrum of animal experiments and toxicity studies with a virus that has such a fear-instilling history, progress to early-phase clinical trials is slow, but it will most likely come in the near future.

The parvovirus H1 is also still in the stage of late animal experimentation and assessment of possible toxicity to humans, which in itself is nonpathogenic to humans and intracerebrally in orthotopic models highly selective oncolytic, so that early-phase human clinical trials should be expected (Geletneky et al. 2005).

9.7
Oncolytic Viruses

Oncolytic viruses have the advantage of being a reagent that self-replicates and therefore overcomes the problem of repeated delivery and half-life. Nevertheless, oncolytic viruses have been very promising but not yet lived up to their expectations because of complex regulatory requirements. The most promising viruses have CNS specificity, no neuronal toxicity, and selective tumor toxicity. Conditionally replicating viruses that need cellular deficiencies in the P53 or RB pathway sounded the most promising (Fueyo et al. 2003) but have not been followed up since the early studies established proof of principle. Advances have also been made in the testing of various oncolytic herpesviruses, which have been engineered to be selectively toxic to tumors. The

9.8
Gene Therapy

The concept of gene therapy had suffered a severe setback with the negative phase III trial using a retroviral strategy for the transduction of the HSV TK gene (Rainov 2000). After years of further development, another phase III clinical trial with the same transgene but based on an adenoviral delivery system is being evaluated based on promising phase II trials showing a sharp increase in survival (Immonen et al. 2004). This approach encompasses direct intraparenchymal injection of the adenovirus at multiple sites (up to 60, at a depth of 1 cm) after a surgical resection cavity is created. The adenovirus is highly infectious and the amount of virus vastly exceeds what was present in the earlier trial, which used not plain virus but rather vector-producing cells that released only very few viral particles per day. The major question around which all gene therapy concepts revolve is the unresolved delivery of any gene therapy reagent to the infiltrating cells and in this context gene therapy and stem cell biology become inseparable because stem cells with their homing capacity are genetically engineered to deliver reagents, as discussed in the next section.

9.9 Stem Cells

Normal neural stem cells derived from the rodent but also human autologous neuroglial stem cells seem to have the capacity to home in to tumor cell accumulations (Aboody et al. 2000; Glass et al. 2005). Knowing that there is a decreasing number of stem cells with age and having some evidence for a direct cytotoxic activity, there is even a hypothesis which proposes that the raised incidence of glioma in the elderly is caused by this decreasing number of stem cells (Glass et al. 2005). Such cells, appropriately modified, could therefore make an ideal vehicle to deliver therapeutics to the individually targeted infiltrating tumor cells (Ehtesham et al. 2002). So far, however, there is mainly proof of principle (homing) but little proof for the efficacious delivery of therapeutic agents. Not surprisingly, one of the early concepts for this approach is again the HSV-TK/ganciclovir system because it has already been so widely used. Using stem cells modified accordingly, ganciclovir-converting stem cells were seen to home in to orthotopically disseminated tumor cells, which also translated into prolonged survival when ganciclovir was given to the animals (Li et al. 2006). Clinical trials will nevertheless be far away because the source of stem cells, their immunological properties, or the methods to rapidly expand autologous stem cells require much more experimentation.

From the technological standpoint of available reagents, it must be expected that the first trials will use murine neural stem cells, but any further development should need to concentrate on autologous stem cells derived form the subventricular zone although other sources have been proposed (Fu et al. 2008; Hunt et al. 2008).

9.10 Final Remarks

Currently, therapy evaluations in clinical trials run parallel to the development of much more rational, discovery-based therapeutic developments. Gene expression profiling provides pathway analyses (Phillips et al. 2006) and thereby targets that are as yet completely unevaluated or underevaluated. In addition, the concept that for each tumor there may be specific tumor stem cells and that there is a persisting stem cell subpopulation (Singh et al. 2003) must lead to a reevaluation of the strategies that are employed to test for new reagents or the efficacy of any reagent, old or new. If it turns out that the genetic instability inherent to tumor cells and the resulting genetic anarchism in tumor cells once they have spun off from the stem cells makes the majority of the tumor cell masses unrepresentative of the root of the disease, then all future testing will need to include the biology of the tumor stem cells, which may be radioresistant, chemoresistant, and very different from the mass.

References

Aboody KS, Brown A, Rainov NG, Bower KA, Liu S, Yang W, Small JE, Herrlinger U, Ourednik V, Black PM, Breakefield XO, Snyder EY (2000) Neural stem cells display extensive tropism for pathology in adult brain: evidence from intracranial gliomas. Proc Natl Acad Sci USA 97: 12846–12851

Brem H, Piantadosi S, Burger PC, Walker M, Selker R, Vick NA, Black K, Sisti M, Brem S, Mohr G, et al. (1995) Placebo-controlled trial of safety and efficacy of intraoperative controlled delivery by biodegradable polymers of chemotherapy for recurrent gliomas. The Polymer-brain Tumor Treatment Group. Lancet 345:1008–1012

Comprehensive genomic characterization defines human glioblastoma genes and core pathways. (2008) Nature 455:1061–1068

de Vleeschouwer S, Rapp M, Sorg RV, Steiger HJ, Stummer W, van Gool S, Sabel M (2006) Dendritic cell vaccination in patients with malignant gliomas: current status and future directions. Neurosurgery 59:988–999; discussion 999–1000

Dickinson PJ, LeCouteur RA, Higgins RJ, Bringas JR, Roberts B, Larson, RF, Yamashita Y, Krauze M, Noble CO, Drummond D, Kirpotin DB, Park JW, Berger MS, Bankiewicz KS (2008) Canine model of convection-enhanced delivery of liposomes investigation. J Neurosurg 108:989–998

Ehtesham M, Kabos P, Kabosova A, Neuman T, Black KL, Yu JS (2002) The use of interleukin 12-secreting neural stem cells for the treatment of intracranial glioma. Cancer Res 62:5657–5663

Friedman HS, Keir S., Pegg AE, Houghton PJ, Colvin OM, Moschel RC, Bigner DD, Dolan ME (2002) O6-benzylguanine-mediated enhancement of chemotherapy. Mol Cancer Ther 1:43–948

Fueyo J, Alemany R, Gomez-Manzano C, Fuller GN, Khan A, Conrad CA, Liu TJ, Jiang H, Lemoine MG, Suzuki K, Sawaya R, Curiel DT, Yung WK, Lang FF (2003) Preclinical characterization of the antiglioma activity of a tropism-enhanced adenovirus targeted to the retinoblastoma pathway. J Natl Cancer Inst 95:652–660

Fu L, Zhu L, Huang Y, Lee TD, Forman SJ, Shih CC (2008) Derivation of neural stem cells from mesenchymal stemcells: evidence for a bipotential stem cell population. Stem Cells Dev 17:1109–1121

Geletneky K, Herrero YCM, Rommelaere J, Schlehofer JR (2005) Oncolytic potential of rodent parvoviruses for cancer therapy in humans: a brief review. J Vet Med B Infect Dis Vet Public Health 52:327–330

Glass R, Synowitz M, Kronenberg G, Walzlein JH, Markovic DS, Wang LP, Gast D, Kiwit J, Kempermann G, Kettenmann H (2005) Glioblastoma-induced attraction of endogenous neural precursor cells is associated with improved survival. J Neurosci 25:2637–2646

Goetz C, Riva P, Poepperl G, Gildehaus FJ, Hischa A, Tatsch K, Reulen HJ (2003) Locoregional radioimmunotherapy in selected patients with malignant glioma: experiences, side effects and survival times. J Neurooncol 62:321–328

Gromeier M, Lachmann S, Rosenfeld MR, Gutin PH, Wimmer E (2000) Intergeneric poliovirus recombinants for the treatment of malignant glioma. Proc Natl Acad Sci USA 97:6803–6808

Hegi ME, Diserens AC, Gorlia T, Hamou MF, de Tribolet N, Weller M, Kros JM, Hainfellner JA, Mason W, Mariani L, Bromberg JE, Hau P, Mirimanoff RO, Cairncross JG, Janzer RC, Stupp R (2005) MGMT gene silencing and benefit from temozolomide in glioblastoma. N Engl J Med 352:997–1003

Hunt DP, Morris PN, Sterling J, Anderson JA, Joannides A, Jahoda C, Compston A, Chandran S (2008) A highly enriched niche of precursor cells with neuronal and glial potential within the hair follicle dermal papilla of adult skin. Stem Cells 26:163–172

Immonen A, Vapalahti M, Tyynela K, Hurskainen H, Sandmair A, Vanninen R, Langford G, Murray N, Yla-Herttuala S (2004) AdvHSV-tk gene therapy with intravenous ganciclovir improves survival in human malignant glioma: a randomised, controlled study. Mol Ther 10:967–972

Kneifel S, Bernhardt P, Uusijarvi H, Good S, Plasswilm L, Buitrago-Tellez C, Muller-Brand J, Macke H, Merlo A (2007) Individual voxelwise dosimetry of targeted (90)Y-labelled substance P radiotherapy for malignant gliomas. Eur J Nucl Med Mol Imaging 34(9):1388–1395

Kuan CT, Wikstrand CJ, Bigner DD (2001) EGF mutant receptor vIII as a molecular target in cancer therapy. Endocr Relat Cancer 8:83–96

Kunwar S (2003) Convection enhanced delivery of IL13-PE38QQR for treatment of recurrent malignant glioma: presentation of interim findings from ongoing phase 1 studies. Acta Neurochir (Suppl 88):105–111

Kunwar S, Prados MD, Chang SM, Berger MS, Lang FF, Piepmeier JM, Sampson JH, Ram Z, Gutin PH, Gibbons RD, Aldape KD, Croteau DJ, Sherman, JW,

Puri RK (2007) Direct intracerebral delivery of cintredekin besudotox (IL13-PE38QQR) in recurrent malignant glioma: a report by the Cintredekin Besudotox Intraparenchymal Study Group. J Clin Oncol 25:837–844

Laske DW, Youle RJ, Oldfield EH (1997) Tumor regression with regional distribution of the targeted toxin TF-CRM107 in patients with malignant brain tumors. Nat Med 3:1362–1368

Li S, Gao Y, Tokuyama T, Yamamoto J, Yokota N, Yamamoto S, Terakawa S, Kitagawa M, Namba H (2006) Genetically engineered neural stem cells migrate and suppress glioma cell growth at distant intracranial sites. Cancer Lett 251(2): 220–227

Markert JM, Parker JN, Buchsbaum DJ, Grizzle WE, Gillespie GY, Whitley RJ (2006) Oncolytic HSV-1 for the treatment of brain tumours. Herpes 13:66–71

Menei P, Capelle L, Guyotat J, Fuentes S, Assaker R, Bataille B, Francois P, Dorwling-Carter D, Paquis P, Bauchet L, Parker F, Sabatier J, Faisant N, Benoit JP (2005) Local and sustained delivery of 5-fluorouracil from biodegradable microspheres for the radiosensitization of malignant glioma: a randomized phase II trial. Neurosurgery 56:242–248; discussion 242–248

Parajuli P, Mathupala S, Mittal S, Sloan AE (2007) Dendritic cell-based active specific immunotherapy for malignant glioma. Expert Opin Biol Ther 7:439–448

Phillips HS, Kharbanda S, Chen R, Forrest WF, Soriano RH, Wu TD, Misra A, Nigro JM, Colman H, Soroceanu L, Williams PM, Modrusan Z, Feuerstein BG, Aldape K (2006) Molecular subclasses of high-grade glioma predict prognosis, delineate a pattern of disease progression, and resemble stages in neurogenesis. Cancer Cell 9:157–173

Pope WB, Lai A, Nghiemphu P, Mischel P, Cloughesy TF (2006) MRI in patients with high-grade gliomas treated with bevacizumab and chemotherapy. Neurology 66:1258–1260

Rainov NG (2000) A phase III clinical evaluation of herpes simplex virus type 1 thymidine kinase and ganciclovir gene therapy as an adjuvant to surgical resection and radiation in adults with previously untreated glioblastoma multiforme. Hum Gene Ther 11:2389–2401

Ram Z, Culver KW, Oshiro EM, Viola JJ, DeVroom HL, Otto E, Long Z, Chiang Y, McGarrity GJ, Muul LM, Katz D, Blaese RM, Oldfield EH (1997) Therapy of malignant brain tumors by intratumoral implantation of retroviral vector-producing cells. Nat Med 3:1354–1361

Ramos TC, Figueredo J, Catala M, Gonzalez S, Selva JC, Cruz TM, Toledo C, Silva S, Pestano Y, Ramos M, Leonard I, Torres O, Marinello P, Perez R, Large A (2006) Treatment of high-grade glioma patients with the humanized anti-epidermal growth factor receptor (EGFR) antibody h-R3: report from a phase I/II trial. Cancer Biol Ther 5:375–379

Reardon DA, Akabani G, Coleman RE, Friedman AH, Friedman HS, Herndon JE, 2nd, Cokgor I, McLendon RE, Pegram CN, Provenzale JM, Quinn JA, Rich JN, Regalado LV, Sampson JH, Shafman TD, Wikstrand CJ, Wong TZ, Zhao XG, Zalutsky MR, Bigner DD (2002) Phase II trial of murine (131)I-labeled antitenascin monoclonal antibody 81C6 administered into surgically created resection cavities of patients with newly diagnosed malignant gliomas. J Clin Oncol 20:1389–1397

Rich JN, Bigner DD (2004) Development of novel targeted therapies in the treatment of malignant glioma. Nat Rev Drug Discov 3:430–446

Riva P, Franceschi G, Arista A, Frattarelli M, Riva N, Cremonini AM, Giuliani G, Casi M (1997) Local application of radiolabeled monoclonal antibodies in the treatment of high grade malignant gliomas: a six-year clinical experience. Cancer 80:2733–2742

Roullin VG, Mege M, Lemaire L, Cueyssac JP, Venier-Julienne MC, Menei P, Gamelin E, Benoit JP (2004) Influence of 5-fluorouracil-loaded microsphere formulation on efficient rat glioma radiosensitization. Pharm Res 21:1558–1563

Sampson JH, Akabani G, Archer GE, Bigner DD, Berger MS, Friedman AH, Friedman HS, Herndon JE, 2nd, Kunwar S, Marcus S, McLendon RE, Paolino A, Penne K, Provenzale J, Quinn J, Reardon DA, Rich J, Stenzel T, Tourt-Uhlig S, Wikstrand C, Wong T, Williams R, Yuan F, Zalutsky MR, Pastan I (2003) Progress report of a Phase I study of the intracerebral microinfusion of a recombinant chimeric protein composed of transforming growth factor (TGF)-alpha and a mutated form of the Pseudomonas exotoxin termed PE-38 (TP-38) for the treatment of malignant brain tumors. J Neurooncol 65:27–35

Sampson JH, Crotty LE, Lee S, Archer GE, Ashley DM, Wikstrand CJ, Hale LP, Small C, Dranoff G, Friedman AH, Friedman HS, Bigner DD (2000) Unarmed, tumor-specific monoclonal antibody effectively treats brain tumors. Proc Natl Acad Sci U S A 97:7503–7508

Schumacher T, Hofer S, Eichhorn K, Wasner M, Zimmerer S, Freitag P, Probst A, Gratzl O, Reubi JC, Maecke R, Mueller-Brand J, Merlo A (2002) Local injection of the 90Y-labelled peptidic vector DOTATOC to control gliomas of WHO grades II and III: an extended pilot study. Eur J Nucl Med Mol Imaging 29:486–493

Shankar S, Vaidyanathan G, Kuan CT, Bigner DD, Zalutsky MR (2006) Antiepidermal growth factor variant III scFv fragment: effect of radioiodination method on tumor targeting and normal tissue clearance. Nucl Med Biol 33:101–110

Singh SK, Clarke ID, Terasaki M, Bonn VE, Hawkins C, Squire J, Dirks PB (2003) Identification of a cancer stem cell in human brain tumors. Cancer Res 63:5821–5828

Stummer W, Pichlmeier U, Meinel T, Wiestler OD, Zanella F, Reulen HJ (2006) Fluorescence-guided surgery with 5-aminolevulinic acid for resection of malignant glioma: a randomised controlled multicentre phase III trial. Lancet Oncol 7:392–401

Stummer W, Reulen HJ, Meinel T, Pichlmeier U, Schumacher W, Tonn JC, Rohde V, Oppel F, Turowski B, Woiciechowsky C, Franz K, Pietsch T (2008) Extent of resection and survival in glioblastoma multiforme: identification of and adjustment for bias. Neurosurgery 62:564–576; discussion 564–576

Stupp R, Mason WP, van den Bent MJ, Weller M, Fisher B, Taphoorn MJ, Belanger K, Brandes AA, Marosi C, Bogdahn U, Curschmann J, Janzer RC, Ludwin SK, Gorlia T, Allgeier A, Lacombe D, Cairncross JG, Eisenhauer E, Mirimanoff RO (2005) Radiotherapy plus concomitant and adjuvant temozolomide for glioblastoma. N Engl J Med 352:987–996

Weingart J, Grossman SA, Carson KA, Fisher JD, Delaney SM, Rosenblum ML, Olivi A, Judy K, Tatter SB, Dolan ME (2007) Phase I trial of polifeprosan 20 with carmustine implant plus continuous infusion of intravenous O6-benzylguanine in adults with recurrent malignant glioma: new approaches to brain tumor therapy CNS consortium trial. J Clin Oncol 25:399–404

Westphal M, Lamszus K, Hilt D (2003) Intracavitary chemotherapy for glioblastoma: present status and future directions. Acta Neurochir Suppl 88:61–67

Yamashita Y, Krauze MT, Kawaguchi T, Noble CO, Drummond DC, Park JW, Bankiewicz KS (2007) Convection-enhanced delivery of a topoisomerase I inhibitor (nanoliposomal topotecan) and a topoisomerase II inhibitor (pegylated liposomal doxorubicin) in intracranial brain tumor xenografts. Neurooncol 9:20–28

Zalutsky MR (2005) Current status of therapy of solid tumors: brain tumor therapy. J Nucl Med 46 (Suppl1):151S–156S

Neurotoxicity of Treatment   10

Pasquale Calabrese and Uwe Schlegel

Abstract With the advent of effective treatment regimes increasing survival rates, delayed treatment-related cognitive dysfunction has been recognized as a significant problem. It is considered the most frequent complication among long-term survivors. WBRT may lead to deep brain atrophy and leukoencephalopathy associated with severe cognitive dysfunction, single-fraction dosages of greater than 2 Gy are related to an increased risk of late neurotoxicity, and other factors such as old age, concomitant chemotherapy and preexisting neurological disease increase this risk. However, the potential of focal radiotherapy (RT) with single dosages of 2 Gy or less to a maximal total dose of 60 Gy to produce significant neurotoxicity is less clear. There is a need for a concise neuropsychological test battery to be included in clinical trials, which should meet the following criteria: assess several domains found to be most sensitive to tumor and treatment effects, have standardized stimuli and administration procedures, have published normative data, have moderate to high test-retest reliability, have alternate forms or be relatively insensitive to practice effects, and therefore be suitable to monitor changes in cognitive function over time, include tests that have been translated into several languages, which can be administered by a trained psychometrician or clinical research associate under supervision of a neuropsychologist, and have a relatively short total administration time. The neuropsychological domains to be evaluated should comprise the cognitive core deficit in brain-tumor patients, namely attention, executive functions (i.e., working memory, processing speed, sequencing abilities), verbal memory, and motor speed.

10.1
Introduction

Neurological complications of RT and chemotherapy in gliomas can affect the central or (with much lesser frequency) the peripheral nervous system. Chemotherapy-related neurotoxicity in glioma treatment – with the exception of vincristine- or platinum-induced peripheral neuropathy – is rare and its incidence is difficult to determine, because chemotherapy often is given in combination with RT. RT-induced intellectual decline may have a profound impact on quality of life and becomes increasingly important because of long-term survival in patients with low-grade gliomas or with tumors of oligodendroglial histology. Therefore, cognitive function, together with response to therapy and survival is increasingly regarded an important outcome

Pasquale Calabrese (✉)
In der Schornau 23-25, 44892 Bochum, Germany
E-mail: pasquale.calabrese@rub.de

measure in patients with brain tumors, in particular in patients living long enough to face these long-term consequences.

10.2
Radiation

Radiation-induced neurological complications are classified as acute, early-delayed, or delayed radiation reaction (Rottenberg 1991). Late complications comprise radionecrosis, deep brain atrophy, and leukoencephalopathy as well as more subtle cognitive dysfunction not necessarily associated with radiomorphological changes (Armstrong et al. 2001).

In pediatric neuro-oncology, RT has long been recognized as the main cause of cognitive decline (Danoff et al. 1982). In long-term surviving patients, RT may indeed lead to cognitive deficits, or even dementia. However, in recent studies, it has been argued that focal RT in adult patients with low-grade gliomas is very well tolerated and possible cognitive dysfunction is not more frequent and not more severe than those resulting from other treatment conditions, such as the administration of antiepileptic drugs (AEDs) (Klein et al. 2002). In the following, some key studies are summarized that relate cognitive deficits as well as quality of life measures to several treatment factors in patients with gliomas.

10.3
Radiation-Induced Neurotoxicity

Timing of RT in the treatment of patients with low-grade glioma is controversial. While some studies advocate early RT, others defer RT because a survival benefit after early RT has not been shown in any randomized trial (Karim et al. 1996, 2002; Shaw et al. 2002; van den Bent et al. 2005). An important reason to delay cerebral RT is the risk of radiation-induced neurotoxicity. This is associated with radiation dose, volume, and the patient's condition as well as age, preexisting vascular disorder, other diseases, etc. (Behin et al. 2004). However, the relationship between radiation and cognitive function still is debatable: While in some studies of patients with low-grade gliomas no differences in cognitive, affective, or psychological status were observed between subjects who had been treated with focal irradiation and those who had not, more recently, leukoencephalopathy, related to deficient cognitive performance as a corollary long-term effect, was observed in patients with LGG treated with whole-brain or focal RT (Swennen et al. 2004). Kleinberg et al. (1993) used Karnofsky Performance Status, employment history, and memory function to determine the long-term impact on function of treatment for primary cerebral gliomas in adults who were alive and disease-free for more than 1 year after cranial irradiation. Of a total of 30 eligible adult patients with gliomas of different grades, 16 received partial-brain irradiation only, 12 whole-brain irradiation with a partial-brain boost, and two whole-brain irradiation only with a total dose of 54–66 Gy, a fraction size of 1.7–2.0 Gy, and the median follow-up was 3.5 years. Eighty-three percent of patients also received adjuvant chemotherapy. After the completion of irradiation, the authors found a stable Karnofsky Performance Status. At 5 years, the actuarial freedom from "performance status decline" after irradiation was 93%; the performance status was found to be increased in two patients, both within several months of completing irradiation. Most patients (68%) returned to work after irradiation: 62% remained at work 1 year later, and 58% were working at the time of the last follow-up. All working patients were employed in a capacity similar to their pre-morbid position. On the basis of this outcome, the authors concluded that in contrast to previously published reports, long-term glioma survivors maintained a relatively good performance status in the absence of recurrence and did not experience a progressive decline in neuropsychologic function after completion of cranial irradiation. However, the number of patients in each subgroup was small and patients treated with partial brain irradiation had a higher and more stable performance status, better memory function, and superior employment history. In another study by North and colleagues (North et al. 1990), 66 out of 77 patients (age range, 7 months to 72 years) with supratentorial grades I and II astrocytoma diagnosed in a 10-year-period (1975–1984), were treated with postoperative radiation therapy. The patients received a tumor dose of 50–55 Gy in 1.8-Gy fractions, five fractions per week, over 5.5–6 weeks. An overall actuarial survival at 2, 5 and 10 years of 71%, 55%, and 43%, respectively, was reported. Progression-free survival at 2, 5, and 10 years was 69%, 50%, and 39%, respectively. Survival for patients receiving postoperative radiation therapy in the range of 45–59 Gy was 78% and 66% at 2 and 5 years, respectively. Quality of life was determined at 1–2 years postoperatively, and at last follow-up (2–12 years postoperatively). The occurrence of mental retardation was specifically addressed in long-term survivors, and was observed in 50% of children. Overall, however, 80% of short-term survivors and 67% of long-term survivors were described as intellectually and physically intact, without major neurologic deficit. Laack and coworkers (Laack et al. 2005) evaluated the effects of cranial RT on cognitive function in 20 adult patients with supratentorial low-grade glioma treated with 50.4 Gy (ten patients) or 64.8 Gy (ten patients) focal RT. The patients were evaluated with an extensive battery of psychometric tests at baseline (before RT) and at approximately 18-month intervals for as long as 5 years after completing RT. To allow patients to serve as their own controls, cognitive performance was evaluated as change in scores over time. All patients underwent at least two evaluations. The baseline test scores were below average compared with age-specific norms. However, at the second evaluation, the groups' mean test scores were higher than their initial performances on all psychometric measures, although this was not statistically significant. No changes in cognitive performance were seen during the evaluation period when test scores were analyzed by age, treatment, tumor location, tumor type, or extent of resection.

10.4
Brain Atrophy

Brain atrophy is a more obvious sequelae of radiation therapy and is associated with cognitive decline. Postma and colleagues (Postma et al. 2002) detected abnormalities on computed tomography (CT) or magnetic resonance imaging (MRI) and neuropsychological performance in patients with low-grade glioma, with ($n = 23$) or without ($n = 16$) prior cerebral RT. In most of the patients receiving RT ($n = 19$), the target volume of RT encompassed the primary tumor site with a 1- to 2-cm margin; in the other four patients, WBRT with a boost to the tumor site was given. They noted cerebral atrophy in 14 of 23 patients (61%) treated with prior RT, and in one of 16 patients (6%) without prior RT. White matter abnormalities were observed in six patients, all of whom were treated with prior RT. The radiological abnormalities were correlated with cognitive performance. Additional retrospective data highlighting the detrimental effects of RT on brain volume and white matter was presented by Swennen and colleagues (Swennen et al. 2004). They evaluated the influence of radiation volume and other risk factors for the development of delayed radiation toxicity in patients treated for low-grade glioma in 41 adult patients treated with focal or WBRT. For all patients, CT and MRI scans were revised to quantify brain atrophy and white matter lesions. Medical data were reviewed concerning baseline and tumor characteristics, treatment, survival, signs, and symptoms of clinical encephalopathy and cardiovascular risk factors. An increased risk was found for brain atrophy in patients treated with WBRT [relative risk (RR), 3.1], white matter lesions (RR, 3.8) and clinical encephalopathy (RR, 4.2). An increased risk of atrophy (RR, 2.2) and white matter lesions (RR, 2.9) was also found in patients aged over 40 years. Furthermore, brain atrophy and white matter lesions were more severe in patients treated with WBRT and in older patients. In conclusion, both the incidence and the severity of abnormalities was found to be greater in patients treated with WBRT and in older patients.

10.5
The Effect of Radiation Dosage

Another variable within the domain of limited field RT is related to the dosage. One of the few prospective studies to assess the neurocognitive effects of cranial RT on patients with low-grade gliomas with high-dose versus low-dose radiation therapy was done by Brown and colleagues (Brown et al. 2003). They analyzed cognitive performance data collected in a prospective, intergroup clinical trial in 203 adults with supratentorial low-grade gliomas randomly assigned to a lower dose (50.4 Gy in 28 fractions) or a higher dose (64.8 Gy in 36 fractions) of localized RT. These authors used the Folstein Mini-Mental State Examination (MMSE) scores to evaluate cognitive function. The median follow-up was 7.4 years in 101 survivors at the time of analysis. The authors considered a change of more than three MMSE points to be clinically significant. In patients without tumor progression, they found significant deterioration from baseline to occur at years 1, 2, and 5 in 8.2%, 4.6%, and 5.3% of patients, respectively. Most patients with an abnormal baseline MMSE score (< 27) experienced significant increases. Baseline variables such as radiation dose, conformal versus conventional RT, number of radiation fields, age, sex, tumor size, neurofunctional status, seizures, and seizure medications had no predictive power for cognitive functions. Taken together, these authors found most of their low-grade glioma patients to maintain a stable neurocognitive status after focal RT as measured by the MMSE. Whereas patients with an abnormal baseline MMSE were more likely to have an improvement in cognitive abilities than deterioration after receiving RT, only a small percentage of patients had cognitive deterioration after RT. However, since the MMSE score gives only a raw picture of the cognitive status it can be argued that more discriminating neurocognitive assessment tools may have identified more subtle cognitive deficits not apparent in the MMSE total score. In this study population, Shaw and colleagues (Shaw et al. 2002) reported on radiation necrosis in seven patients, with one fatality in each treatment arm. The 2-year actuarial incidence of radiation necrosis was 2.5% with low-dose RT and 5% with high-dose RT. Taken together, the authors found somewhat lower survival and slightly higher incidence of radiation necrosis in the high-dose RT arm.

10.6
Neuropsychological Deficits Associated with Radiotherapy

In a study by Klein and co-workers (Klein et al. 2002), the authors aimed to identify the specific effects of RT on objective and self-reported cognitive function, and on cognitive deterioration over time. In their study, 195 patients with low-grade glioma (104 of whom had received RT 1–22 years previously) were compared with 100 patients harboring hematological malignancies not affecting the CNS and with 195 healthy controls. The aim of their analyses was to differentiate between the effects of the tumor (e.g., disease duration, lateralization) and treatment effects (neurosurgery, RT, AEDs) on cognitive function and on relative risk of cognitive disability. As a group, low-grade glioma patients had lower ability in all cognitive domains than did low-grade hematological patients, and did less well in comparison to healthy controls. The use of RT to the brain was associated with poorer cognitive function; however, cognitive disability in the memory domain was found only in RT patients who received single-fraction doses exceeding 2 Gy. Moreover, additional AED use was also strongly associated with disability in attentional and executive function. The authors interpreted their findings imputing the tumor itself to have the most deleterious effect on cognitive function and that RT mainly resulted in additional long-term cognitive disability only when high-fraction doses are used. In addition, the effects of other medical factors, especially AED use, were prone to have additional detrimental effects on cognition. However, an extended observation of this study group with repeated measurements over a 6-year period revealed that irradiated patients showed a significant long-term decline in cognitive functions in nearly all domains investigated, a finding not restricted to patients treated with greater than 2-Gy fraction doses (Klein et al. 2006). Thus, in contrast to their previous notion, the authors concluded that neurocognitive deterioration might not be restricted to a subpopulation of patients who received high-fraction doses of brain irradiation.

10.7
Quality of Life After Radiotherapy

Another study examining the impact of RT on quality of life in long-term survivors of biopsy-proven low-grade gliomas without signs of tumor recurrence was conducted by Taphoorn and coworkers (Taphoorn et al. 1994). Twenty patients (age range, 18–66 years) were treated with early focal RT; the other 21 patients (age range, 19–65 years) underwent surgery or biopsy only. The interval from diagnosis to testing ranged from 1 to 12 years (mean, 3.5 years). Nineteen patients with low-grade hematological malignancies, surviving 1–15 years without central nervous system involvement, served as control subjects. Besides neurological and functional status, the patients were also examined neuropsychologically. None of the survivors was found to have significant neurological impairment and the Karnofsky index for them was at least 70. However, more subtle tests indicated that, compared to the control subjects, the patients with low-grade gliomas had significantly more cognitive disturbances and suffered more frequently from fatigue and depressed moods. Moreover, the two groups with low-grade gliomas (with RT vs. no RT) did not differ significantly on any of these measures. The authors concluded that RT did not cause these disturbances and had no negative impact on quality of life in these patients.

The beneficial effects concerning focused irradiation and the masking effect of shorter study periods are corroborated by a prospective study of Vigliani and co-workers (1996) conducted on 17 patients who underwent conventional limited-field RT for a low-grade glioma or for good-prognosis anaplastic glioma. The results were compared with 14 control patients with low-grade gliomas who did not receive RT. The authors found a significant transient decrease of reaction-time performances at 6 months in the irradiated group with return to baseline values 12 months after RT. Subsequently, no other significant changes were observed over a 48-month follow-up period in the irradiated and nonirradiated groups. However, when the scores of each patient were considered longitudinally, one irradiated patient (5.8%) experienced progressive deterioration, while two irradiated patients

(11.7%) improved. Individual changes did not occur in the control group. The results were interpreted as being suggestive of a transient early-delayed drop of neuropsychological performances at 6 months after limited-field conventional RT and an overall low risk of long-term cognitive dysfunction after irradiation when it is administered alone in young adults.

By using more extended time points of behavioral analysis, Armstrong and colleagues (Armstrong et al. 1995) were able to identify some early-delayed effects and to separate those from late-delayed effects of partial-brain RT for patients with supratentorial brain tumors with favorable histology. This was achieved by including baseline measures and the use of subjects as their own controls on a wide range of neurobehavioral domains. Ten neuropsychologic domains were measured in 12 patients at baseline (after surgery and immediately before initiation of RT), and followed every 3 months for 1 year. Four to six patients were examined at 2 and 3 years after baseline. Patients were impaired at baseline compared with controls only in visual memory and sentence recall, but demonstrated significant improvement in visual memory by 2 years after baseline. Speed of processing information also showed a slope of improvement over 2 years. Retrieval from verbal long-term memory was impaired at 1.5 months after completion of RT, but recovered to baseline levels by 1 year. Interestingly, when looking at 2 years after baseline, long-term memory retrieval demonstrated a decline, but remained unchanged at 3 years. Taken together, by considering sensitive neurobehavioral measures the authors were able to demonstrate differential effects of RT, namely a decrement with rebound during the early-delayed period followed by a long-term decline again at 2 years after baseline. The authors discuss their findings with reference to demyelination followed by remyelination. Moreover, their neuropsychological approach suggests that memory retrieval may be the earliest marker of late-delayed effects. Their findings were corroborated by a consecutive study on a total of 26 patients (Armstrong et al. 2002) with an extended follow-up period. While seven of 37 neuropsychological indices showed an improvement over a 6-year period, there were selective cognitive declines in the memory domain after 5 years. Again, these findings were interpreted on the basis of a selective hippocampal vulnerability to late-delayed RT effects.

10.8 Other Treatment-Related Parameters Influencing Cognitive Function

The effect of other treatment-related factors was further substantiated in an additional analysis by Klein and associates (Klein et al. 2003). One hundred fifty-six low-grade glioma patients without clinical or radiological signs of tumor recurrence for at least 1 year after histological diagnosis and with an epilepsy burden (based on seizure frequency and AED use) ranging from none to severe were compared with healthy controls. The association between epilepsy burden and cognition/health-related quality of life (HRQoL) was also investigated. Eighty-six percent of the patients had epilepsy and 50% of those using AEDs actually were seizure-free. Compared with healthy controls, glioma patients had significant reductions in information processing speed, psychomotor function, attentional functioning, verbal and working memory, executive functioning, and HRQoL. In their analysis, the increase in epilepsy burden that was associated with significant reductions in all cognitive domains except for attentional and memory functioning could primarily be attributed to the use of AEDs, whereas the decline in HRQoL could be ascribed to the lack of complete seizure control. The authors concluded that low-grade glioma patients show multiple cognitive problems that are aggravated by the severity of epilepsy and by the intensity of the treatment.

apy, disease duration, and antiepileptic treatment contributed to mild cognitive difficulties in LGG patients.

10.9 Radiotherapy and Chemotherapy

Controversial results have been reported concerning the role of RT and chemotherapy in the treatment of low-grade gliomas and their effect on survival and the development of neurotoxicity. This issue was addressed in a recent study conducted by Correa and co-workers (Correa et al. 2006). They assessed cognitive functioning in 40 patients with low-grade gliomas who received conformal radiation therapy (RT), chemotherapy, or no treatment; 16 patients had RT ± chemotherapy, and 24 patients had no treatment. All patients underwent a neuropsychological evaluation. APOE genotype was obtained in 36 patients who were classified in two groups based on the presence or absence of at least one apolipoprotein E ε4 (APOE ε4) allele. The authors found that treated patients had lower scores than untreated patients on several cognitive domains; patients who completed treatment at intervals greater than 3 years and had long disease duration had significantly lower scores on the nonverbal memory domain. Moreover, antiepileptic multitherapy, treatment history, and disease duration jointly contributed to low psychomotor domain scores. While 62% of treated patients showed white matter confluence on MRI, such changes were only apparent in 9% of the untreated patients. Preliminary comparisons between APOE ε4 carriers ($n = 9$) and noncarriers ($n = 27$) on cognitive domain scores revealed no statistically significant differences, but APOE ε4 carriers had lower mean scores on the verbal memory domain than did non-ε4 carriers. The authors concluded that RT ± chemother-

10.10 Conclusions

Cognitive disturbances have been described in most studies analyzing long-term outcomes of patients with low-grade gliomas. While there is little doubt that WBRT may lead to deep brain atrophy and leukoencephalopathy associated with severe cognitive dysfunction, that single fraction dosages over 2 Gy are related to an increased risk of late neurotoxicity and that other factors such as old age, concomitant chemotherapy and preexisting neurological disease increase this risk, the potential of focal RT with single dosages of 2 Gy or less to a maximal total dose of 60 Gy to produce significant neurotoxicity is less clear. Studies aimed at analyzing the specific cognitive deficits in this population report that the main effects are exerted in the areas of cognitive speed, memory, and flexibility. These disturbances are related to multiple factors including the effects of the tumor itself, age, and the delayed effects of treatment with WBRT and chemotherapy, either combined or alone. With the advent of effective treatment regimes increasing survival rates, delayed treatment-related cognitive dysfunction has been recognized as a significant problem. Neurotoxicity is considered the most frequent complication among long-term survivors, and may interfere with the patient's ability to function at premorbid levels professionally and socially, despite adequate disease control. However, the specific contribution of the disease itself and various treatment modalities to cognitive dysfunction remains to be elucidated, as the neurotoxic potential of combined treatments is difficult to determine since each can produce CNS damage alone. Although it is argued that studies on the cognitive effects of treatment of these patients with a good prognosis should be strongly encouraged, caution is warranted against the overuse of cognitive batteries not specifically designed to tap the cognitive core deficit of these patient groups. This argument might be exemplified by the above-mentioned study of Brown and colleagues (Brown et al. 2003) using the Mini-Mental Status Examination to screen for cognitive dysfunctions in low-grade glioma patients. Since the MMSE was intended to assist older psychiatric residents in the cognitive part of the mental status exam and was meant to be used for the diagnosis of more advanced stages of dementia, it is not surprising that more subtle cognitive deterioration in tumor patients were not detected or were not detectable. In addition, variables such as formal education and language problems must also be considered since differences in educational level or in the incidence of aphasia between patient groups may substantially influence the outcomes if not corrected for these factors in their statistical analyses. Conversely, when using tests not specifically constructed to address the cognitive core deficit expressed by these patients, subjects who are highly educated may get a maximum score even though clinically they are severely affected. Furthermore, some studies used several scales that assess neurologic function as well as cognition (e.g., language and visuospatial abilities) to describe cognitive domains. This argument can again be exemplified in the study by Brown et al. (2003). Since in this study, at each key evaluation, patients were classified as progressors or non-progressors according to their neurologic status, predictably, Brown et al. reported the worst neurologic status in patients with abnormal MMSE scores. In fact, this was the only patient characteristic that showed a statistically significant difference between the two groups. Consequently, Brown et al. found evidence for cognitive deterioration after RT in only a small percentage of patients. Given its limited sensitivity, their documented declines on the MMSE may be underestimates of the proportion of patients with true declines: potential subtle negative effects of RT on cognition, if present at all, may have been missed. RT in glioma patients may give rise to subcortical white matter changes that are associated with behavioral slowing. If cognitive items that have no time constraints are used, this effect might also have contributed to the lack of a clear trend toward cognitive worsening after RT in a significant proportion of patients or might at least have led to an underestimation of the actual radiation effects. These aspects call for using more sophisticated and discriminating neurocognitive assessment tools.

10.11 Proposed Neuropsychological and Quality of Life Test Battery

Recognizing the relevance of cognition and quality of life in tumor patients, there is a need for a concise neuropsychological test battery to be included in clinical trials. This battery should meet the following criteria:

1. Assess several domains found to be most sensitive to tumor and treatment effects
2. Have standardized materials and administration procedures
3. Have published normative data
4. Have moderate to high test-retest reliability
5. Have alternate forms or be relatively insensitive to practice effects, and therefore be suitable to monitor changes in cognitive function over time
6. Include tests that have been translated into several languages
7. Can be administered by a trained psychometrician or clinical research associate under supervision of a neuropsychologist
8. Have a relatively short total administration time

The neuropsychological domains to be evaluated should include those areas that represent the cognitive core deficit in brain-tumor patients, namely attention, executive functions (i.e., working memory, processing speed, sequencing abilities), verbal memory, and motor speed. By doing so, it is important to include tests that are not confounded by motor difficulties, since a significant number of tumor patients have psychomotor slowing. According to an expert consensus, the suggested definition of cognitive impairment to be used in clinical trials is a test score ≥ 1.5 standard deviations worse than the mean of a given test's normative age-adjusted distribution, and if possible gender- and education-adjusted distribution.

An estimate of premorbid intellectual ability is relevant, as neuropsychological test results are often interpreted in the context of premorbid capacity. This can be derived from educational level and occupation status, and regression formulas based on demographic variables can be used in circumstances in which estimates based on literacy are not appropriate. In addition, self-report scales to assess the impact of disease and treatment on the patient's quality of life and activities of daily living are important components of the evaluation. Time points for assessment intervals for patients enrolled in prospective clinical trials should be standardized. If possible, the initial cognitive evaluation should be performed at diagnosis and prior to initiation of treatment. Follow-up assessments should be conducted in patients with a CR at approximately 6-month intervals following treatment completion for the initial 2 years. Subsequent to year 2, evaluations can be performed on an annual basis. These intervals are suggested in part to minimize patient attrition and the impact of practice effects, and to have consistency across studies for purposes of comparison. Patients should not be assessed during treatment unless there is evidence of acute psychiatric disturbances. In case of relapse, the follow-up cognitive assessment should be postponed to approximately 6 months after a CR to the salvage treatment.

In conclusion, the administration of the same test-battery at comparable follow-up time intervals to a large number of patients involved in collaborative trials would allow for a more accurate assessment of both disease and treatment effects on cognition.

References

Armstrong CL, Ruffer J, Corn B, et al. (1995) Biphasic patterns of memory deficits following moderate-dose partial-brain irradiation: neuropsychologic outcome and proposed mechanisms. J Clin Oncol 13:2263–2271

Armstrong CL, Stern CH, Corn BW (2001) Memory performance used to detect effects on cognitive functioning. Appl Neuropsych 8:129–139

Behin A, Delattre JY (2004) Complications of radiation therapy on the brain and spinal cord. Semin Neurol 24:405–17

Brown PD, Buckner JC, Uhm JH (2003) The neurocognitive effects of radiation in adult low-grade glioma patients. Neurooncology 5:161–167

Brown PD, Buckner JC, O'Fallon JR, et al. (2003) Effects of radiotherapy on cognitive function in patiens with low-grade glioma measured by the Folstein Mini-Mental State examination. J Clin Oncol 21:2519–2524

Byrne T (2005) Cognitive sequelae of brain tumor treatment. Curr Opin Neurol 18:662–666

Correa DD, De Angelis LM, Shi W, et al. (2006) Cognitive functions in low-grade gliomas: disease and treatment effects. J Neurooncol Jul 19; [Epub ahead of print]

Danoff BF, Cowchock S, Marquette C, et al. (1982) Assessment of the long-term effects of primary radiation therapy for brain tumours in children. Cancer 49:1580–1586

Gregor A, Cull A, Traynor E, et al. (1996) Neuropsychometric evaluation of adult brain tumours: relationship with tumour and treatment parameters. Radiother Oncol 41:55–59

Karim AB, Maat B, Hatlevoll R, et al. (1996) A randomized trial on dose-response in radiation therapy of low-grade cerebral glioma: European Organization for Research and Treatment of Cancer (EORTC) Study 22844. Int J Radiat Oncol Biol Phys 36:549–556

Karim AB, Afra D, Cornu P, et al. (2002) Randomized trial on the efficacy of radiotherapy for cerebral low-grade glioma in the adult: European Organization for research and treatment of Cancer Study 22845 with the Medical Research Council study BRO4: an interim analysis. Int J Radiat Oncol Biol Phys 52:316–324

Klein M, Heimans JJ, Aaronson NK, et al. (2002) Effect of radiotherapy and other treatment- related factors on mid-term to long-term cognitive sequelae in low-grade gliomas: a comparative study. Lancet 360:1361–1368

Klein M, Engelberts NHJ, van der Ploeg HM et al. (2003) Epilepsy in low-grade gliomas: the impact on cognitive function and quality of life. Ann Neurol 54:514–520

Klein M, Fagel S, Taphoorn MJB, et al. (2006) Neurocognitive functioning in long-term low-grade glioma survivors: a six-year follow-up study. Presented at the 7th congress of the European Association for Neurooncology (EANO), Vienna, Austria

Kleinberg L, Wallner K, Malkin MG (1993) Good performance status of long-term disease-free survivors of intracranial gliomas. Int J Radiat Oncol Biol Phys 26:129–133

Laack NN, Brown PD, Ivnik RJ, et al. (2005) Cognitive function after radiotherapy for supratentorial low-grade glioma: a north central cancer treatment group prospective study. Int J Radiat Oncol Biol Phys 63:1175–1183

North CA, North RB, Epstein JA, et al. (1990) Low grade cerebral astrocytomas. Cancer 66:6–14

Postma TJ, Klein M, Verstappen CC, et al. (2002) Radiotherapy-induced cerebral abnormalities in patients with low-grade glioma. Neurology 59:121–123

Rottenberg D (1991) Acute and chronic effects of radiation therapy on the nervous system. In: Rottenberg D (ed) Neurological complications of cancer treatment. Butterworth-Heineman, Boston, pp 3–18

Shaw E, Arusell R, Scheithauer B, et al. (2002) Prospective randomized trial of low- versus high-dose radiation therapy in adults with supratentorial low-grade glioma: initial report of a North Central Cancer Treatment Group/Radiation Therapy Oncology Group/Eastern Cooperative Oncology Group study. J Clin Oncol 20:2267–2276

Taphoorn MJB, Klein M, Schiphorst A, et al. (1994) Cognitive functions and quality of life in Patients with low-grade gliomas: the impact of radiotherapy. Ann Neurol 36:48–54

Van den Bent MJ, Afra D, de Witte O et al. (2005) Long-term efficacy of early versus delayed radiotherapy for low-grade astrocytoma and oligodendroglioma in adults: the EORTC 22845 randomised trial. Lancet 366:985–990

Vigliani MC, Sichez N, Poisson M, Delattre JY (1996) A prospective study of cognitive functions following conventional radiotherapy for supratentorial gliomas in young adults: 4-year results. Int J Rad Oncol Biol Phys 35:527–533

Neuroimaging

R. Klingebiel and G. Bohner

Abstract Neuroimaging plays a crucial role in establishing the diagnosis, planning the therapy, as well as evaluating therapeutic effects and detecting early recurrence in brain tumors. It has evolved from a morphology-driven discipline to the multimodal assessment of CNS lesions, incorporating biochemistry (e.g., indicators of cell membrane synthesis) as well as physiologic parameters (e.g., hemodynamic variables).

Tumor cellularity, metabolism, and angiogenesis are important predictors for tumor grading, therapy, and prognosis, all of which are provided by dedicated use of advanced magnetic resonance imaging (MRI) techniques by the neuroradiologist.

Unprecedented views of tumor-affected brain cytoarchitecture are yielded by diffusion tensor imaging and tractography, discriminating between displacement and infiltration of highly relevant white matter tracts and guiding the neurosurgeon's CNS approach.

Functional MRI (fMRI) visualizes the spatial relationship between functionally important areas and the tumor site.

Many of these techniques use superimposition on high-anatomic-resolution MR images within the submillimeter range, in order to assure precise stereotactic proceedings. Yet, the borders of neuroimaging are subject to constant updating.

Molecular imaging has become one of the most promising research areas, as the molecular fingerprint of the tumor is required for targeting chemotherapy-resistant, migrating glial tumor cells.

11.1
Introduction

Of all imaging devices available to the neuroradiologist such as conventional x-ray, color Doppler sonography, digital subtraction angiography (DSA), and the two major cross-sectional imaging modalities, magnetic resonance imaging (MRI) and computed tomography (CT), MRI and CT are by far the most important imaging techniques with respect to glioma assessment.

With the advent of MRI, computed tomography of the central nervous system has lost its importance, mainly because of the superior soft tissue contrast provided by MRI (Fig. 11.1), enabling detailed and sensitive evaluation of various CNS pathologies.

Since CNS lesions of different origins may show similar morphological changes in MRI, morphology does not necessarily predict the type of lesion, histological grading, and/or tumor growth; thus so-called advanced MRI techniques have gained increasing importance (Fig. 11.2).

R. Klingebiel (✉)
Department of Neuroradiology
Charité-Universitätsmedizin Berlin
Charitéplatz 1
10117 Berlin
Germany
E-mail: Randolf.klingebiel@charite.de

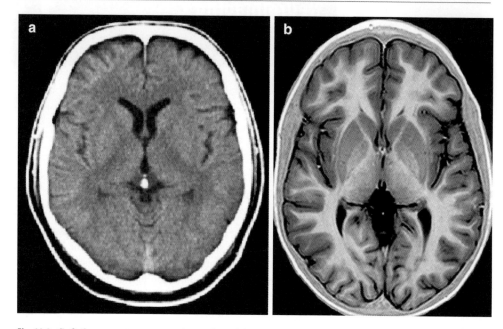

Fig. 11.1 Soft tissue contrast comparison of cranial CT (**a**) and MRI (**b**) at corresponding levels. MRI (TIR sequence) clearly shows superior gray to white matter differentiation, as compared to CT, and closely approximates that of an anatomic specimen

These techniques comprise MR spectroscopy, diffusion- and perfusion-weighted imaging, and diffusion tensor imaging, among others.

With respect to tumor imaging, CT has regained some importance with the introduction of multi-slice CT (MSCT) at the turn of the century. MSCT, compared to single-slice CT, provides technically improved perfusion imaging as well as detailed cerebrovascular imaging, both available in an emergency room setting (Fig. 11.3). Yet, MRI remains the first-line modality for basic and advanced tumor imaging and will be discussed in more detail in the following sections.

11.2
MRI and CT – Technique

11.2.1
MRI – General Aspects

As mentioned above, the superior soft tissue contrast of MRI has made this technique the first-line modality for brain-tumor imaging. The major goals of this technique are the detection and characterization of CNS lesions, their differentiation, predominantly with respect to their potentially ischemic, neoplastic, or inflammatory pathogenesis, their intracerebral and intra- and extracranial extension, therapeutic tumor control, and assessment of therapy-associated parenchymal side effects.

Yet, challenges to brain-tumor imaging have changed as much as therapeutic options and tumor targeting have progressed. With the increasing precision of radiotherapeutic and neurosurgical modalities, i.e., stereotactic radiation as well as brain biopsy, the accurate definition of various histologically different tumor areas (i.e., low- and high-grade malignant tumors) has become an important issue. Moreover, recently introduced dose-modulated radiation therapy combines the option of high-dose therapy in dedifferentiated tumor areas and moderate- to low-dose radiation in the tumor border zone, thus increasing therapeutic success and decreasing

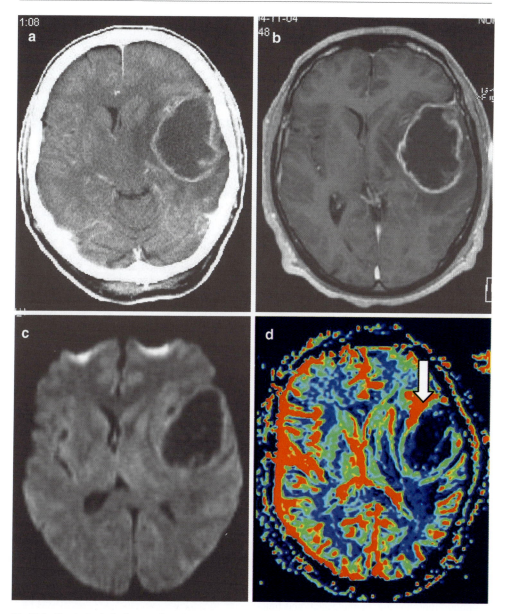

Fig. 11.2 Cystic brain lesion, easily mistaken for an abscess on contrast-enhanced CT (**a**) and MR (**b**) scans. Yet, advanced MR techniques such as diffusion imaging (**c**) and perfusion imaging (cerebral blood volume map; CBV) exclude an abscess. The CBV map shows the hypervascularized margin (*arrow*) of this CNS neoplasm (supratentorial PNET)

side effects that might further compromise quality of life in tumor patients.

Advanced MRI techniques can assess regional differences in cerebral blood volume (reflecting neoangiogenesis), permeability of tumor vessels (indicating the degree of tumor growth), cellular density (corresponding to the grade of tumor differentiation), regional distribution of bio-

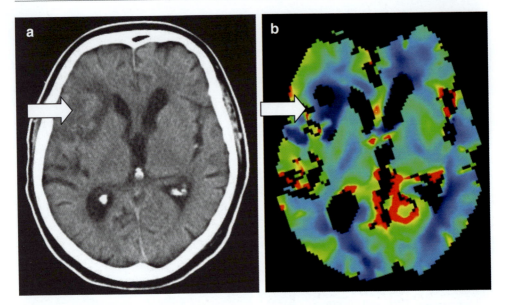

Fig. 11.3 Unenhanced CT (**a**) in this 72-year-old patient shows irregular densities in the right frontal lobe (*arrow*), along with an equivocal clinical history compatible with a neoplastic process as well as an ischemia. Perfusion CT (**b**; cerebral blood volume map) clarifies the issue by showing a hypovascularized process, indicating ischemia

chemical markers (i.e., choline as a marker for cell membrane synthesis) and the spatial relationship between functionally relevant areas (such as cortical speech areas or the corticospinal tract) and the tumor-infiltrated brain parenchyma.

Questions that arise once the diagnosis has been established and tumor therapy has been accomplished are not less demanding: differentiation of therapy-associated side effects such as radiation necrosis with reactive border zone inflammation from peripheral tumor recurrence or even tumor persistence is another major challenge to the neuroradiologist.

Therefore, up-to-date CNS tumor imaging combines morphologic, biomolecular, and functional imaging to meet the requirements raised by advances at all stages of glioma management.

Since nuclear medicine is not a genuine neuroradiologic imaging modality, it will only be briefly addressed in this chapter.

Positron emission tomography (PET) has been clinically proven in the context of glioma management, using scintigraphic markers bound to glucose to assess lesion metabolism. This technique with a high sensitivity for metabolically active lesions is hampered by limitations in specificity and spatial resolution.

PET-CT, a recently introduced combined scanner modality, provides exact coupling of scintigraphic and computer tomographic images, thus counteracting the resolution limitations of PET.

Following a short introduction into the various principles and techniques applied in cross-sectional glioma imaging, the major clinical questions and neuroradiologic proceedings will be addressed with respect to detection, diagnosis, therapy planning, and posttherapeutic CNS assessment.

11.2.2
Imaging Technique

11.2.2.1
Computed Tomography

The history of CT in CNS imaging dates back to the 1970s, when this technique was introduced into clinical imaging. Since CT is based on the attenuation of x-rays, it suffers from methodological restrictions with respect to soft tissue contrast.

In 1999, multislice CT (MSCT) renewed the interest in computed tomography because higher resolution, increased scan speed, and extended scan length were all provided by this technique, opening up new diagnostic fields to CT. In glioma imaging, MSCT might be of use for perfusion imaging purposes (Fig. 11.3), detection of calcifications or tumor hemorrhage (Fig. 11.4a, b), cellular density (Fig. 11.4c), and characteristic tumor morphology, as in the case of a butterfly glioblastoma (Fig. 11.4d), evaluation of tumor-adherent osseous changes, arterial tumor supply, and short-term follow-up subsequent to neurosurgical and/or radiosurgical intervention.

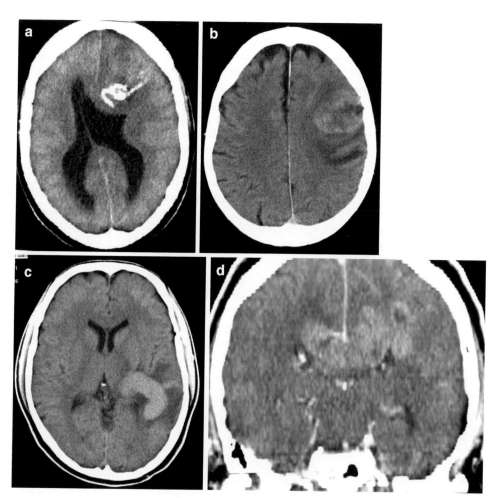

Fig. 11.4 Various aspects in CNS tumor assessment which are covered by MSCT. **a** Unenhanced CT scan of a left frontal tumor with calcifications and extension into the callosal genu, suggesting oligidendroglioma. **b** Glioblastoma showing hemorrhagic transformation. **c** Unenhanced scan of a left-sided hyperdense lesion with perifocal edema, suggesting lymphoma (high cellularity) rather than glioma (biopsy proven). **d** Coronal CT reconstruction, showing the virtually pathognomonic morphology of a butterfly glioblastoma, extending across the callosal body

As most health systems across Europe face increasing economic pressures, appropriate use of MSCT might significantly accelerate diagnostic and therapeutic processes in patients with equivocal clinical history and physical examination, thus cutting down individual healthcare costs.

11.2.2.2
Magnetic Resonance Tomography

MRI today comprises numerous data acquisition and postprocessing techniques, the detailed presentation of which is beyond the scope of this chapter. Although all signals are derived from hydrogen protons, protons may respond differently to the so-called pulse sequences depending on their molecular environment. A pulse sequence is a precisely defined sequence of electromagnetic waves applied by a coil, which usually also serves as a receiver, and the corresponding signal read-out.

Gradients allow the spatial localization of the receiver signal, the strength of which (signal intensity) depends on the tissue examined by the chosen sequences and transferred into gray-scaled picture elements (pixels).

Two sequences are most widely used, T1- and T2-weighted, meaning that these measurements are tailored to receive a strong signal from tissues depending on their T1/T2 constant. T1 and T2 are time constants defining the tendency of tissue to return to its former state of magnetization, once the exciting pulse is turned off.

Introducing inversion recovery sequences made it possible to suppress free water protons, for example in CSF or cystic lesions, and enhance the visualization of interstitial water, such as within the tumor as well as the perifocal edema (Fig. 11.5a, b).

Gradient-echo sequences considerably shorten acquisition times and allow 3D imaging, meaning contiguous high-resolution imaging of a lesion rather than slice-by-slice visualization (Fig. 11.5c). These 3D measurements are now indispensable for diagnostic and therapeutic stereotactic interventions.

Pre- and post-contrast-enhanced scans are mandatory for visualizing blood–brain barrier breakdown in various CNS pathologies, such as high-grade gliomas. The contrast media applied (i.e., gadolinium) increase local T1 tissue relaxivity subsequent to vessel leakage, thus requiring T1-weighed scans before and after i.v. contrast medium application for appropriate lesion depiction.

As far as differentiation of morphologically and clinically equivocal CNS lesions are concerned from non-neoplastic lesions as well as the approximative glioma grading, MR spectroscopy has proven to be of considerable value. Again, protons respond slightly differently to

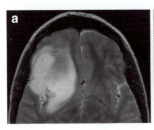 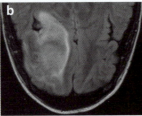 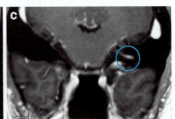

Fig. 11.5 Supplementary MRI techniques for improved and detailed morphologic tumor depiction (**a, b**) T2-weighted compared to fluid-attenuated inversion recovery image (FLAIR). FLAIR does allow better differentiation of CSF (*arrow*) and perifocal edema. **c** High-resolution T1-weighted gradient echo image in a patient with glioblastoma seeding into the subarachnoidal space. Subtle enhancement within the internal acoustic meatus on the right side (circle) as well as ependymal enhancement in the fourth ventricle are noted

the electromagnetic excitation, depending on their molecular environment. Using these differences, the resonance of specific marker molecules (choline, n-acetyl-aspartate, lactate, etc.) can be differentiated, like taking a noninvasive brain sample and analyzing its biomolecular content.

With aggressive, rapidly growing neoplastic lesions, the high cell membrane synthesis rate is essential, leading to an increase in choline in the tissue (Fig. 11.6a–c). Choline can thus be used as a marker molecule for neoplastic lesions and the degree of choline increase has been suggested to reflect the degree of histologic tumor grading. Typically, gliomas show an increase in the choline-to-creatine ratio (creatine is used as a reference value because it remains stable in most disease processes). In contrast, inflammatory CNS and ischemic lesions tend to show prominent lactate peaks.

MR spectroscopy (MRS) might be performed using different repetition times as well as single- or multivoxel techniques. Multivoxel imaging might be viewed as rolling out a voxel carpet at the very brain level and is more suitable when infiltrative lesion extension has to be assessed in otherwise normal-looking brain parenchyma (Fig. 11.7a, b). So-called parameter maps which color-code the concentrations of the target mol-

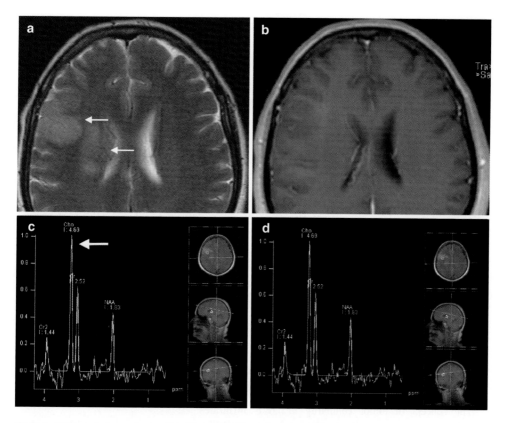

Fig. 11.6 MR spectroscopy in an astrocytoma (WHO grade III). An ill-defined lesion is depicted in the right frontal lobe (**a**; T2-weighted) without significant enhancement in the T1-weighted image (**b**). **c** MR spectroscopy clearly shows a tumor spectrum with a marked increased in choline (*arrow*) as compared to the reference voxel from the same hemisphere in the same patient (**d**)

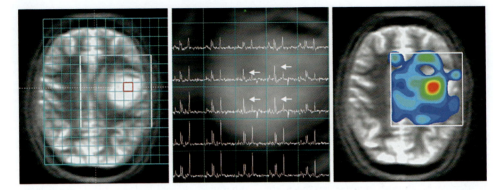

Fig. 11.7 MR spectroscopy, using the multivoxel technique (chemical shift imaging). **a** Multivoxel rectangle placed across the lesion. **b** Magnified lesion voxels, showing increased choline levels (*arrows*). **c** Choline/creatine ratio map, outlining intralesional areas of increased metabolism with respect to cell membrane synthesis

ecule enable visualization of areas of increased tumor metabolism (Fig. 11.7c).

Diffusion-weighted imaging (DWI) is well known for its ability to nearly immediately visualize irreversible brain ischemia, in other words stroke. The reason for this is that in irreversible hypoxic tissue damage, the cell membrane ion pump breaks down due to ATP deficiency and water influx causes a cytotoxic edema. Cytotoxic edema increases the total intracellular space and decreases the volume of the extracellular space, which in turn keeps the hydrogen protons from following their random movement (Brownian motion). Since freely moving protons are suppressed in DWI, only protons with restricted Brownian motion yield a signal, outlining the infarct core.

With respect to glioma imaging, DWI, including its derived parameter maps (the so-called apparent diffusion coefficient), has been suggested for evaluating tumor cellularity, differentiating postoperative injury from tumor recurrence and separating vasogenic from infiltrative edema.

The concept of tumor cellularity in DWI resembles that used for explaining DWI changes in stroke; higher cellularity means less extracellular space and subsequent diffusion restriction. Whereas this hypothesis was supported in non-glial, well-circumscribed tumors such as lymphomas (Fig. 11.8a), gliomas, especially WHO grade III–IV tumors (Fig. 11.8b), do not seem to be a useful target for DWI-driven assessment, largely because of their heterogeneous histological constitution.

Recent studies suggest that immediate collection of DWI data in the postoperative phase differentiate later-appearing contrast enhancement from tumor recurrence. Restricted diffusion postoperatively in this context is considered as a sequela of direct surgical trauma, retraction, and tumor devascularization. In this area of diffusion restriction, enhancing parenchyma in follow-up studies represents a physiologic process and is not a sign of therapy failure that could prompt more aggressive therapy.

Given that high-grade gliomas are particularly well known for their infiltrative growth, it has been speculated that diffusion should be restricted in T2-hyperintense areas of pure vasogenic edema as compared to edematous tissue with interposed tumor cells. Yet, spatial resolution of DWI is clearly not high enough to detect sometimes microscopically subtle tumor infiltrates.

Diffusion tensor imaging (DTI), including white matter tractography (Fig. 11.9) is different from DWI because directionally dependent diffusion, for example along the long axes of axonal bundles such as the corticospinal tract, is the

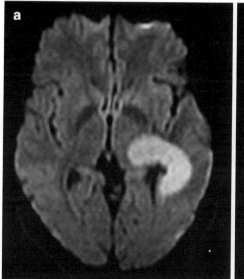 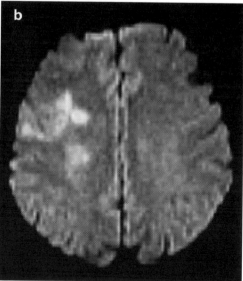

Fig. 11.8 Tumor cellularity assessed by DWI (b = 1000). Lymphoma (**a**) with high cellularity and diffusion restriction as compared to WHO grade III astrocytoma (**b**) The more aggressive tumor shows less intense and less homogeneous diffusion restriction than the lymphoma

target of imaging. This directional diffusion, also called anisotropic diffusion, seems to be caused by the myelin sheath as well as axonal components (neurofilaments, etc.) and is defined on a pixel-by-pixel basis with respect to direction and magnitude (Fig. 11.9a). Color-coding direction and magnitude (Fig. 11.9b) creates unprecedented images of the cerebral cytoarchitecture (Fig. 11.9c) and has proven to be of significant clinical value in visualizing white matter tract affection by neoplastic lesions, i.e., differentiating displaced from infiltrated tracts (Fig. 11.9d). Furthermore, undesirable injury to functionally important, dislocated tracts might be avoided by feeding these data into high-resolution 3D MRI data of the brain for stereotactic guidance.

Finally, brain perfusion imaging, referring to one of the key concepts in tumor research, i.e., tumor angiogenesis, has gained tremendous attention. Malignancy, grading, and prognosis in gliomas all are to some degree reflected by the degree of angiogenesis and capillary permeability. Several studies have underlined that a statistically relevant correlation exists between histopathologic tumor grading of astrocytomas and the most relevant perfusion parameter in this context, the regional cerebral blood volume (rCBV).

Elucidation of the complex representation of cerebral perfusion dynamics within various models applied is beyond the scope of this chapter. Basically, two methods have to be differentiated, the dynamic susceptibility contrast (DSC) MR perfusion and the dynamic contrast-enhanced perfusion (DCE) technique, the latter one derived from a T1-weighted signal increase using contrast medium-induced T1 shortening, the first one based on a signal decrease on $T2^*$ weighted images by contrast medium-induced susceptibility effect.

The most widely used MRI perfusion parameters are rCBV and the transfer constant K^{trans}, the latter being a marker of neovascular permeability derived from DCE MRI.

Quantitative estimates of endothelial permeability have been shown to correlate with tumor

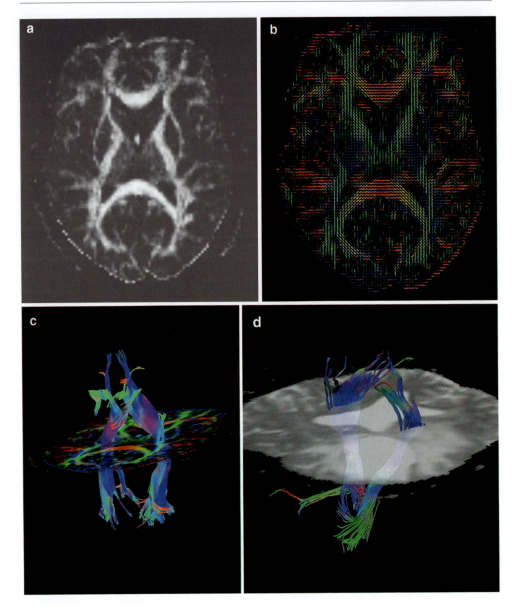

Fig. 11.9 Diffusion tensor imaging and tractography. Directional diffusion maps are established (**a**) and color-coded according to the diffusion direction (**b**). By following axonal bundles of the same color-coding, i.e., direction, tractographic images are obtained (**c**). **d** Clinical DTI application in a patient with glioblastoma preceding neurosurgical intervention. The corticospinal tract is displaced anteromedially rather than infiltrated and glioma cells

grade in several studies. Apart from tumor grading, detecting higher malignant focal spots for brain biopsy, evaluating new antiangiogenic drugs, and differentiating therapy-induced necrosis from recurrent tumor are potential further applications for MRI permeability imaging.

11.3
Indications

The following sections focus on cerebral gliomas that differ from spinal gliomas with respect to their imaging representation. For example, low-grade medullary astrocytomas tend to show contrast enhancement, whereas cerebral astrocytomas up to grade III are often nonenhancing.

11.3.1
Differential Diagnosis of Cerebral Tumors

The primary task of imaging-based CNS lesion assessment is to differentiate neoplastic lesions from ischemic, inflammatory, developmental, or other types of lesions.

Although quite often clinical history, physical examination, and paraclinical studies other than cross-sectional imaging (blood and CSF studies, electrophysiology, etc.) are helpful in narrowing the differential diagnosis, there remains a considerable number of patients in whom imaging plays a crucial role for establishing the diagnosis and guiding therapy.

Various CNS lesion qualities can be assessed by imaging, as mentioned above.

These include:

- Gross morphologic appearance (clearly differentiated or poorly defined, single or multifocal lesions, butterfly appearance, hemorrhage, calcification, etc.)
- Tumor site (intra-axial or extra-axial, cortical, subcortical, callosal involvement)
- Lesion- to- (perifocal) edema ratio
- Quality of growth (rate, infiltration, perineural extension)
- Involvement of adjacent compartments (vessels, skull base)
- Tumor cellularity
- Tumor angiogenesis
- Tumor metabolism
- Therapy response

With respect to gliomas, there are well-known look-alikes that might mislead diagnosis and therapy, such as tumefactive multiple sclerosis, lymphoma, abscess, etc. Even an ischemic lesion might be mistaken for a glioma when the clinical history is incomplete or erroneous.

Moreover, tumor grade and imaging representation do not always match. Particularly glioblastomas may show an atypical appearance, such as a predominantly cystic morphology (mimicking an abscess or low-grade cystic glioma, Fig. 11.10a), subarachnoidal as well as ependymal spread (mimicking carcinomatous meningitis, Fig. 11.10b), lack of enhancement (resembling a low-grade astrocytoma or leukoencephalopathy, Fig. 11.10c, d) and lack of regressive signal alterations (again pointing to low-grade glioma).

On the other hand, some morphologic characteristics of CNS tumors are virtually diagnostic, not requiring sophisticated imaging techniques for advancing a meaningful differential diagnosis, such as the butterfly glioma, symmetrically spreading across the callosal body (Fig. 11.4d).

Oligodendrogliomas are often calcified and show callosal involvement (Fig. 11.4a). Lymphomas in immunocompetent patients are usually dense (CT; Fig. 11.4c) and gray matter-isointense (MRI) lesions with avid enhancement and smooth borders. Meningiomas, also known for high cellularity, show a broad contact zone with the dura and tend to cause sclerotic changes in adjacent bone. Nevertheless, tumor biopsy might be required for histological confirmation and treatment planning.

Most often, CT is the initial imaging modality in patients whose symptoms and/or clinical state require emergency evaluation. This might be a generalized seizure in a patient without a clinical history of epilepsy as well as severe quantitative impairment of the state of consciousness.

Whenever a small CNS lesion is suspected but cannot be assessed because of partial volume effects, multislice CT might be helpful in

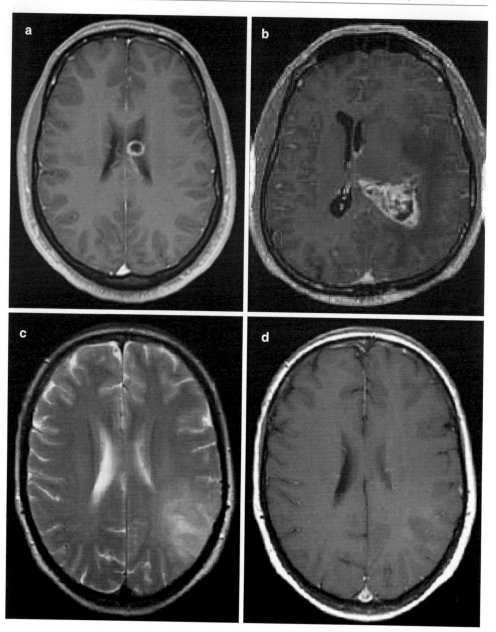

Fig. 11.10 Misleading imaging findings in glioblastomas. **a** Small cystic morphology, mimicking an inflammatory lesion. **b** Predominantly intraventricular glioblastoma with subsequent arachnoidal and ependymal spread. **c, d** Glioblastoma without significant enhancement, initially mistaken for a low-grade astrocytoma

providing helical scans with multiplanar image reformations.

As mentioned above, unenhanced CT already provides information on cellularity, hemorrhage, calcification, and adjacent bone alterations.

When a glioma is included in the differential diagnosis, perfusion imaging should be added, providing information on angiogenesis and permeability. When a vascular malformation or sinus vein thrombosis as well as an ischemic lesion are part of the diagnostic spectrum, CT angiography is mandatory and may answer most of these questions right away. Thus, a wealth of relevant and even sophisticated information is provided within no more than 30 min of data acquisition and postprocessing by an experienced neuroradiologist at the time of admission, just by performing CT.

This might be an economically relevant factor, since unnecessary costly or invasive diagnostic procedures might be avoided. The patients can be directly forwarded from the ER to a referral center, when specialized treatment (stroke unit, neurosurgery) is required.

At this time, MRI has to be considered for further lesion characterization, if other circumstances (age, pregnancy, iodine allergy) do not require MRI right away. The wealth of potential MRI-based information with respect to tumor characterization has already been described.

As far as outpatients are concerned, the referral to a neuroradiologic department should be considered whenever time-consuming, specialized MR studies are necessary (cranial nerve imaging, high-resolution 3D sequences, MR spectroscopy, diffusion/perfusion imaging, DTI, flow measurements in hydrocephalic tumor patients, etc.), because of the high economic pressure which forces radiologists in private offices to tightly limit their investigational time per patient.

In summary, detection and characterizing of glioma-resembling CNS lesions does not always require the full armory of CT and MRI.

Although cross-sectional imaging modalities available at present, together with the MR techniques currently under investigation, such as molecular imaging, promise abundant imaging-based information, substantial neuroradiologic expertise may help to tremendously shorten the diagnostic algorithms and increase efficiency in these times of limited health system resources.

Invasive diagnostic procedures, such as brain biopsy or tumor resection, should not be tackled without an interdisciplinary case approach in neuro-oncologic centers, involving advanced neuroimaging procedures whenever necessary.

11.3.2
Peritherapeutic Imaging

Peritherapeutic imaging is used for biopsy guidance, definition of target areas for radiotherapeutic therapy, and/or neurosurgical intervention as well as the detection and follow-up of therapy-induced side effects.

11.3.2.1
Biopsy Guidance

Brain biopsy by itself is an invasive procedure with potentially hazardous side effects, such as bleeding and infection, even if properly performed from a technical point of view, thus making any attempt to minimize unfruitful interventions reasonable.

High-grade gliomas typically are heterogeneous and show various stages of dedifferentiated glial tissue in areas of necrotic and unspecific granulomatous alterations. In addition, the space-occupying tumor, grossly distorting local cytoarchitecture, together with its infiltrative growth, put the neurosurgeon, and consequently the patient, at risk, such that instead of a meaningful biopsy, unspecific or even misleading low-grade tumor tissue is harvested, with the additional risk of damaging important functional tracts and areas that have unexpectedly been displaced into the biopsy access route.

Areas of increased angiogenesis and vascular permeability as well as areas of high metabolic activity should be targeted by biopsy. MR perfusion imaging and spectroscopy provide this highly relevant information. Functionally important areas might be recognized by tractography and by fMRI using paradigms such as finger tapping. Melted into high-resolution anatomic 3D MRI data sets, these data might be used for stereotactic guidance and significantly increase interventional efficacy and safety.

11.3.2.2
Radiosurgery

The situation is comparable when radiation therapy, especially stereotactic radiosurgery, is scheduled. Dose-modulated radiation, possibly increasing toxicity in high-grade tumor areas, while sparing the uninvaded but vasogenically affected peritumoral tissue, requires high-quality tumor tissue evaluation. Given the infiltrative growth of high-grade gliomas, conventional MR techniques are unable and unsuitable for directing radiotherapy.

11.3.3
Posttherapeutic Imaging

In this section, the sequela of interventional procedures for diagnostic as well as therapeutic purposes are addressed.

11.3.3.1
Diagnostic Interventions

Following brain biopsy, the occurrence and extension of intracranial bleeding and potential mass effects are the major concern. CT is cost-efficient, demonstrating these phenomena clearly, and can also be used for ventricle drainage placement. In the rare case of a subsequent infection, such as meningoencephalitis, ventriculitis, abscess, or empyema, MR should be the method of choice.

If subsequent to diagnostic lumbar taps the patient develops an intracranial hypotension, MRI typically shows low-lying cerebellar tonsils and strong dural enhancement, whereas CT myelography may be helpful in defining the site of CSF leakage and guiding the epidural patching.

11.3.3.2
Therapeutic Interventions

More recently, diffusion-weighted imaging has been suggested following neurosurgery so that the neuroradiologist can differentiate granulation tissue and tumor recurrence on follow-up scans. Contrast medium uptake beyond this surgically manipulated border zone on follow-up scans should raise the suspicion of tumor recurrence.

Sometimes subtle T1-hyperintense signals caused by minor hemorrhage persist at the resection edges and might mislead the evaluation of post-contrast scans as showing questionable enhancement. Particularly with infratentorial tumors, saturation of the (sigmoid) sinus is essential, because flow artifacts can also mimic contrast enhancement.

With radiotherapy, imaging assessment is more complex. Usually the exact area of tissue radiation is not known to the neuroradiologist reading post-radiation scans. Additionally, sequela of neurosurgery, radiotherapy, and chemotherapy might be superimposed. Whereas the clarification of whether posttherapeutic leukoencephalopathy is induced by radiation or chemotherapy might be looked upon as somewhat academic, late-onset radiation necrosis is difficult to separate from tumor recurrence on the basis of conventional MR imaging. In these cases, advanced MRI including perfusion and spectroscopy are indispensable tools for further lesion assessment.

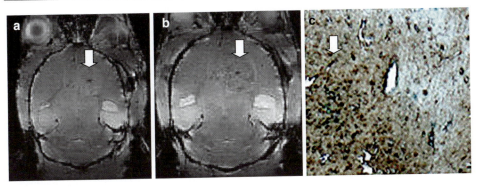

Fig. 11.11 Molecular imaging, using iron oxide particles (VSOP). MRI of the brain in mice, subsequent to experimental glioblastoma inoculation. **a** The tumor is depicted in the periventricular region. **b** Subsequent to injection of very small iron oxide particles (VSOP), tumor-associated T2* signal reduction is noted. **c** Histologic specimen showing iron deposits within the tumor (Iba1iron staining). (Images courtesy of Prof. Dr. Endres, Charité, Berlin, Germany)

11.4 Perspectives

Although tremendous progress in imaging-based tumor evaluation has been achieved in the last decade, especially by integrating morphologic, biochemical, and physiologic data provided by MRI, clinical prognosis in high-grade gliomas remains poor.

Obviously some glioma cells are migrating and resistant to proapoptotic insults such as chemotherapy. These cells might be responsible for the almost invariable tumor recurrence in WHO grade IV gliomas. Evidence has been shown that signaling pathways on a molecular level are responsible for recruitment of these cells, yet they differ in their activation according to the tumor's molecular profile.

Although the term "molecular imaging" is not precisely defined, it is often associated with one of its key techniques, the MR labeling of superparamagnetic iron oxide particles (SPIOs). Macrophages in the inflammatory glioma border zone are prone to phagocytosis of SPIOs, thus allowing perception of true tumor extension in an experimental setting (Fig. 11.11). These highly relaxive particles can be coated with specific antibodies and are then phagocytosed by antigen-expressing cells, such as specific glioma cells in vitro and in vivo, which are depicted on MR scans as areas of strong negative T2 contrast. Since this requires particle extravasation into the interstitial space, this technique also has been used to assess vessel permeability.

Further potential applications include targeted drug delivery to the glioma cells of interest, allowing tailored therapy regimens with respect to the glioma's molecular fingerprint.

Optical imaging is another technique with promising results in animal experiments because of its high spatial resolution. Yet, the shallow penetration depth is a significant methodological limitation.

11.5 Summary

More than ever, neuroimaging serves as a key discipline in glioma management, from lesion detection, lesion description, biopsy, and therapy guidance to evaluation of therapeutic efficacy, side effects, and tumor recurrence. Tumor morphology, cellularity, vascularization, and metabolism all are assessable, at least to some extent, in a clinical setting.

Where are we heading then?

The issue of therapy resistance in high-grade gliomas seems to require therapeutic strategies on a molecular level. The contribution of neuroimaging at this level presently focuses on iron oxide particles, serving several purposes such as outlining the tumor borders by phagocytic uptake or cell-targeted delivery of specific drugs in an experimental setting.

Thus neuroimaging not only is keeping pace with progress in glioma research and therapy, but it also remains one of the major promoters in this multidisciplinary neuroscientific challenge.

Suggested Reading

The following articles are recommended for further literature review.

Aronen HJ, Perkio J (2002) Dynamic susceptibility contrast MRI of gliomas. Neuroimaging Clin N Am 12(4):501–523

Behin A, Hoang-Xuan K, Carpentier AF, Delattre JY (2003) Primary brain tumours in adults. Lancet 361(9354):323–331

Benard F, Romsa J, Hustinx R (2003) Imaging gliomas with positron emission tomography and single-photon emission computed tomography. Semin Nucl Med 33(2):148–162

Bogler O, Mikkelsen T (2003) Angiogenesis in glioma: molecular mechanisms and roadblocks to translation. Cancer J 9(3):205–213

Buschmann U, Gers B, Hildebrandt G (2003) Pilocytic astrocytomas with leptomeningeal dissemination: biological behavior, clinical course, and therapeutical options. Childs Nerv Syst 19(5–6):298–304. Epub 2003 May 2022

Cha S (2003) Perfusion MR imaging: basic principles and clinical applications. Magn Reson Imaging Clin N Am 11(3):403–413

de Wit MC, de Bruin HG, Eijkenboom W, Sillevis Smitt PA, van den Bent MJ (2004) Immediate post-radiotherapy changes in malignant glioma can mimic tumour progression. Neurology 63(3):535–537

Fiveash JB, Spencer SA (2003) Role of radiation therapy and radiosurgery in glioblastoma multiforme. Cancer J 9(3):222–229

Hartmann M, Heiland S, Sartor K (2002) [Functional MRI procedures in the diagnosis of brain tumours: Perfusion- and diffusion-weighted imaging]. Rofo 174(8):955–964

Jacobs AH, Dittmar C, Winkeler A, Garlip G, Heiss WD (2002) Molecular imaging of gliomas. Mol Imaging 1(4):309–335

Jacobs AH, Li H, Winkeler A, Hilker R, Knoess C, Ruger A, et al. (2003) PET-based molecular imaging in neuroscience. Eur J Nucl Med Mol Imaging 30(7):1051–1065. Epub 2003 May 1023

Jacobs AH, Voges J, Kracht LW, Dittmar C, Winkeler A, Thomas A, et al. (2003) Imaging in gene therapy of patients with glioma. J Neurooncol 65(3):291–305

Levivier M, Wikler D, Jr., Massager N, David P, Devriendt D, Lorenzoni J, et al. (2002) The integration of metabolic imaging in stereotactic procedures including radiosurgery: a review. J Neurosurg 97(5 Suppl):542–550

McKnight TR (2004) Proton magnetic resonance spectroscopic evaluation of brain tumour metabolism. Semin Oncol 31(5):605–617

Miles KA (2002) Functional computed tomography in oncology. Eur J Cancer 38(16): 2079–2084

Mitchell DA, Fecci PE, Sampson JH (2003) Adoptive immunotherapy for malignant glioma. Cancer J 9(3):157–166

Nelson SJ, Graves E, Pirzkall A, Li X, Antiniw Chan A, Vigneron DB, et al. (2002) In vivo molecular imaging for planning radiation therapy of gliomas: an application of 1H MRSI. J Magn Reson Imaging 16(4):464–476

Nelson SJ, McKnight TR, Henry RG (2002) Characterization of untreated gliomas by magnetic resonance spectroscopic imaging. Neuroimaging Clin N Am 12(4):599–613

Nelson SJ, Cha S (2003) Imaging glioblastoma multiforme. Cancer J 9(2):134–145

Rees JH (2002) Low-grade gliomas in adults. Curr Opin Neurol 15(6):657–661

See SJ, Gilbert MR (2004) Anaplastic astrocytoma: diagnosis, prognosis, and management. Semin Oncol 31(5):618–634

Spence AM, Muzi M, Krohn KA (2002) Molecular imaging of regional brain tumour biology. J Cell Biochem Suppl 39:25–35

Weber MA, Risse F, Giesel FL, Schad LR, Kauczor HU, Essig M (2005) [Perfusion measurement using the $T2^*$ contrast media dynamics in neuro-oncology. Physical basics and clinical applications]. Radiologe 45(7):618–632

Wick W, Kuker W (2004) Brain edema in neurooncology: radiological assessment and management. Onkologie 27(3):261–266

Part III
Concepts

Angiogenesis in Gliomas

Marcia Machein and Lourdes Sánchez de Miguel

Abstract Angiogenesis, the sprouting of new blood vessels from preexisting blood vessels, is a hallmark of glioma progression. Malignant gliomas are among the most lethal tumors with a very dismal prognosis, despite advances in standard therapy, including surgery, radiation, and chemotherapy. The median survival of patients with malignant gliomas has changed little in the last few years and is still measured in months. In an attempt to develop new therapeutic strategies and identify the molecular mechanism involved in glioma growth and progression, there has been extraordinary scientific interest in the past 2 decades in angiogenic responses associated with gliomas. This chapter focuses on the molecular mechanism of glioma angiogenesis and summarizes some of the therapeutic approaches based on antiangiogenesis.

12.1 Introduction

The concept of the "angiogenic switch" driving tumor growth and malignant progression was introduced by Folkman in the early 1970s (Folkman 1985). This concept presumed that only tumors with angiogenic activity might grow beyond size of 2 mm, a size that tumor cells could no longer be nourished by mere diffusion. It is widely accepted that most tumors and metastases originate as small avascular structures. This growth pattern seems to be typical for epithelial tumors but is not applicable to gliomas. Evidence suggests that glioma may not initially grow in an avascular fashion, but tumor cells co-opted to the existing native brain capillaries in order to obtain nutrients and oxygen (Holash et al. 1999). In the second phase, there is a angiogenic response with new capillaries sprouting from preexisting blood vessels. This angiogenic response is a multistep process characterized by proteolytic breakdown of the vascular membrane and extracellular matrix, proliferation, directional migration of microvascular cells, formation of vascular lumina, and finally the coverage of the new vessels by pericytes. In the third stage, vascular regression through endothelial cell apoptosis might occur, depending on the interaction between endothelial cells and smooth muscle cells. Also, the presence of growth factors within the tumor microenvironment mediates the survival of the newly formed vessels (Zagzag et al. 2000a; Jain et al. 2007). The resulting vascular network provides a conduit for blood flow to deliver nutrients and to meet the metabolic demands of the growing tumor.

The progression from a low-grade astrocytoma to a highly vascularized glioblastoma involves profound changes in the vascular phenotype.

Marcia Machein (✉)
Department of Neurosurgery
University of Freiburg Medical School
Breisacher Str. 64
79106 Freiburg
Germany
E-mail: marcia.machein@uniklinik-freiburg.de

Neovascularization in gliomas correlates directly with their biological aggressiveness and inversely with clinical outcome. Microvascular proliferation is not observed in low-grade astrocytomas, where the vascularization patterns resemble that of normal brain (Burger and Fuller 1991). On the other hand, glioblastoma capillaries are characterized by increased endothelial proliferation, chaotic association with pericytes, and intravascular occlusion. Newly formed glioma vessels lack blood–brain barrier properties contributing to the formation of peritumoral edema and arterious-venous shunting without cerebrovascular autoregulation.

A typical feature of glioblastomas is necrotic foci surrounded by pseudopalisading cells (Rong et al. 2006). These cells express high amounts of hypoxia inducible factor-1 (HIF-1), a nuclear transcription factor that orchestrates the adaptive response to low levels of oxygen (Semenza and Wang 1992; Kaur et al. 2005; Zagzag et al. 2000b). HIF-1 is a heterodimeric protein composed of two subunits (alpha and beta). The regulation of HIF-1 protein is mediated either by several proteins that promote its stability or by the ability to induce its transcriptional activation by low levels of oxygen. HIF-1 acts as a potent stimulator of angiogenesis by induction of angiogenic factors such as vascular endothelial growth factor (VEGF). In situ hybridization analysis has shown that VEGF mRNA was found expressed at relatively low levels in normal brain, up-regulated in low-grade gliomas and highly expressed in glioblastomas. In globalstomas, VEGF mRNA is up to 50-fold overexpressed when compared with normal brain tissue (Plate et al. 1992; Shweiki et al. 1992) and remarkably spatially restricted to pseudopalisading cells (Plate et al. 1992). The association of VEGF mRNA producer cells with necrotic areas strongly support the hypothesis that hypoxia is in vivo the major driving force that regulates angiogenesis in glioblastomas.

HIF-1 also controls the expression of other pro-angiogenic molecules such as angiopoietins, platelet-derived growth factor (PDGF), placenta growth factor (PlGF) and interleukin-8 (IL-8), stroma-derived factor 1 (SDF-1, also referred as CXCL12), as well as the expression of proteases such cathepsins and metalloproteases (Semenza and Wang 1992; Acker et al. 2005). The hypoxic cells expressing high amounts of extracellular matrix metalloproteases enable them to migrate away from the hypoxic zone, creating a pro-angiogenic wave that amplifies the neovascularization in tumors and promotes tumor invasion (Sato et al. 1994).

Apart from metabolic demands, genetic mutations have been identified in the induction of a robust angiogenic response in malignant glial tumors. The link between these genetic events and angiogenesis is only partly understood; however, evidence suggests that they are crucial for the development of an angiogenic phenotype. Recent attention has been focused on the role of the p53 tumor-suppressor gene in angiogenesis. The p53 gene is inactivated in over 50% of all human cancers including malignant gliomas. Mutant p53 correlates with reduced expression of thrombospondin-1 (an endogenous inhibitor of angiogenesis) and with increased levels of VEGF, leading to angiogenesis and malignant progression (Tenan et al. 2000). Moreover, exogenous expression of wild type p53 inhibits angiogenesis in vivo, resulting in the formation of dormant tumors (Van Meir et al. 1994).

Other genetic alterations found in malignant gliomas are the amplification of epithelial growth factor receptors (EGFR) and inactivation of the phosphatase and tensin homolog, also referred as to the PTEN tumor suppression gene. EGFR belongs to a large family of tyrosine kinase receptors named HER, which are surface transmembrane receptors important in cell growth, survival, motility, and resistance to chemotherapy and radiotherapy. In glioblastomas, EGFR is overexpressed and truncated, giving rise to a chronically activated mutant receptor called EGFRviii. PTEN functions as a negative regulator of the phosphatidylinositol 3′ kinase/AKT (PIK3/AKT) pathway (Gomez-Manzano et al. 2003). Loss of function of PTEN as well as amplification of EGFR lead to a persistent activation of the downstream signaling PI3K/AKT pathway (Maity et al. 2000). Subsequently, an up-regulation of VEGF expression occurs, probably by enhancing HIF-1 activity. Moreover, PTEN loss of function during glioma progression leads to up-regulation of the tissue factor (TF), the catalyst of extrinsic hemostasis (Rong et al. 2005). The prothrombotic effect of TF may induce vascular occlusion and enhance tumor tissue hypoxia.

Recent studies of glioblastomas identified a subpopulation of tumor cells that shares characteristics with normal neural stem cells. These cells express stem cell markers and are capable of self-renewal as well as differentiating into several lineages from the nervous system like oligodendrocytes, astrocytes, and neurons. These cells, termed cancer stem cells, express high levels of VEGF and when implanted into immunocompromised mice give rise to the formation of tumors with more vessels than glioma cells that do not have stem cell characteristics (Bao et al. 2006). The up-regulation of VEGF by cancer stem cells in glioblastomas is most probably mediated by HIF-1 alpha. Together these data indicate that stem cell-like tumor cells can be a crucial source of key angiogenic factors in gliomas.

Table 12.1 Summary of the main angiogenic molecules involved in the regulation of angiogenesis in gliomas (Modified from "Angiogenesis and cancer control: from concept to therapeutic trial," Steven Brem, www.moffitt.usf.edu)

	Activators	Inhibitors
Growth factors	Vascular endothelial growth factor	Angiopoietin-2
		Transforming growth factor-beta
	Fibroblast growth factor (acid and basic)	
	Granulocyte stimulating growth factor	
	Hepatocyte growth factor	
	Angiopoietin-1	
	Angiopoietin-2	
	Placenta growth factor	
	Platelet-derived growth factor	
	Transforming Growth factor (alpha and beta)	
	Tumor necrosis factor	
	SDF-1	
Endogenous modulators		Endostatin
		Angiostatin
		Thrombospondin
		Prolactin 16kD
		Platelet factor-4
		PEX
Matrix enzymes	MMP-2 and MMP-9	Metalloprotease inhibitors (TIMPs)
	Cathepsin	Plasminogen activator inhibitor
	Urokinase-type plasminogen activator	
Cytokines	Interleukin-1	Interleukin 10
	Interlukin-6	Interleukin 12
	Interleukin-8	Interferons (alpha and beta)
Genetic changes	EGFR-amplification	p53
	Ras-raf mutation	PTEN
		VHL

12.2
The Angiogenic Factors in Gliomas

The list of angiogenic and antiangiogenic molecules identified from both normal and neoplastic tissue is still growing (Table 12.1) (Jain et al. 2007). These factors interact in a highly complex and coordinate manner to produce and maintain normal vessels in physiological conditions. Angiogenesis during adulthood is regulated by a tight balance between proangiogenic and antiangiogenic factors. During tumor growth, angiogenic activators are produced in excess with respect to angiogenic inhibitors. The balance between pro- and antiangiogenic molecules is tipped in favor of blood vessel growth (angiogenic switch).

Among the factors driving endothelial cell proliferation in gliomas, the best characterized are VEGF, bFGF, and hepatocyte growth factor/scatter factor (HGF/SC) (Machein and Plate 2000; Bian et al. 2000; Lamszus et al. 2003; Plate et al. 1994). Other important regulators of angiogenesis are angiopoietins, granulocyte colony-stimulating factor (GCSF), interleukin-1 (IL-1), interleukin-6 (IL-6), interleukin-8 (IL-8) (Brat et al. 2005; Desbaillets et al. 1999), platelet-derived growth factor (PDGF) (Shih and Holland 2006b) and SDF-1. Some factors such as tumor necrosis factor-alpha (TNF-alpha) and transforming growth factor-beta (TGF-beta) are bifunctional factors; their role in inducing or inhibiting angiogenesis may vary depending on the microenvironment, spatial and temporal expression, and interaction with other factors. Matrix proteins such as fibronectin, laminin, tenascin C, vitronectin, collagen, and heparin sulphate proteoglycans are critical to angiogenesis because they promote phosphorylation of the focal adhesion kinase (Vitolo et al. 1996; Zagzag et al. 1995, 2002). Several proteolytic enzymes play an essential role in the degradation of vascular membrane, and extracellular matrix to angiogenesis and tumor spread includes the participation of metalloproteases (MMPs), cathepsin, and urokinase-type plasminogen activator (Lakka et al. 2004; Thorns et al. 2003).

Angiogenesis is physiologically suppressed by endogenous inhibitors, including angiostatin, endostatin, tumstatin, arresten, cantastin, interferon-alfa, kringle-5, platelet factor-4, prolactin (16-kD fragment), thrombospondin, and tissue inhibitors of metalloproteinase (TIMP-1, TIMP-2, and TIMP-3). Some of these molecules are produced by tumor or stroma cells, others are generated by proteolytic cleavage of plasma-derived or extracellular proteins. In particular, pigment epithelial-derived factor (PEDF), thrombospondin (TSP)-1 and 2, angiostatin, and endostatin appear to mediate antiangiogenic effects in glioma. This assumption is based on the fact that these molecules are either expressed in malignant glioma or because in animal models their administration induces tumor regression (reviewed in (Nyberg et al. 2005)).

12.3
Growth Factors and Their Cognate Receptors

12.3.1
VEGF

The VEGF and VEGF-receptor family constitute one of the most important and well-studied systems in physiological and pathological angiogenesis. VEGF belongs to a large family of secreted growth factors that includes placenta growth factor (PlGF-1, PlGF-2, PlGF-3, and PlGF-4), VEGF-B, VEGF-C, VEGF-D, VEGF-E, and VEGF-F. VEGF-A, the prototype of the VEGF family, is denominated VEGF. VEGF mRNA generates by alternative splicing six isoforms (VEGF-121, -145, -165, -183, -189, -206) with VEGF-165 being the most abundant in human brains in physiological and pathological conditions (Ferrara et al. 2003). VEGF-B is expressed mostly in the heart, brain, and kidney. Like PlGF, VEGF-B binds only to VEGFR-1 and appears to be involved in coronary vascularization. VEGF-C and VEGF-D activate VEGFR-2 and -3. VEGF-C and VEGF-D have been identified as regulators of lymph angiogenesis.

The production of VEGF in gliomas is significant. VEGF has been found in fluids of cystic glial tumors (Weindel et al. 1994). In glioblastomas, necrotic areas are typically surrounded by pseudopalisading cells, which express high amounts of VEGF (Plate et al. 1992). VEGF expression under hypoxia is mediated by two main mechanisms: hypoxia response elements (HRE) are present in the 5' and 3' regulatory sequences of the VEGF gene. The 5' HRE binding domain is necessary for hypoxia transactivation, whereas the 3' regulatory sequence is responsible for stabilization of the mRNA (Damert et al. 1997). Posttranslational regulation, such as secretion and protein export, seems to be controlled by oxygen tension.

Similar to VEGF, PlGF is expressed in high-grade gliomas (Nomura et al. 1998). The role of PlGF in the vascularization is still not fully understood. PlGF stimulates endothelial cell growth, migration, and survival signaling directly through VEGFR-1 and overexpression of PlGF in glioma cells lead to an increase in tumor growth and angiogenesis (Adini et al. 2002). PlGF genetic deletion is not lethal and PlGF-deficient mice develop normally (Carmeliet et al. 2001). In tumor vascularization, PlGF acts synergically with VEGF and induces mobilization of hematopoietic precursors to tumor bed (Carmeliet et al. 2001). Furthermore, overexpression of PlGF through an inducible system increases tumor growth and anti-PlGF therapy has shown an efficient ability to inhibit the growth of resistant tumors by targeting macrophage infiltration and hypoxia activation (Fischer et al. 2007).

VEGF-C and VEGF-D are lymphangiogenic factors and their potential role in glioma biology is still poorly understood, since normal brain and brain tumors are devoid of lymphatics (Su et al. 2007).

VEGF acts through activation of its cognate receptors VEGFR-1 (flt-1) and VEGF-R2, VEGFR-3, and neuropilin receptors (NRP-1 and NRP-2) (Olsson et al. 2006; Ferrara et al. 2003). VEGFR-1 is expressed in endothelial cells, but also in myeloid cells – predominantly monocytes and macrophages – and is involved in the monocyte migration upon VEGF activation (Clauss et al. 1996). The exact function of VEGFR-1 in supporting angiogenesis is still not completely elucidated. At least in developmental angiogenesis, VEGFR-1 seems to have a negative regulatory function possibly by acting as a decoy receptor with a strong VEGF-trapping activity (Shibuya 2006). In tumor angiogenesis, VEGFR-1 is thus involved in the recruitment of accessory cells such as macrophages amplifying the angiogenic loop (M. Machein and L. de Sánchez de Miguel, personal data; Kerber et al. 2008). VEGFR-1 is expressed as full length receptor and as soluble form that carries only the extracellular domain. VEGFR-1 binds VEGF with a tenfold higher affinity than VEGFR-2, although its tyrosine kinase activity is weaker compared to that of VEGFR-2. VEGFR-2 is expressed in endothelial cells but also in a subset of hematopoietic stem cells (Witmer et al. 2001; Millauer et al. 1993; Kabrun et al. 1997) and is the major receptor that mediates VEGF function on endothelial cells. VEGFR-2 tyrosine kinase activity induces a downstream cascade of signaling leading to migration, proliferation, and survival of endothelial cells. Ligation of VEGF family members to their receptors results in autophosphorylation of the intracellular domain and activation of their kinase moieties. VEGF, VEGFR-1, and VEGFR-2 mRNA are highly expressed in gliomas and their expression correlates with the degree of malignancy (Plate et al. 1993). VEGFR-3 is expressed in lymphatic vessels and was thought to be primarily involved in lymphangiogenesis (Witmer et al. 2001). VEGFR-3 is up-regulated in tumor microvasculature (Valtola et al. 1999) and its expression correlates with glioma tumor grade (Grau et al. 2007). Blocking of VEGFR-3 or its genetic targeting decreases vascular density, and when combined with an anti-VEGFR-2 therapy, this inhibited tumor angiogenesis (Tammela et al. 2008). In a recent study, it has been shown that VEGFR-3 is expressed in glioblastomas. Their localization in macrophages points to a possible role in tumor-associated inflammation (Jenny et al. 2006).

12.3.2
Angiopoietins

Another family of growth factors is the angiopoeitin-Tie-2 system, which acts as crucial regulator of vessel maturation and quiescence. Tie-2, a tyrosine kinase receptor, binds two major ligands: angiopoietin-1 (ang-1) and angiopoietin-2 (ang-2) (Schnurch and Risau 1993; Sato et al. 1995; Fiedler and Augustin 2006). Upon binding to Tie-2, ang-1 is involved in pericyte recruitment, leading to a vessel stabilization and antipermeability effects; on the other hand, by binding to Tie-2, ang-2 provides an example of naturally occurring antagonist: ang-2 blocks the effect of ang-1, thereby disrupting the contact between endothelial cells and perivascular cells (smooth muscle cells and pericytes), exposing the endothelial cells to the effect of angiogenic factors such as VEGF. In addition, Tie-2 regulates several aspects of endothelial biology such as survival, migration, and remodeling of initial vascular network.

In malignant gliomas, ang-2 is expressed by endothelial cells in very early stages during glioma angiogenesis (Zagzag et al. 1999), particularly in the sprouting vessels localized at the tumor periphery (Stratmann et al. 1998; Holash et al. 1999). Ang-2 is highly induced in co-opted vessels even before VEGF induction. Hypoxic up-regulation of VEGF and ang-2 is associated with robust angiogenic response and increased vessel permeability, both hallmarks of malignant gliomas (Zagzag et al. 2000a). In the absence of VEGF, ang-2 induces endothelial cell apoptosis and vessel regression (Holash et al. 1999; Reiss et al. 2005). Ang-2 expression is still present in glioma vessels in later stages. Increased ang-2 expression is found in hyperplastic vessels, but not in sclerotic vessels (Stratmann et al. 1998; Zagzag et al. 2000a). Furthermore, ang-2 induces glioma invasion through the activation of metalloprotesases (Hu et al. 2003). Glioblastomas express high levels of ang-1 compared to a healthy brain and low-grade gliomas (Audero et al. 2001). Overexpression of ang-1 by glioma cells induces a more functional vascular network, which leads to enhanced tumor growth, whereas ang-2 overexpression leads to less intact tumor vessels, inhibited capillary sprouting, and impaired tumor growth (Machein et al. 2004).

12.3.3
Other Angiogenic Growth Factors

Other molecules such as TNF-alpha, TGF-β, FGF, PDFG, and HGF/SF have also been shown to mediate angiogenic response in gliomas (Dunn et al. 2000).

The family of fibroblast growth factors comprises 23 FGFs. The best characterized are the acidic FGF (FGF-1) and basic-FGF (FGF-2), the latter being the first proangiogenic molecule identified. Regarding the role of FGF-2 in glioma, the results presented in the literature are quite contradictory. While Zagzag et al. showed that the immunoreactivity for FGF-2 correlates with histological grade (Zagzag et al. 1990), other authors (Schmidt et al. 1999; Samoto et al. 1995) did not find a correlation between FGF-2 expression and degree of malignancy and vascularity in brain tumors (Bian et al. 2000). Strong expression of FGF-2 has been reported in the perivascular space. Diminished expression of FGFR-2 and increased levels of FGFR-1 were found in malignant gliomas. There are still conflicting results regarding the status of FGFR expression on tumor endothelial cells. Some studies suggest that FGF-2 might stimulate glioma angiogenesis by stimulating VEGF secretion by glioma cells (Tsai et al. 1995).

A second way by which FGF-2 might participate in angiogenesis is by mediating the proteolytic degradation of extracellular matrix by invading endothelial cells (Mignatti et al. 1991; Dunn et al. 2000).

The scatter factor, also known as the hepatocyte growth factor (SF/HGF) is a multifunctional heterodimeric growth factor, which through its receptor c-met regulates developmental, regenerative, and neoplastic processes. SF/HGF and c-met are up-regulated in gliomas and their expression pattern correlates with microvessel density (Lamszus et al. 1999). The effect of SF/HGF in stimulating angiogenesis is likely to be mediated by up-regulation of VEGF and down-regulation of TSP-1 (Jeffers et al. 1996).

Platelet-derived growth factor (PDGF) is a 30-kDa protein consisting of disulfide-bonders dimers of A, B C, and D chains. The homodimers PDGF AA, BB, CC, and DD and the heterodimer AB bind to two receptor types, PDFGR-alpha and beta, which are activated by ligand-induced dimerization, leading to phosphorylation of tyrosine residues. PDGFR stimulation activates the Raf-Ras signaling cascade (Risau et al. 1992). PDGF is a potent mitogen and chemoattractant for mesenchymal cells and fibroblasts. Plentiful evidence suggests that PDGF plays an important role in angiogenesis. PDGF-B and its receptor PDFGR-β are responsible for recruiting periendothelial cells to vessels (Board and Jayson 2005). However, PDGF-B also plays a major role in gliomagenesis (Shih and Holland 2006b). Human gliomas express high levels of PDGF ligands and corresponding receptors. Robust expression of PDGF-B and PDGFR-β was reported in hyperplastic tumor endothelial cells in glioblastomas. (Board and Jayson 2005). Mice transgenic for neural progenitor-driven expression of PDGF-B resulted in the formation of oligodendrogliomas (Dai et al. 2001).

Transforming growth factor-β (TGF-β) is a member of a superfamily that consists of at least of 26 closely related proteins. TGF-β is involved in an extraordinary range of biological processes, including embryonic development and angiogenesis. TGF-β is secreted as an inactive protein that is activated by enzymatic cleavage. At least three genes encode the latent TGF-β (TGFβ-1, TFG-β2, and TGFβ-3). TGF-β binds to its serine/threonine kinase receptors, which induces phosphorylation of SMAD proteins (Wick et al. 2001). TGF-β is expressed in gliomas and its expression has been correlated with either tumor-suppressive as well as tumor-promoting effects (Platten et al. 2001). TGF-β has been shown to be a mitogen for several glioma cell lines (Yamada et al. 1995). TGF-β might support angiogenesis by influencing the expression of other proteins and growth factors (Breier et al. 2002; Kaminska et al. 2005).

12.4
Guidance Molecules

Several families of molecules involved in axon and neural network formation may regulate vessel pathfinding and vascular branching in tumor angiogenesis (Carmeliet and Tessier-Lavigne 2005)

12.4.1
Ephrins

The ephrin family is involved in various developmental processes as guidance molecules not only in neuronal development but also in the regulation of the blood's vascular system (Cheng et al. 2002; Klein 2001; Augustin and Reiss 2003). This large family is formed by at least 16 receptors and 9 ligands. Gene-targeting studies suggest that ephrins play a critical role in arteriovenous differentiation and vascular assembly. The ephrin receptors comprise the largest group of tyrosine kinase receptor with two main subgroups: EphA (1–10) and EphB (1–6) (Yancopoulos et al. 1998). Interaction of EphB receptors with corresponding ephrin ligands differs from the classical binding of a secreted ligand. Both receptors and ligands are transmembrane receptors and signaling occurs only if the expressing cells are in juxtapositional contact. Like other tyrosine kinase receptors, ephrin receptors initiate signal transduction by autophosphorylation after ligand–receptor binding, which is termed forward signaling. Ephrins are also capable of receptor-like active signaling (reverse signaling). Ephrin B2 and Eph-receptor B4 are co-expressed by blood vessels of human and experimental malignant gliomas. Emerging data suggest that alterations in ephrin signaling in tumor endothelial cells affect the morphogenesis and remodeling of the tumor vascular system (Erber et al. 2006). Some studies demonstrate that Ephrin B3 promotes glioma invasion by activating Rac-1 (Nakada et al. 2006) and that ephrin B2 inhibits glioma cell adhesion and promotes cell growth and invasion through R-Ras signaling (Nakada et al. 2005).

12.4.2
Delta-Like 4 Ligand-Notch

The Delta-like 4 ligand (Dll-4)-Notch pathway is another pivotal regulator of angiogenesis and development (Gridley 2007; Benedito and Duarte 2005). Dll4-Notch signaling regulates guide vessel-sprouting and branching in the tip cells from the vessels (Noguera-Troise et al. 2007). It comprises several receptors (Notch-1, -2, -3, -4) that bind specific transmembrane ligands known as jagged 1, jagged 2, and Dll1, Dll3, and Dll-4 present in adjacent cells. Notch receptors are heterodimeric proteins composed of one intracellular and one extracellular monomeric protein. These receptors are expressed in the cell surface and ligand binding stimulates the interaction between adjacent cells. Notch receptors are expressed in various cell types but Dll-4 is exclusively present in endothelial cells. Dll4 genetic deletion is lethal for the embryo (Gale et al. 2004). Dll-4 is up-regulated in the tumor vessels (Li et al. 2007) and blockade of Dll4 inhib-

its tumor growth by a mechanism that involves a first stage of angiogenic stimulation and creation of abnormal and nonfunctional vessels. Paradoxically, this process leads to a second stage of severe hypoxia and poor perfusion that finally decrease tumor growth (Noguera-Troise et al. 2006). Notch receptor and its ligands are expressed in glioblastoma (Purow et al. 2005; Shih and Holland 2006a), playing a critical role in cell survival and proliferation of glioma through EGFR.

12.4.3
ROBO/Slit

Another group of guidance molecules is the receptor family of the roundabouts (ROBO: robo-1, robo-2, robo3/rig-1, and robo4/Magic Roundabout) and their ligands (slit1, slit2, and slit3). They were first identified as chemorepellent in axon guidance and neuronal migration, and by acting as repellents also inhibit leukocyte chemotaxis (Wong et al. 2002). Tumor cells may secrete slit2, which attracts robo-1-expressing endothelial cells. Neutralization of robo-1 reduced vessel density and tumor growth (Wang et al. 2003). Moreover, interaction between robo-1 and slit2 in glioma cell lines mediated chemorepulsive effects involved in tumor cell migration (Mertsch et al. 2008). Other studies suggest that slit2 recombinant protein did not inhibit glioma invasion (Werbowetski-Ogilvie et al. 2006). Slit2 also may have activity as a tumor suppressor and it is epigenetically inactivated in different types of glioma (Dallol et al. 2003).

12.4.4
Netrins and DCC/UNC Receptors

Netrins are chemotropics that belong to the laminin-related secreted protein family. Three members of the netrin gene family, netrin-1, netrin-3, and β-netrin/netrin-4, have been identified in mammals. Netrins are expressed in the brain and peripheral tissues and have a critical role in determining the direction and extent of cell migration and axon outgrowth in the developing nervous system (Forcet et al. 2002). Axon attraction and repulsion are mediated via activation of receptors of the deleted in colorectal cancer (DCC) and the type 1 transmembrane receptors from the uncoordinated (UNC) family, respectively. UNC5H1, UNC5H2, and UNC5H3 mediate the chemorepulsive activity of netrin-1 (Hong et al. 1999). They are dependence receptors. They may act as tumor suppressors by inducing apoptosis in the absence of their ligand netrin-1, whereas they act as anti-apoptotic molecules, promoting tumorigenesis and inhibiting cell death when they are engaged by a ligand. DCC is also considered a tumor constraint for tumor growth (Fearon et al. 1990). Netrin and their receptors also regulate diverse processes such as cell adhesion, motility, proliferation, differentiation, and cell survival (Cirulli and Yebra 2007). Netrin-1 and netrin receptors control morphogenesis of endothelial cells and vascular smooth muscle cells and are implicated in the reorganization of the cytoskeleton, epithelial cell adhesion, and migration (Shekarabi and Kennedy 2002). Moreover, activation of UNC5 via netrin-1 inhibits sprouting angiogenesis (Larrivee et al. 2007). The netrin-1 and its receptors are implicated in cancer cell invasion and tumor progression (Rodrigues et al. 2007; Meyerhardt et al. 1999). A decrease in netrin-1 transcription has been shown in brain tumor and neuroblastoma (Meyerhardt et al. 1999).

semaphorins belonging to the class 3 subfamily (SEMA-3) are expressed in mammals. The activation of plexins by semaphorins modulates cell adhesion and induces changes in the organization of the cytoskeleton of target cells (Neufeld and Kessler 2008). The function of semaphorins in tumor progression is still controversial. Semaphorin 3B and semaphorin 3F have been characterized as tumour suppressors (Kuroki et al. 2003), but they can further inhibit tumor proliferation in vitro and in vivo (Tomizawa et al. 2001). Some studies have found that SEMA3B expression inhibited tumor growth, whereas metastatic dissemination was surprisingly increased (Rolny et al. 2008). In the brain, semaphorin-6B expression decreases after antitumor treatment in some glioma cell lines (Correa et al. 2001).

The neuropilins also function as receptors for several pro-angiogenic factors. Neuropilin-1 (NRP-1) was first identified as a neuronal receptor that mediates repulsive growth guidance. Further studies identified NRP-1 as a co-receptor of VEGFR-2 in endothelial cells (Soker et al. 1998). The precise role of NRP in supporting glioma angiogenesis remains to be clarified. NRP may play a role facilitating the presentation and binding of $VEGF_{165}$ isoform to its VEGFR-2 (Soker et al. 2002). Neuropilins, semaphorins, and plexins are expressed in malignant gliomas by endothelium and glioma cells, and their expression has been linked to cancer invasion and correlated with patient's poor prognosis (Broholm and Laursen 2004; Osada et al. 2004; Rieger et al. 2003).

12.4.5
Semaphorins

Semaphorins are another large family of secreted and membrane anchored proteins initially characterized as axon guidance factors that have been implicated in angiogenesis, immune function, and cancer (Kruger et al. 2005). Semaphorins are divided into eight subfamilies that bind to the plexin and the neuropilin receptors, but only the

12.5
Endogenous Inhibitors

The concept of tumor dormancy suggests that tumor cells undergo a prolonged period of latency before they grow further (Folkman 1996). Malignant gliomas are generally considered nonmetastatic, although they are able to spread into all parts of the brain. Pathological observations provide evidence that glioma cells might persist into a dormant stage in sites far away from the primary tumor. Given the extent of spread of glioma cells into the brain, multifocal lesions would be expected to be more frequently observed in malignant glioma patients. This phenomenon also supports the concept of dormancy in the brain. Several endogenous inhibitors are expressed in gliomas (Kirsch et al. 2000). A number of endogenous inhibitors have been identified; some of them arise by proteolytic cleavage of extracellular proteins (for review, see Nyberg et al. 2005).

12.5.1
Thrombospondin 1 and 2

Thrombospondin (TSP) 1 and 2 are components of the extracellular matrix involved in cell adhesion, cell–cell interaction, migration, and activation of TGF-β. TSPs are produced by different types of cells, including endothelial cells, smooth muscle cells, fibroblasts, monocytes, and macrophages, platelets, and tumor cells. Thrombospondins are potent inhibitors of angiogenesis, most probably by interacting with the specific receptor CD36, which mediates the antiangiogenic response (Rege et al. 2005). In gliomas, expression of thrombospondin-2 correlated inversely with the degree of tumor vascularization (Kazuno et al. 1999). Hypoxia down-regulated the expression of TSP-1, suggesting that low levels of oxygen can promote angiogenesis not only by inducing the expression of VEGF and other angiogenic molecules, but also by reducing the production of inhibitors (Tenan et al. 2000).

12.5.2
Angiostatin

Angiostatin is an internal fragment of plasminogen originated by proteolytic cleavage (O'Reilly et al. 1994). The potential receptors for angiostatin are integrin αvβ3, ATP synthetase, NG2 condroitin sulfate proteoglycan, and angiomotion. In the rat C6 and 9L and in the U87MG glioma model, angiostatin exerted a dose-dependent growth suppressive effect by reducing substantially the tumor vascularity and increasing the apoptotic rate (Kirsch et al. 1998).

12.5.3
Endostatin

Endostatin is a 22-kDa peptide derived from the carboxy-terminal proteolytic cleavage of collagen type XV and XVIII. Endostatin inhibits the proliferation of bovine capillary endothelial cells and reduces angiogenesis in a chick chorioallantoic membrane model. The current hypothesis is that endostatin interacts with heparin sulfate proteoglycans (HSPGs) and subsequently inhibits the signaling of bFGF, which requires interaction with HSPGs. (O'Reilly et al. 1997). Another proposed mechanism for the antiangiogenic effect of endostatin is the interaction of endostatin with several proangiogenic molecules such as VEGF, VEGFR-2, and MMP. Increased endostatin expression is found in grade IV gliomas in hyperplastic vessels (Morimoto et al. 2002). This study suggested that endostatin expression is up-regulated in response to increased angiogenic response. In another study, the authors detected decreased endostatin expression in high-grade tumors (Strik et al. 2001). Local delivery of endostatin by microencapsulated producer cells to experimental gliomas leads to apoptosis of tumor vessels with an increased survival of the animals (Read et al. 2001).

12.5.4
Pigment Epithelial-Derived Factor

Pigment epithelial-derived factor (PEDF) belongs to the family of serpins and is involved in neuronal differentiation and survival. The mechanism by which PEDF inhibits angiogenesis is probably associated with its ability to bind collagen. In addition, PEGF might induce Fas-mediated apoptosis of endothelial cells. PEDF expression inversely correlated with the glioma grade (Guan et al. 2004).

12.5.5
PEX

PEX is a naturally occurring 210-amino-acid fragment of metalloprotease-2 (MMP-2) that has significant antiproliferative, anti-invasive, and antiangiogenic properties in glioblastoma cells in vitro and in vivo (Kim et al. 2005). PEX binds integrin $\alpha v \beta 3$ and blocks cell surface activation of MMP-2 (Brooks et al. 1998).

12.6
Strategies for Therapeutic Angiogenesis Inhibition in Glioma Treatment

Malignant gliomas are among the most vascularized and invasive neoplasms. The present treatment of gliomas is plagued by three main problems: (a) given the diffuse infiltrative nature of gliomas, a complete resection is nearly impossible; (b) the blood–brain barrier impairs the delivery of therapeutic agents in optimal quantity, and (c) clonal evolution gives rise to more aggressive and resistant tumor cells. The little improvement in the survival of brain tumor patients with conventional cytotoxic agents has stimulated neuro-oncologists to search for new therapeutic options. Antiangiogenic therapy has the potential to overcome these problems with different promising strategies. To date over 70 individual drugs with antiangiogenic properties have been tested in gliomas, some of them are in clinical trials. Preclinical data have demonstrated that angiogenesis inhibition can reduce glioma growth in various syngeneic and xenographs models (Izumi et al. 2003; Jain et al. 2006; Albini et al. 1999; Drevs et al. 2002). While preclinical experiments demonstrate that glioma growth and progression is angiogenesis-dependent, the evidence that glioblastomas patients can benefit from antiangiogenic therapy is still awaited. The enthusiasm for antiangiogenic approaches in glioma therapy has been restrained by the preliminary results and published integrin analysis from clinical trials using antiangiogenic drugs as monotherapy, indicating that angiogenesis inhibition alone has little efficacy in tumor control. Moreover, the reports that anti-VEGF agents could result in fatal intracranial hemorrhage further increases the skepticism (Duda 2006; Kerbel 2008).

An explanation for the lack of robust effect of antiangiogenic monotherapies in malignant gliomas is that by reducing vessel density, antiangiogenic agents may further increase hypoxia in the remaining tumor, perpetuating the cycles of hypoxia, and continued angiogenesis and tumor growth. Thus, combined regimes with antiangiogenic substances and either radiation or chemotherapy might result at least in long-lasting glioma growth control. However, how antiangiogenic therapy can augment the response to cytotoxic or radiation therapy still remains a matter of debate. Several reports point out that combined therapy of antiangiogenic substances and cytotoxic therapies increases their effect (Baumann et al. 2004; Arrieta et al. 2002; Chang et al. 2004); other data showed that these might be antagonistic (Ma et al. 2001; Murata et al. 1997; Fenton et al. 2004). How can antiangiogenic therapy increase the response to cytotoxic agents, which require blood vessels for drug delivery if these approaches disrupt the vascular network? New evidence suggests that tumor blood vessel normalization can be induced by antiangiogenic approaches. Blocking VEGFR-2 by the monoclonal antibody DC101 can induce structural and functional changes in the tumor vasculature, culminating in remodeling imma- ture and inefficient vessels, probably because of increased recruitment of pericytes to the tumor vasculature. The transient stabilization of vessels prevents edema and tumor hemorrhage and increases tumor perfusion, creating a therapeutic window for improved drug penetration and tissue oxygenation and thus enhancing sensitivity to radiation treatment (Jain 2005).

Another reason for the modest effect of antiangiogenic therapy in clinical trials is our incomplete understanding of the mechanisms that regulate angiogenesis. Most therapies are based on a single agent. It is well known that more than a single factor orchestrates the angiogenic response in solid tumors. Once a factor is blocked by a particular substance, other growth factors might sustain the angiogenic response. A cocktail of antiangiogenic agents may very well be needed to block important pathways (Carmeliet and Jain 2000).

Moreover, antiangiogenic intervention efficacy cannot be primarily evaluated by the classical readout parameters used in clinical tumor trials, namely progression time and median survival time. These parameters do not allow an assessment of the angiogenic status of a given tumor. Complementary techniques with reliable biomarkers need to be included in antiangiogenic trials. In this regard, dynamic contrast-enhanced magnetic resonance imaging (MRI) may evolve to be a useful marker to evaluate the response to antiangiogenic therapies.

Basically, four general strategies have been proposed for angiosuppression: (a) inhibition of endothelial cell proliferation and inhibition of adhesion molecules, (b) blocking of stimulatory factors, (c) amplification of endogenous inhibitors of angiogenesis, and (d) blockade of invasive activity. Several other target-specific drugs can indirectly inhibit the angiogenic response such as EGFR inhibitors (Tacerva or Iressa), inhibitors of the Pl3K/Akt cascade (Rapamycin) or Ras pathway (Farnesyl transferase inhibitors), proteasome inhibitors, and cyclooxygenase inhibitors (Celebrex).

The next section will briefly outline the antiangiogenic tumor therapies, already under clinical evaluation in patients with malignant gliomas (reviewed in (Jouanneau 2008)).

12.6.1
Inhibition of Endothelial Cell Proliferation and Adhesion Cell Molecules

Thalidomide (Celgene Pharmaceuticals, Warren, NJ, USA), originally described as a sedative, has a potent antiangiogenic effect. The mechanism of action of thalidomide is not completely understood, but it has been postulated that thalidomide interferes with the expression of adhesion molecules such as integrins and inhibits the action of growth factors such as bFGF and VEGF (Cohen 2000; D'Amato et al. 1994). Several phase II clinical trials with thalidomide as a single agent have been published. These data showed that thalidomide is well tolerated and has as monotherapy little antitumor activity. A phase II study showed that thalidomide in combination with BCNU is well tolerated and has antitumor activity in patients with recurrent high-grade combination disease (Fine et al. 2000; Fine et al. 2003). Overall, the early trials with thalidomide conducted primarily in glioblastoma patients yielded disappointing results.

AGM-1470 (TNP-470) is a synthetic analog of fumagillin, a compound secreted by *Aspergillus fumigates*. AGM-1470 inhibits proliferation and migration of endothelial cells and showed potent antiangiogenic activity in preclinical studies (Kragh et al. 1999; Lund et al. 2000; Takamiya et al. 1994). In trials with this substance, patients have attained disease stabilization. However at the high dose necessary for tumor stabilization, many patients experienced neurotoxicity. Other major clinical limitation is the poorly oral availability of this substance (Benny et al. 2008)

Integrins are a large family of transmembrane molecules that mediate cell–cell contact and cell adhesion, migration, and invasion. It has been discovered that the $\alpha v\beta 3$ integrin is a critically important adhesion molecule in the regulation of angiogenesis and that it promotes endothelial and tumor cell survival (Bello et al. 2001; McDonald et al. 2004). A role of integrins in tumor angiogenesis is supported by the observation that integrins are up-regulated in tumor endothelium. It has been suggested that the block of integrin induces apoptosis in tumor capillaries by preventing the interaction with extracellular matrix component tenascin. EMD 121974 (Cilengitide, Merck, Darmstadt, Germany) is a selective inhibitor of $\alpha v \beta 3$ integrin receptor suppressed the growth of glioblastomas implanted orthotopically in nude mice (Taga et al. 2002). The efficacy of antagonizing integrins in inhibiting glioma angiogenesis and growth is being evaluated in combination with alkylating agents in a multicenter phase III study.

12.6.2
Blocking Stimulatory Factors

VEGF and its receptors have been identified as essential mediators of angiogenesis in gliomas and are promising targets for antiangiogenic therapies (Machein and Plate 2000; Stratmann et al. 1997). There is compelling evidence that inhibition of VEGF and its receptor signaling not only blocks angiogenesis but leads to regression of existing vessels. This knowledge is based on the use of multiple different approaches to inhibit VEGF signaling, including neutralizing antibodies, antisense VEGF, conditional expression of the VEGF gene, dominant inhibition of VEGFR-2, small molecules that inhibited VEGFR phosphorylation (Kim et al. 1993; Millauer et al. 1994; Machein et al. 1999; Heidenreich et al. 2004; Sasaki et al. 1999).

Bevacizumab (Avastin, Roche, Switzerland) is a genetically engineered antibody that blocks VEGF. Blocking VEGF activity in experimental gliomas augments tumor radiation response under normoxic and hypoxic conditions in glioblastoma xenographs (Lee et al. 2000). The efficacy of bevacizumab was tested in combination with the chemotherapeutic agent Irinotecan in recurrent malignant gliomas and the results are encouraging: The 6-month progression-free survival among all 35 patients was 46% with a partial response rate of 57% (Vredenburgh et al. 2007a, b). Although the high response rates might partly result from a decrease in the vascular permeability and contrast enhancement in MRI studies, the 6-month progression free interval suggests a real antitumor effect. However, some preclinical results suggest that by decreasing VEGF activity in experimental gliomas, tumor cells became more invasive (Rubenstein et al. 2000). Moreover, a more proinvasive adaptation has been inferred from MRI imaging of patients treated with bevacizumab. These results suggest that combining antiangiogenic therapy and chemotherapy may be clinically useful and effective; however, simultaneous block of invasion might improve current antiangiogenic approaches with bevacizumab.

VEGF-Trap (Aflibercept, Regeneron, Tarrytown, NJ, USA) is a soluble hybrid receptor composed of portions of VEGFR-1 and VEGFR-2 fused to an immunoglobulin. Like bevacizumab, VEGF-Trap has been designed to deplete VEGF, but it has a greater affinity than bevacizumab itself. A phase II trial aiming to determine the efficacy of VEGF Trap in patients with temozolomide-resistant malignant gliomas at first recurrence is ongoing.

PTK787/ZK222584 (Novartis, Basel, Switzerland) is a new synthesized compound that selectively inhibited VEGFR-2, with weaker blocking activity on PDGFR. In experimental models of gliomas, PTK87/ZK222584 treatment leads to significantly delayed tumor growth (Goldbrunner et al. 2004). In a phase I clinical trial, preliminary results suggested that PTK787/ZK222584 showed antitumor activity, which correlated with changes in the vascular permeability as measured by dynamics. Clinical trials investigating the efficacy of PTK787 in combination with chemotherapy in colon carcinoma showed very disappointing results so that these trials were discontinued. Whether PTK787 efficacy will be further pursued by Novartis is uncertain.

Imantinib mesylate (Gleevec, Novartis, Basel, Switzerland) has been shown to inhibit PDGFR. In combination with Hydrourea, an antitumor activity was observed in some patients, but the overall results of phase II and phase III studies were disappointing.

There are, however, encouraging results with inhibitors of VEGF receptors. A recent trial of AZD2117 (Recentin™, Astra Zeneca, London, UK) a multikinase inhibitor, demonstrated a reduction in contrast-enhanced tumor volume, a decrease in peritumoral edema, and an approximately 25% increase in the 6-month progression-free interval in patients with recurrent glioblastomas (Batchelor et al. 2007). This effect most probably results from reconstitution of the blood–brain barrier through vessel normalization. SU11248 (Sunitinib, Sutent, Pfizer, New York, NY, USA) is a new oral generation of multitargeted tyrosine kinase inhibitor, which blocks VEGF, PDGF, Flt-3, and cKit receptors. In vivo SU11248 blocks vascularization and tumor growth of syngeneic glioma models (Schueneman et al. 2003). Several trials with Sunitinib in treatment of patients with malignant gliomas are ongoing. Studies with other inhibitors of VEGF such as sorafenib (Nexavar®, Bayer AG Leverkusen, Germany), vandetanib (ZD6474, Zactima, Astra Zeneca) for glioblastoma patients are in progress.

Protein kinases are downstream targets of several receptor tyrosine kinases, including EGFR and PDGFR. Furthermore, there is evidence that a link exists between PKC and the Pl3K/Akt pathway. A novel PKC-β inhibitor (Enzastaurin, Eli Lilly, Indianapolis, USA) has been tested as monotherapy in glioblastoma multiforme (GBM). This trial was terminated earlier because of the lack of evidence in recurrent tumors. A new trial in primary glioblastomas is being conducted in combination with radiotherapy in tumors resistant to temozolomide. There are also several Pl3K inhibitors under development and are expected to enter into clinical trial for glioblastoma patients soon.

12.6.3 Increase of Endogenous Inhibitors of Angiogenesis

A number of endogenous inhibitors of angiogenesis are expressed in gliomas. These inhibitors appear to mediate an antiangiogenic effect through protein–protein interaction, which blocks the function of proangiogenic molecules. However, how these endogenous inhibitors counteract the action of proangiogenic growth factors and cytokines is not yet fully understood. Several reports have suggested that the amplification of endogenous inhibitors is effective in inhibiting tumor growth in animal models of malignant glioma. Two broad experimental strategies have been used to deliver endogenous inhibitors to solid tumors: (a) delivery of purified or recombinant protein by systemic injection or intracerebral microperfusion and (b) transgene overexpression by adenovirus or packing cells. The potential therapeutic application of endogenous inhibitors is being considered in clinical trials for malignant gliomas (reviewed in (Janson and Oberg 2002)).

12.6.4 Inhibition of Invasive Activity

The matrix metalloproteases (MMPs) are zinc-dependent endopeptidases that degrade the basement membrane and compounds of extracellular matrix. Anaplastic gliomas depend on matrix metalloproteinases for tumor cell invasion and angiogenesis. Experimental studies have demonstrated that in glioma models MMP inhibitors (MMPIs) can restrict the growth and regional spread of solid tumors and block the process of tumor neovascularization. MMPs (especially MMP-2 and MMP-9) are up-regulated in malignant gliomas and correlate with their malignant progression (Tonn et al. 1999). MMP inhibitors such as marimastat, metastat, and prinomastat have entered clinical development in combination with chemotherapy. The results of the phase II trials suggested that marimastat as a single agent does not improve survival following surgery and radiotherapy but in combination with chemotherapy there was an improved overall survival in patients treated with marimastat (Groves et al. 2006).

12.7
Perspectives and Unanswered Questions

Glioma progression requires the acquisition of an angiogenic phenotype. Rapid progress has been made in the identification of target molecules that modulate the angiogenic response in gliomas. Similar efforts in the development of antiangiogenic therapies have been made in the recent years. The role of antiangiogenic therapies in clinical settings for the treatment of malignant gliomas still remains to be defined. Whereas eradication of tumor cells is the primary goal of anti-cancer therapies, at least for patients with malignant gliomas, arresting tumor growth and significantly prolonging the survival of these patients might be an achievable goal for the future and will require systemic as well as local therapies. Meanwhile, it is believed that future therapies should be a tailored treatment based on molecular features of individual tumors. This treatment should combine specific antiangiogenic agents with chemo- and radiotherapy.

Several challenges in the field still remain. One of the major efforts of research should be the development of molecular features that predict sensitivity to a particular inhibitor. Since successful therapy will require simultaneous administration of multiple substances, a better understanding of the interaction between the molecules involved in glioma angiogenesis is necessary. A molecularly complex disease such as GBM requires the development of reliable animal models, which better resemble human brain cancers, in order to provide suitable settings for testing antiangiogenic therapies in preclinical studies. Finally, the future of antiangiogenic therapies will involve the inclusion of imaging techniques and surrogate markers to evaluate the efficacy of antiangiogenic approaches.

Acknowledgments

Our work is supported by grants from Deutsche Krebshilfe (grant 10–2224-Ma2) and from Deutsche Forschunggemeischaft (SFB-TR 23; Projects C4). We are gratefully to Prof. H. Augustin (Division of Vascular Oncology and Metastasis; German Cancer Research Center, Heidelberg) for critical reading of this review.

References

Acker T, Diez-Juan A, Aragones J, Tjwa M, Brusselmans K, Moons L, Fukumura D, Moreno-Murciano MP, Herbert JM, Burger A, Riedel J, Elvert G, Flamme I, Maxwell PH, Collen D, Dewerchin M, Jain RK, Plate KH, Carmeliet P (2005) Genetic evidence for a tumor suppressor role of HIF-2alpha. Cancer Cell. 8:131–141

Adini A, Kornaga T, Firoozbakht F, Benjamin LE (2002) Placental growth factor is a survival factor for tumor endothelial cells and macrophages. Cancer Res. 62 2749–2752

Albini A, Noonan D, Santi L (1999) Angiogenesis at the interface between basic and clinical research. Int J Biol Markers 14:202–206

Arrieta O, Guevara P, Tamariz J, Rembao D, Rivera E, Sotelo J (2002) Antiproliferative effect of thalidomide alone and combined with carmustine against C6 rat glioma. Int J Exp Pathol 83:99–104

Audero E, Cascone I, Zanon I, Previtali SC, Piva R, Schiffer D, Bussolino F (2001) Expression of angiopoietin-1 in human glioblastomas regulates tumor-induced angiogenesis: in vivo and in vitro studies. Arterioscler Thromb Vasc Biol 21:536–541

Augustin HG, Reiss Y (2003) EphB receptors and ephrinB ligands: regulators of vascular assembly and homeostasis. Cell Tissue Res 314:25–31

Bao S, Wu Q, Sathornsumetee S, Hao Y, Li Z, Hjelmeland AB, Shi Q, McLendon RE, Bigner DD, Rich JN (2006) Stem cell-like glioma cells promote tumor angiogenesis through vascular endothelial growth factor. Cancer Res 66:7843–7848

Batchelor TT, Sorensen AG, di Tomaso E, Zhang WT, Duda DG, Cohen KS, Kozak KR, Cahill DP, Chen PJ, Zhu M, Ancukiewicz M, Mrugala MM, Plotkin S, Drappatz J, Louis DN, Ivy P, Scadden DT, Benner T, Loeffler JS, Wen PY, Jain RK (2007) AZD2171, a pan-VEGF receptor tyrosine kinase inhibitor, normalizes tumor vasculature and alleviates edema in glioblastoma patients. Cancer Cell 11:83–95

Baumann F, Bjeljac M, Kollias SS, Baumert BG, Brandner S, Rousson V, Yonekawa Y, Bernays RL (2004) Combined thalidomide and temozolomide treatment in patients with glioblastoma multiforme. J Neurooncol 67:191–200

Bello L, Francolini M, Marthyn P, Zhang J, Carroll RS, Nikas DC, Strasser JF, Villani R, Cheresh DA, Black PM (2001) Alpha(v)beta3 and alpha(v)beta5 integrin expression in glioma periphery. Neurosurgery 49:380–389

Benedito R, Duarte A (2005) Expression of Dll4 during mouse embryogenesis suggests multiple developmental roles. Gene Expr Patterns 5:750–755

Benny O, Fainaru O, Adini A, Cassiola F, Bazinet L, Adini I, Pravda E, Nahmias Y, Koirala S, Corfas G, D'Amato RJ, Folkman J (2008) An orally delivered small-molecule formulation with antiangiogenic and anticancer activity. Nat Biotechnol 26(7):799–807

Bian XW, Du LL, Shi JQ, Cheng YS, Liu FX (2000) Correlation of bFGF, FGFR-1 and VEGF expression with vascularity and malignancy of human astrocytomas. Anal Quant Cytol Histol 22:267–274

Board R, Jayson GC (2005) Platelet-derived growth factor receptor (PDGFR): a target for anticancer therapeutics. Drug Resist Updat 8:75–83

Brat DJ, Bellail AC, Van Meir EG (2005) The role of interleukin-8 and its receptors in gliomagenesis and tumoral angiogenesis. Neurooncol 7:122–133

Breier G, Blum S, Peli J, Groot M, Wild C, Risau W, Reichmann E (2002) Transforming growth factor-beta and Ras regulate the VEGF/VEGF-receptor system during tumor angiogenesis. Int J Cancer 97:142–148

Broholm H, Laursen H (2004) Vascular endothelial growth factor (VEGF) receptor neuropilin-1's distribution in astrocytic tumors. APMIS 112:257–263

Brooks PC, Silletti S, von Schalscha TL, Friedlander M, Cheresh DA (1998) Disruption of angiogenesis by PEX, a noncatalytic metalloproteinase fragment with integrin binding activity. Cell 92:391–400

Burger PC, Fuller GN (1991) Pathology–trends and pitfalls in histologic diagnosis, immunopathology, and applications of oncogene research. Neurol Clin 9:249–271

Carmeliet P, Jain RK (2000) Angiogenesis in cancer and other diseases. Nature 407:249–257

Carmeliet P, Moons L, Luttun A, Vincenti V, Compernolle V, De Mol M, Wu Y, Bono F, Devy L, Beck H, Scholz D, Acker T, DiPalma T, Dewerchin M, Noel A, Stalmans I, Barra A, Blacher S, Vandendriessche T, Ponten A, Eriksson U, Plate KH, Foidart JM, Schaper W, Charnock-Jones DS, Hicklin DJ, Herbert JM, Collen D, Persico MG (2001) Synergism between vascular endothelial growth factor and placental growth factor contributes to angiogenesis and plasma extravasation in pathological conditions. Nat Med 7:575–583

Carmeliet P, Tessier-Lavigne M (2005) Common mechanisms of nerve and blood vessel wiring. Nature 436:193–200

Chang SM, Lamborn KR, Malec M, Larson D, Wara W, Sneed P, Rabbitt J, Page M, Nicholas MK, Prados MD (2004) Phase II study of temozolomide and thalidomide with radiation therapy for newly diagnosed glioblastoma multiforme. Int J Radiat Oncol Biol Phys 60:353–357

Cheng N, Brantley DM, Chen J (2002) The ephrins and Eph receptors in angiogenesis. Cytokine Growth Factor Rev 13:75–85

Cirulli V, Yebra M (2007) Netrins: beyond the brain. Nat Rev Mol Cell Biol 8:296–306

Clauss M, Weich H, Breier G, Knies U, Rockl W, Waltenberger J, Risau W (1996) The vascular endothelial growth factor receptor Flt-1 mediates biological activities. Implications for a functional role of placenta growth factor in monocyte activation and chemotaxis. J Biol Chem 271:17629–17634

Cohen MH (2000) Thalidomide in the treatment of high-grade gliomas. J Clin Oncol 18:3453

Correa RG, Sasahara RM, Bengtson MH, Katayama ML, Salim AC, Brentani MM, Sogayar MC, de Souza SJ, Simpson AJ (2001) Human semaphorin 6B [(HSA)SEMA6B], a novel human class 6 semaphorin gene: alternative splicing and all-trans-retinoic acid-dependent downregulation in glioblastoma cell lines. Genomics 73:343–348

D'Amato RJ, Loughnan MS, Flynn E, Folkman J (1994) Thalidomide is an inhibitor of angiogenesis. Proc Natl Acad Sci USA 91:4082–4085

Dai C, Celestino JC, Okada Y, Louis DN, Fuller GN, Holland EC (2001) PDGF autocrine stimulation dedifferentiates cultured astrocytes and induces oligodendrogliomas and oligoastrocytomas from neural progenitors and astrocytes in vivo. Genes Dev 15:1913–1925

Dallol A, Krex D, Hesson L, Eng C, Maher ER, Latif F (2003) Frequent epigenetic inactivation of the SLIT2 gene in gliomas. Oncogene 22:4611–4616

Damert A, Machein M, Breier G, Fujita MQ, Hanahan D, Risau W, Plate KH (1997) Up-regulation of vascular endothelial growth factor expression in a rat glioma is conferred by two distinct hypoxia-driven mechanisms. Cancer Res 57:3860–3864

Desbaillets I, Diserens AC, de Tribolet N, Hamou MF, Van Meir EG (1999) Regulation of interleukin-8 expression by reduced oxygen pressure in human glioblastoma. Oncogene 18:1447–1456

Drevs J, Laus C, Medinger M, Schmidt-Gersbach C, Unger C (2002) Antiangiogenesis: current clinical data and future perspectives. Onkologie 25:520–527

Duda DG (2006) Antiangiogenesis and drug delivery to tumors: bench to bedside and back. Cancer Res 66:3967–3970

Dunn IF, Heese O, Black PM (2000) Growth factors in glioma angiogenesis: FGFs, PDGF, EGF, and TGFs. J Neurooncol 50:121–137

Erber R, Eichelsbacher U, Powajbo V, Korn T, Djonov V, Lin J, Hammes HP, Grobholz R, Ullrich A, Vajkoczy P (2006) EphB4 controls blood vascular morphogenesis during postnatal angiogenesis. EMBO J 25:628–641

Fearon ER, Cho KR, Nigro JM, Kern SE, Simons JW, Ruppert JM, Hamilton SR, Preisinger AC, Thomas G, Kinzler KW, (1990) Identification of a chromosome 18q gene that is altered in colorectal cancers. Science 247:49–56

Fenton BM, Paoni SF, Ding I (2004) Effect of VEGF receptor-2 antibody on vascular function and oxygenation in spontaneous and transplanted tumors. Radiother Oncol 72:221–230

Ferrara N, Gerber HP, LeCouter J (2003) The biology of VEGF and its receptors. Nat Med 9:669–676

Fiedler U, Augustin HG (2006) Angiopoietins: a link between angiogenesis and inflammation. Trends Immunol 27:552–558

Fine HA, Figg WD, Jaeckle K, Wen PY, Kyritsis AP, Loeffler JS, Levin VA, Black PM, Kaplan R, Pluda JM, Yung WK (2000) Phase II trial of the antiangiogenic agent thalidomide in patients with recurrent high-grade gliomas. J Clin Oncol 18:708–715

Fine HA, Wen PY, Maher EA, Viscosi E, Batchelor T, Lakhani N, Figg WD, Purow BW, Borkowf CB (2003) Phase II trial of thalidomide and carmustine for patients with recurrent high-grade gliomas. J Clin Oncol 21:2299–2304

Fischer C, Jonckx B, Mazzone M, Zacchigna S, Loges S, Pattarini L, Chorianopoulos E, Liesenborghs L, Koch M, De Mol M, Autiero M, Wyns S, Plaisance S, Moons L, van Rooijen N, Giacca M, Stassen JM, Dewerchin M, Collen D, Carmeliet P (2007) Anti-PlGF inhibits growth of VEGF(R)-inhibitor-resistant tumors without affecting healthy vessels. Cell 131:463–475

Folkman J (1985) Tumor angiogenesis. Adv Cancer Res 43:175–203

Folkman J (1996) Endogenous inhibitors of angiogenesis. Harvey Lect. 92:65–82

Forcet C, Stein E, Pays L, Corset V, Llambi F, Tessier-Lavigne M, Mehlen P (2002) Netrin-1-mediated axon outgrowth requires deleted in colorectal cancer-dependent MAPK activation. Nature 417:443–447

Gale NW, Dominguez MG, Noguera I, Pan L, Hughes V, Valenzuela DM, Murphy AJ, Adams NC, Lin HC, Holash J, Thurston G, Yancopoulos GD (2004) Haploinsufficiency of delta-like 4 ligand results in embryonic lethality due to major defects in arterial and vascular development. Proc Natl Acad Sci USA 101:15949–15954

Goldbrunner RH, Bendszus M, Wood J, Kiderlen M, Sasaki M, Tonn JC (2004) PTK787/ZK222584, an inhibitor of vascular endothelial growth factor receptor tyrosine kinases, decreases glioma growth and vascularization. Neurosurgery 55:426–432

Gomez-Manzano C, Fueyo J, Jiang H, Glass TL, Lee HY, Hu M, Liu JL, Jasti SL, Liu TJ, Conrad CA, Yung WK (2003) Mechanisms underlying PTEN regulation of vascular endothelial growth factor and angiogenesis. Ann Neurol 53:109–117

Grau SJ, Trillsch F, Herms J, Thon N, Nelson PJ, Tonn JC, Goldbrunner R (2007) Expression of VEGFR3 in glioma endothelium correlates with tumor grade. J Neurooncol 82:141–150

Gridley T (2007) Notch signaling in vascular development and physiology. Development 134:2709–2718

Groves MD, Puduvalli VK, Conrad CA, Gilbert MR, Yung WK, Jaeckle K, Liu V, Hess KR, Aldape KD, Levin VA (2006) Phase II trial of temozolomide plus marimastat for recurrent anaplastic gliomas: A relationship among efficacy, joint toxicity and anticonvulsant status. J Neurooncol 80:83–90

Guan M, Pang CP, Yam HF, Cheung KF, Liu WW, Lu Y (2004) Inhibition of glioma invasion by overexpression of pigment epithelium-derived factor. Cancer Gene Ther 11:325–332

Heidenreich R, Machein M, Nicolaus A, Hilbig A, Wild C, Clauss M, Plate KH, Breier G (2004) Inhibition of solid tumor growth by gene transfer of VEGF receptor-1 mutants. Int J Cancer 111:348–357

Holash J, Maisonpierre PC, Compton D, Boland P, Alexander CR, Zagzag D, Yancopoulos GD, Wiegand SJ (1999) Vessel cooption, regression, and growth in tumors mediated by angiopoietins and VEGF. Science 284:1994–1998

Hong K, Hinck L, Nishiyama M, Poo MM, Tessier-Lavigne M, Stein E (1999) A ligand-gated association between cytoplasmic domains of UNC5 and DCC family receptors converts netrin-induced growth cone attraction to repulsion. Cell 97:927–941

Hu B, Guo P, Fang Q, Tao HQ, Wang D, Nagane M, Huang HJ, Gunji Y, Nishikawa R, Alitalo K, Cavenee WK, Cheng SY (2003) Angiopoietin-2 induces human glioma invasion through the activation of matrix metalloprotease-2. Proc Natl Acad Sci USA 100:8904–8909

Izumi Y, di Tomaso E, Hooper A, Huang P, Huber J, Hicklin DJ, Fukumura D, Jain RK, Suit HD (2003) Responses to antiangiogenesis treatment of spontaneous autochthonous tumors and their isografts. Cancer Res 63:747–751

Jain RK (2005) Normalization of tumor vasculature: an emerging concept in antiangiogenic therapy. Science 307:58–62

Jain RK, di Tomaso E, Duda DG, Loeffler JS, Sorensen AG, Batchelor TT (2007) Angiogenesis in brain tumours. Nat Rev Neurosci 8:610–622

Jain RK, Duda DG, Clark JW, Loeffler JS (2006) Lessons from phase III clinical trials on anti-VEGF therapy for cancer. Nat Clin Pract Oncol 3:24–40

Janson, ET, Oberg K (2002) Malignant neuroendocrine tumors. Cancer Chemother. Biol Response Modif 20:463–470

Jeffers M, Rong S, Woude GF (1996) Hepatocyte growth factor/scatter factor-Met signaling in tumorigenicity and invasion/metastasis. J Mol Med 74:505–513

Jenny B, Harrison JA, Baetens D, Tille JC, Burkhardt K, Mottaz H, Kiss JZ, Dietrich PY, de Tribolet N, Pizzolato GP, Pepper MS (2006) Expression and localization of VEGF-C and VEGFR-3 in glioblastomas and haemangioblastomas. J Pathol 209:34–43

Jouanneau E (2008) Angiogenesis and gliomas: current issues and development of surrogate markers. Neurosurgery 62:31–50

Kabrun N, Buhring HJ, Choi K, Ullrich A, Risau W, Keller G (1997) Flk-1 expression defines a population of early embryonic hematopoietic precursors. Development 124:2039–2048

Kaminska B, Wesolowska A, Danilkiewicz M (2005) TGF beta signalling and its role in tumour pathogenesis. Acta Biochim Pol 52:329–337

Kaur B, Khwaja FW, Severson EA, Matheny SL, Brat DJ, Van Meir EG (2005) Hypoxia and the hypoxia-inducible-factor pathway in glioma growth and angiogenesis. Neurooncol 7:134–153

Kazuno M, Tokunaga T, Oshika Y, Tanaka Y, Tsugane R, Kijima H, Yamazaki H, Ueyama Y, Nakamura M (1999) Thrombospondin-2 (TSP2) expression is inversely correlated with vascularity in glioma. Eur J Cancer 35:502–506

Kerbel RS (2008) Tumor angiogenesis. N Engl J Med 358:2039–2049

Kerber M, Reiss Y, Wickersheim A, Jugold M, Kiessling F, Heil M, Tchaikovski, V, Waltenberger J, Shibuya M, Plate KH, Machein MR (2008) Flt-1 signaling in macrophages promotes glioma growth in vivo. Cancer Res 68(18):7342–7351

Kim KJ, Li B, Winer J, Armanini M, Gillett N, Phillips HS, Ferrara N (1993) Inhibition of vascular endothelial growth factor-induced angiogenesis suppresses tumour growth in vivo. Nature 362:841–844

Kim SK, Cargioli TG, Machluf M, Yang W, Sun Y, Al Hashem R, Kim SU, Black PM, Carroll RS (2005) PEX-producing human neural stem cells inhibit tumor growth in a mouse glioma model. Clin Cancer Res 11:5965–5970

Kirsch M, Schackert G, Black PM (2000) Angiogenesis, metastasis, and endogenous inhibition. J Neurooncol 50:173–180

Kirsch M, Strasser J, Allende R, Bello L, Zhang J, Black PM (1998) Angiostatin suppresses malignant glioma growth in vivo. Cancer Res 58:4654–4659

Klein R (2001) Excitatory Eph receptors and adhesive ephrin ligands. Curr Opin Cell Biol 13:196–203

Kragh M, Spang-Thomsen M, Kristjansen PE (1999) Time until initiation of tumor growth is an effective measure of the anti-angiogenic effect of TNP-470 on human glioblastoma in nude mice. Oncol Rep 6:759–762

Kruger RP, Aurandt J, Guan KL (2005) Semaphorins command cells to move. Nat Rev Mol Cell Biol 6:789–800

Kuroki T, Trapasso F, Yendamuri S, Matsuyama A, Alder H, Williams NN, Kaiser LR, Croce CM (2003) Allelic loss on chromosome 3p21.3 and promoter hypermethylation of semaphorin 3B in non-small cell lung cancer. Cancer Res 63:3352–3355

Lakka SS, Gondi CS, Yanamandra N, Olivero WC, Dinh DH, Gujrati M, Rao JS (2004) Inhibition of cathepsin B and MMP-9 gene expression in glioblastoma cell line via RNA interference reduces tumor cell invasion, tumor growth and angiogenesis. Oncogene 23:4681–4689

Lamszus K, Laterra J, Westphal M, Rosen EM (1999) Scatter factor/hepatocyte growth factor (SF/HGF) content and function in human gliomas. Int J Dev Neurosci 17:517–530

Lamszus K, Ulbricht U, Matschke J, Brockmann MA, Fillbrandt R, Westphal M (2003) Levels of soluble vascular endothelial growth factor (VEGF) receptor 1 in astrocytic tumors and its relation to malignancy, vascularity, and VEGF-A. Clin Cancer Res 9:1399–1405

Larrivee B, Freitas C, Trombe M, Lv X, Delafarge B, Yuan L, Bouvree K, Breant C, Del Toro R, Brechot N, Germain S, Bono F, Dol F, Claes F, Fischer C, Autiero M, Thomas JL, Carmeliet P, Tessier-Lavigne M, Eichmann A (2007) Activation of the UNC5B receptor by Netrin-1 inhibits sprouting angiogenesis. Genes Dev 21:2433–2447

Lee CG, Heijn M, di Tomaso E, Griffon-Etienne G, Ancukiewicz M, Koike C, Park KR, Ferrara N, Jain RK, Suit HD, Boucher Y (2000) Anti-vascular endothelial growth factor treatment augments tumor radiation response under normoxic or hypoxic conditions. Cancer Res 60:5565–5570

Li JL, Sainson RC, Shi W, Leek R, Harrington LS, Preusser M, Biswas S, Turley H, Heikamp E, Hainfellner JA, Harris AL (2007) Delta-like 4 Notch ligand regulates tumor angiogenesis, improves tumor vascular function, and promotes tumor growth in vivo. Cancer Res 67:11244–11253

Lund EL, Bastholm L, Kristjansen PE (2000) Therapeutic synergy of TNP-470 and ionizing radiation: effects on tumor growth, vessel morphology, and angiogenesis in human glioblastoma multiforme xenografts. Clin Cancer Res 6:971–978

Ma J, Pulfer S, Li S, Chu J, Reed K, Gallo JM (2001) Pharmacodynamic-mediated reduction of temozolomide tumor concentrations by the angiogenesis inhibitor TNP-470. Cancer Res 61:5491–5498

Machein MR, Knedla A, Knoth R, Wagner S, Neuschl E, Plate KH (2004) Angiopoietin-1 promotes tumor angiogenesis in a rat glioma model. Am J Pathol 165:1557–1570

Machein MR, Plate KH (2000) VEGF in brain tumors. J Neurooncol 50:109–120

Machein MR, Risau W, Plate KH (1999) Antiangiogenic gene therapy in a rat glioma model using a dominant-negative vascular endothelial growth factor receptor 2. Hum Gene Ther 10:1117–1128

Maity A, Pore N, Lee J, Solomon D, O'Rourke DM (2000) Epidermal growth factor receptor transcriptionally up-regulates vascular endothelial growth factor expression in human glioblastoma cells via a pathway involving phosphatidylinositol 3-kinase and distinct from that induced by hypoxia. Cancer Res 60:5879–5886

McDonald DM, Teicher BA, Stetler-Stevenson W, Ng SS, Figg WD, Folkman J, Hanahan D, Auerbach R, O'Reilly M, Herbst R, Cheresh D, Gordon M, Eggermont A, Libutti SK (2004) Report from the society for biological therapy and vascular biology faculty of the NCI workshop on angiogenesis monitoring. J Immunother 27:161–175

Mertsch S, Schmitz N, Jeibmann A, Geng JG, Paulus W, Senner V (2008) Slit2 involvement in glioma cell migration is mediated by Robo1 receptor. J Neurooncol 87:1–7

Meyerhardt JA, Caca K, Eckstrand BC, Hu G, Lengauer C, Banavali S, Look AT, Fearon ER (1999) Netrin-1: interaction with deleted in colorectal cancer (DCC) and alterations in brain tumors and neuroblastomas. Cell Growth Differ 10:35–42

Mignatti P, Morimoto T, Rifkin DB (1991) Basic fibroblast growth factor released by single, isolated cells stimulates their migration in an autocrine manner. Proc Natl Acad Sci USA 88:11007–11011

Millauer B, Shawver LK, Plate KH, Risau W, Ullrich A (1994) Glioblastoma growth inhibited in vivo by a dominant-negative Flk-1 mutant. Nature 367:576–579

Millauer B, Wizigmann-Voos S, Schnurch H, Martinez R, Moller NP, Risau W, Ullrich A (1993) High affinity VEGF binding and developmental expression suggest Flk-1 as a major regulator of vasculogenesis and angiogenesis. Cell 72:835–846

Morimoto T, Aoyagi M, Tamaki M, Yoshino Y, Hori H, Duan L, Yano T, Shibata M, Ohno K, Hirakawa K, Yamaguchi N (2002) Increased levels of tissue endostatin in human malignant gliomas. Clin Cancer Res 8:2933–2938

Murata R, Nishimura Y, Hiraoka M (1997) An antiangiogenic agent (TNP-470) inhibited reoxygenation during fractionated radiotherapy of murine mammary carcinoma. Int J Radiat Oncol Biol Phys 37:1107–1113

Nakada M, Drake KL, Nakada S, Niska JA, Berens ME (2006) Ephrin-B3 ligand promotes glioma invasion through activation of Rac1. Cancer Res 66:8492–8500

Nakada M, Niska JA, Tran NL, McDonough WS, Berens ME (2005) EphB2/R-Ras signaling regulates glioma cell adhesion, growth, and invasion. Am J Pathol 167:565–576

Neufeld G, Kessler O (2008) The semaphorins: versatile regulators of tumour progression and tumour angiogenesis. Nat Rev Cancer 8:632–645

Noguera-Troise I, Daly C, Papadopoulos NJ, Coetzee S, Boland P, Gale NW, Lin HC, Yancopoulos GD, Thurston G (2006) Blockade of Dll4 inhibits tumour growth by promoting non-productive angiogenesis. Nature 444:1032–1037

Noguera-Troise I, Daly C, Papadopoulos NJ, Coetzee S, Boland P, Gale NW, Lin HC, Yancopoulos GD, Thurston G (2007) Blockade of Dll4 inhibits tumour growth by promoting non-productive angiogenesis. Novartis Found Symp 283:106–120

Nomura M, Yamagishi S, Harada S, Yamashima T, Yamashita J, Yamamoto H (1998) Placenta growth factor (PlGF) mRNA expression in brain tumors. J Neurooncol 40:123–130

Nyberg P, Xie L, Kalluri R (2005) Endogenous inhibitors of angiogenesis. Cancer Res 65:3967–3979

O'Reilly MS, Boehm T, Shing Y, Fukai N, Vasios G, Lane WS, Flynn E, Birkhead JR, Olsen BR, Folkman J (1997) Endostatin: an endogenous inhibitor of angiogenesis and tumor growth. Cell 88:277–285

O'Reilly MS, Holmgren L, Shing Y, Chen C, Rosenthal RA, Cao Y, Moses M, Lane WS, Sage EH, Folkman J (1994) Angiostatin: a circulating endothelial cell inhibitor that suppresses angiogenesis and tumor growth. Cold Spring Harb Symp Quant Biol 59:471–482

Olsson AK, Dimberg A, Kreuger J, Claesson-Welsh L (2006) VEGF receptor signalling - in control of vascular function. Nat Rev Mol Cell Biol 7:359–371

Osada H, Tokunaga T, Nishi M, Hatanaka H, Abe Y, Tsugu A, Kijima H, Yamazaki H, Ueyama Y, Nakamura M (2004) Overexpression of the neuropilin 1 (NRP1) gene correlated with poor prognosis in human glioma. Anticancer Res 24:547–552

Plate KH, Breier G, Millauer B, Ullrich A, Risau W (1993) Up-regulation of vascular endothelial growth factor and its cognate receptors in a rat glioma model of tumor angiogenesis. Cancer Res 53:5822–5827

Plate KH, Breier G, Weich HA, Mennel HD, Risau W (1994) Vascular endothelial growth factor and glioma angiogenesis: coordinate induction of VEGF receptors, distribution of VEGF protein and possible in vivo regulatory mechanisms. Int J Cancer 59:520–529

Plate KH, Breier G, Weich HA, Risau W (1992) Vascular endothelial growth factor is a potential tumour angiogenesis factor in human gliomas in vivo. Nature 359:845–848

Platten M, Wick W, Weller M (2001) Malignant glioma biology: role for TGF-beta in growth, motility, angiogenesis, and immune escape. Microsc Res Tech 52:401–410

Purow BW, Haque RM, Noel MW, Su Q, Burdick MJ, Lee J, Sundaresan T, Pastorino S, Park JK, Mikolaenko I, Maric D, Eberhart CG, Fine HA (2005) Expression of Notch-1 and its ligands, Delta-like-1 and Jagged-1, is critical for glioma cell survival and proliferation. Cancer Res 65:2353–2363

Read TA, Sorensen DR, Mahesparan R, Enger PO, Timpl R, Olsen BR, Hjelstuen MH, Haraldseth O, Bjerkvig R (2001) Local endostatin treatment of gliomas administered by microencapsulated producer cells. Nat Biotechnol 19:29–34

Rege TA, Fears CY, Gladson CL (2005) Endogenous inhibitors of angiogenesis in malignant gliomas: nature's antiangiogenic therapy. Neurooncol 7:106–121

Reiss Y, Machein MR, Plate KH (2005) The role of angiopoietins during angiogenesis in gliomas. Brain Pathol 15:311–317

Rieger J, Wick W, Weller M (2003) Human malignant glioma cells express semaphorins and their receptors, neuropilins and plexins. Glia 42:379–389

Risau W, Drexler H, Mironov V, Smits A, Siegbahn A, Funa K, Heldin CH (1992) Platelet-derived growth factor is angiogenic in vivo. Growth Factors 7:261–266

Rodrigues S, De Wever O, Bruyneel E, Rooney RJ, Gespach C (2007) Opposing roles of netrin-1 and the dependence receptor DCC in cancer cell invasion, tumor growth and metastasis. Oncogene 26:5615–5625

Rolny C, Capparuccia L, Casazza A, Mazzone M, Vallario A, Cignetti A, Medico E, Carmeliet P, Comoglio PM, Tamagnone L (2008) The tumor suppressor semaphorin 3B triggers a prometastatic program mediated by interleukin 8 and the tumor microenvironment. J Exp Med 205:1155–1171

Rong Y, Durden DL, Van Meir EG, Brat DJ (2006) 'Pseudopalisading' necrosis in glioblastoma: a familiar morphologic feature that links vascular pathology, hypoxia, and angiogenesis. J Neuropathol Exp Neurol 65:529–539

Rong Y, Post DE, Pieper RO, Durden DL, Van Meir EG, Brat DJ (2005) PTEN and hypoxia regulate tissue factor expression and plasma coagulation by glioblastoma. Cancer Res 65:1406–1413

Rubenstein JL, Kim J, Ozawa T, Zhang M, Westphal M, Deen DF, Shuman MA (2000) Anti-VEGF antibody treatment of glioblastoma prolongs survival but results in increased vascular cooption. Neoplasia 2:306–314

Samoto K, Ikezaki K, Ono M, Shono T, Kohno K, Kuwano M, Fukui M (1995) Expression of vascular endothelial growth factor and its possible relation with neovascularization in human brain tumors. Cancer Res 55:1189–1193

Sasaki M, Wizigmann-Voos S, Risau W, Plate KH (1999) Retrovirus producer cells encoding antisense VEGF prolong survival of rats with intracranial GS9L gliomas. Int J Dev Neurosci 17:579–591

Sato H, Takino T, Okada Y, Cao J, Shinagawa A, Yamamoto E, Seiki M (1994) A matrix metalloproteinase expressed on the surface of invasive tumour cells. Nature 370:61–65

Sato TN, Tozawa Y, Deutsch U, Wolburg-Buchholz K, Fujiwara Y, Gendron-Maguire M, Gridley T, Wolburg H, Risau W, Qin Y (1995) Distinct roles of the receptor tyrosine kinases Tie-1 and Tie-2 in blood vessel formation. Nature 376:70–74

Schmidt NO, Westphal M, Hagel C, Ergun S, Stavrou D, Rosen EM, Lamszus K (1999) Levels of vascular endothelial growth factor, hepatocyte growth factor/scatter factor and basic fibroblast growth factor in human gliomas and their relation to angiogenesis. Int J Cancer 84:10–18

Schnurch H, Risau W (1993) Expression of tie-2, a member of a novel family of receptor tyrosine kinases, in the endothelial cell lineage. Development 119:957–968

Schueneman AJ, Himmelfarb E, Geng L, Tan J, Donnelly E, Mendel D, McMahon G, Hallahan DE (2003) SU11248 maintenance therapy prevents tumor regrowth after fractionated irradiation of murine tumor models. Cancer Res 63:4009–4016

Semenza GL, Wang GL (1992) A nuclear factor induced by hypoxia via de novo protein synthesis binds to the human erythropoietin gene enhancer at a site required for transcriptional activation. Mol Cell Biol 12:5447–5454

Shekarabi M, Kennedy TE (2002) The netrin-1 receptor DCC promotes filopodia formation and cell spreading by activating Cdc42 and Rac1. Mol Cell Neurosci 19:1–17

Shibuya M (2006) Vascular endothelial growth factor receptor-1 (VEGFR-1/Flt-1): a dual regulator for angiogenesis. Angiogenesis 9:225–230

Shih AH, Holland EC (2006a) Notch signaling enhances nestin expression in gliomas. Neoplasia 8:1072–1082

Shih AH, Holland EC (2006b) Platelet-derived growth factor (PDGF) and glial tumorigenesis. Cancer Lett 232:139–147

Shweiki D, Itin A, Soffer D, Keshet E (1992) Vascular endothelial growth factor induced by hypoxia may mediate hypoxia-initiated angiogenesis. Nature 359:843–845

Soker S, Miao HQ, Nomi M, Takashima S, Klagsbrun M (2002) VEGF165 mediates formation of complexes containing VEGFR-2 and neuropilin-1 that enhance VEGF165-receptor binding. J Cell Biochem 85:357–368

Soker S, Takashima S, Miao HQ, Neufeld G, Klagsbrun M (1998) Neuropilin-1 is expressed by endothelial and tumor cells as an isoform-specific receptor for vascular endothelial growth factor. Cell 20;92:735–745

Stratmann A, Machein MR, Plate KH (1997) Anti-angiogenic gene therapy of malignant glioma. Acta Neurochir (Suppl. 68):105–110

Stratmann A, Risau W, Plate KH (1998) Cell type-specific expression of angiopoietin-1 and angiopoietin-2 suggests a role in glioblastoma angiogenesis. Am J Pathol 153:1459–1466

Strik HM, Schluesener HJ, Seid K, Meyermann R, Deininger MH (2001) Localization of endostatin in rat and human gliomas. Cancer 91:1013–1019

Su JL, Yen CJ, Chen PS, Chuang SE, Hong CC, Kuo IH, Chen HY, Hung MC, Kuo ML (2007) The role of the VEGF-C/VEGFR-3 axis in cancer progression. Br J Cancer 96:541–545

Taga T, Suzuki A, Gonzalez-Gomez I, Gilles FH, Stins M, Shimada H, Barsky L, Weinberg KI, Laug WE (2002) Alpha v-integrin antagonist EMD 121974 induces apoptosis in brain tumor cells growing on vitronectin and tenascin. Int J Cancer 98:690–697

Takamiya Y, Brem H, Ojeifo J, Mineta T, Martuza RL (1994) AGM-1470 inhibits the growth of human glioblastoma cells in vitro and in vivo. Neurosurgery 34:869–875

Tammela T, Zarkada G, Wallgard E, Murtomaki A, Suchting S, Wirzenius M, Waltari M, Hellstrom M, Schomber T, Peltonen R, Freitas C, Duarte A, Isoniemi H, Laakkonen P, Christofori G, Yla-Herttuala S, Shibuya M, Pytowski B, Eichmann A, Betsholtz C, Alitalo K (2008) Blocking VEGFR-3 suppresses angiogenic sprouting and vascular network formation. Nature 454:656–660

Tenan M, Fulci G, Albertoni M, Diserens AC, Hamou MF, Atifi-Borel M, Feige JJ, Pepper MS, Van Meir EG (2000) Thrombospondin-1 is downregulated by anoxia and suppresses tumorigenicity of human glioblastoma cells. J Exp Med 191:1789–1798

Thorns V, Walter GF, Thorns C (2003) Expression of MMP-2, MMP-7, MMP-9, MMP-10 and MMP-11 in human astrocytic and oligodendroglial gliomas. Anticancer Res 23:3937–3944

Tomizawa Y, Sekido Y, Kondo M, Gao B, Yokota J, Roche J, Drabkin H, Lerman MI, Gazdar AF, Minna JD (2001) Inhibition of lung cancer cell growth and induction of apoptosis after reexpression of 3p21.3 candidate tumor suppressor gene SEMA3B. Proc Natl Acad Sci USA 98:13954–13959

Tonn JC, Kerkau S, Hanke A, Bouterfa H, Mueller JG, Wagner S, Vince GH, Roosen K (1999) Effect of synthetic matrix-metalloproteinase inhibitors on invasive capacity and proliferation of human malignant gliomas in vitro. Int J Cancer 80:764–772

Tsai JC, Goldman CK, Gillespie GY (1995) Vascular endothelial growth factor in human glioma cell lines: induced secretion by EGF, PDGF-BB, and bFGF. J Neurosurg 82:864–873

Valtola R, Salven P, Heikkila P, Taipale J, Joensuu H, Rehn M, Pihlajaniemi T, Weich H, deWaal R, Alitalo K (1999) VEGFR-3 and its ligand VEGF-C are associated with angiogenesis in breast cancer. Am J Pathol 154:1381–1390

Van Meir EG, Polverini PJ, Chazin VR, Su Huang HJ, de Tribolet N, Cavenee WK (1994) Release of an inhibitor of angiogenesis upon induction of wild type p53 expression in glioblastoma cells. Nat Genet 8:171–176

Vitolo D, Paradiso P, Uccini S, Ruco LP, Baroni CD (1996) Expression of adhesion molecules and extracellular matrix proteins in glioblastomas: relation to angiogenesis and spread. Histopathology 28:521–528

Vredenburgh JJ, Desjardins A, Herndon JE, Dowell JM, Reardon DA, Quinn JA, Rich JN, Sathornsumetee S, Gururangan S, Wagner M, Bigner DD, Friedman AH, Friedman HS (2007a) Phase II trial of bevacizumab and irinotecan in recurrent malignant glioma. Clin Cancer Res 13:1253–1259

Vredenburgh JJ, Desjardins A, Herndon JE, Marcello J, Reardon DA, Quinn JA, Rich JN, Sathornsumetee S, Gururangan S, Sampson J, Wagner M, Bailey L, Bigner DD, Friedman AH, Friedman HS (2007b) Bevacizumab plus irinotecan in recurrent glioblastoma multiforme. J Clin Oncol 20;25:4722–4729

Wang B, Xiao Y, Ding BB, Zhang N, Yuan X, Gui L, Qian KX, Duan S, Chen Z, Rao Y, Geng JG (2003) Induction of tumor angiogenesis by Slit-Robo signaling and inhibition of cancer growth by blocking Robo activity. Cancer Cell 4:19–29

Weindel K, Moringlane JR, Marme D, Weich HA (1994) Detection and quantification of vascular endothelial growth factor/vascular permeability factor in brain tumor tissue and cyst fluid: the key to angiogenesis? Neurosurgery 35: 439–448

Werbowetski-Ogilvie TE, Seyed SM, Jabado N, Angers-Loustau A, Agar NY, Wu J, Bjerkvig R, Antel JP, Faury D, Rao Y, Del Maestro RF (2006) Inhibition of medulloblastoma cell invasion by Slit. Oncogene 25:5103–5112

Wick W, Platten M, Weller M (2001) Glioma cell invasion: regulation of metalloproteinase activity by TGF-beta. J Neurooncol 53: 177–185

Witmer AN, van Blijswijk BC, Dai J, Hofman P, Partanen TA, Vrensen GF, Schlingemann RO (2001) VEGFR-3 in adult angiogenesis. J Pathol 195:490–497

Wong K, Park HT, Wu JY, Rao Y (2002) Slit proteins: molecular guidance cues for cells ranging from neurons to leukocytes. Curr Opin Genet Dev 12:583–591

Yamada N, Kato M, Yamashita H, Nister M, Miyazono K, Heldin CH, Funa K (1995) Enhanced expression of transforming growth factor-beta and its type-I and type-II receptors in human glioblastoma. Int J Cancer 62:386–392

Yancopoulos GD, Klagsbrun M, Folkman J (1998) Vasculogenesis, angiogenesis, and growth factors: ephrins enter the fray at the border. Cell 93:661–664

Zagzag D, Amirnovin R, Greco MA, Yee H, Holash J, Wiegand SJ, Zabski S, Yancopoulos GD, Grumet M (2000a) Vascular apoptosis and involution in gliomas precede neovascularization: a novel concept for glioma growth and angiogenesis. Lab Invest 80:837–849

Zagzag D, Friedlander DR, Miller DC, Dosik J, Cangiarella J, Kostianovsky M, Cohen H, Grumet M, Greco MA (1995) Tenascin expression in astrocytomas correlates with angiogenesis. Cancer Res 55:907–914

Zagzag D, Hooper A, Friedlander DR, Chan W, Holash J, Wiegand SJ, Yancopoulos GD, Grumet M (1999) In situ expression of angiopoietins in astrocytomas identifies angiopoietin-2 as an early marker of tumor angiogenesis. Exp. Neurol 159:391–400

Zagzag D, Miller DC, Sato Y, Rifkin DB, Burstein DE (1990) Immunohistochemical localization of basic fibroblast growth factor in astrocytomas. Cancer Res 50:7393–7398

Zagzag D, Shiff B, Jallo GI, Greco MA, Blanco C, Cohen H, Hukin J, Allen JC, Friedlander DR (2002) Tenascin-C promotes microvascular cell migration and phosphorylation of focal adhesion kinase. Cancer Res 62:2660–2668

Zagzag D, Zhong H, Scalzitti JM, Laughner E, Simons JW, Semenza GL (2000b) Expression of hypoxia-inducible factor 1alpha in brain tumors: association with angiogenesis, invasion, and progression. Cancer 88:2606–2618

Gene Regulation by Methylation

13

Wolf C. Mueller and Andreas von Deimling

Abstract Epigenetic gene regulation of specific genes strongly affects clinical outcome of malignant glioma. *MGMT* is the best studied gene for the connection of promoter methylation and clinical course in glioblastoma. While *MGMT* promoter methylation analysis currently does not alter treatment of glioblastoma patients, mainly because of a lack of convincing therapy to radiotherapy and concomitant administration of alkylating drugs, there is increasing interest on the part of patients and physicians in having this molecular parameter assessed.

This chapter gives a short overview of the physiological characteristics of the epigenome in normal cells and tissues and the changes in epigenetic gene regulation following malignant transformation. It discusses the technical aspects, advantages, and shortcomings of currently used approaches for single-gene and genome-wide methylation analyses. Finally, an outlook is given on potential therapeutic avenues and targets to overcome tumor-suppressor gene silencing by aberrant promoter methylation in gliomas.

Wolf C. Mueller (✉)
Department of Neuropathology
Institute of Pathology
Im Neuenheimer Feld 220/221
69120 Heidelberg
Germany
E-mail: Wolf.Mueller@med.uni-heidelberg.de

13.1
Epigenetics

13.1.1
Methylation in Normal Cells and Tissues

DNA methylation as a mechanism to regulate transcription is most important and best studied at CpG dinucleotides. The overall number of CpG dinucleotides is substantially lower than expected if randomly distributed. Furthermore, CpG dinucleotide distribution is asymmetric, with overrepresentation in promoter regions and underrepresentation in coding sequence. Clusters of CpG dinucleotides are termed CpG islands. Approximately 70–80% of CpG dinucleotides resides outside of CpG islands and is usually methylated in normal tissues. Only 7% of all CpG dinucleotides are part of the estimated 15,000 CpG islands (Antequera and Bird 1993) in highly conserved promoter regions of the human genome, and most of the CpG islands in promoter regions are unmethylated in normal tissues. In most genes, this is independent of whether or not the gene is being transcribed (Bird 2002). However, few genes, for example,

Maspin, are silenced in normal tissues in a cell-type specific manner by promoter methylation (Costello and Vertino 2002). This finding indicates that promoter methylation does not only occur aberrantly in tumors, but may help to maintain cell-type-specific gene expression patterns in normal tissues. The haploid human genome contains approximately 28,000 CpG dinucleotides in promoter regions. CpG dinucleotide depletion in coding sequence is explained by spontaneous deamination of methylated cytosine and consecutive replacement by thymidine. This mechanism also underlies the most common type of genetic polymorphism in human population: the cytidine to thymidine transition (Rideout et al. 1990).

During DNA methylation, DNA methyltransferases (*DNMTs*) transfer methyl groups to cytosine residues in CpG dinucleotides. In humans, three *DNMTs* can be distinguished. Of these *DNMT3A* and *DNMT3B* create de novo and *DNMT1* maintains methylation patterns. This is of particular importance during embryogenesis because specific methylation patterns are created. The maintenance enzyme *DNMT1* adds methyl groups to sites in which one DNA strand is already methylated. Thus, the methylation pattern, created by de novo *DNMTS* during embryogenesis, is maintained.

In humans only cytosines preceding a guanosine in the DNA sequence (CpG dinucleotide) are affected by this modification. In animal models, the elimination of any one of these methyltransferases from the germline is lethal.

CpG methylation outside of CpG islands may help maintain noncoding DNA in human cells in a transcriptionally inert state and may help to prevent the transcription of potentially harmful sequences embedded in parts of the noncoding genome (Antequera and Bird 1993; Bird and Wolffe 1999). Examples for such sequences are repeat elements, inserted viral sequences, and transposons. In addition, methylation of pericentromeric heterochromatin appears crucial for maintaining the conformation and integrity of the chromosome.

A special mechanism of silencing genes by methylation is imprinting. Imprinted genes are active and dependent on their parental origin. Imprinting has been shown to be involved in tumorigenesis of the Wilms tumor. Recently paternal inactivation of the maternally imprinted *DIRAS3* gene has been proposed as a mechanism contributing to the formation of oligodendroglial tumors (Riemenschneider et al. 2008).

Inactivation of one copy of the X chromosome in human females is maintained by methylation of CpGs in promoter regions. It is noteworthy silencing of the genes precedes their promoter methylation and is facilitated by X inactive specific transcript (XIST) followed by hypoacetylation of histones. The XIST gene itself remains unmethylated and is transcribed from the otherwise inactivated X chromosome (Goto et al. 2002). This mechanism serves the purpose of ensuring roughly similar transcription levels of X chromosomal genes independent of the presence of one or two X chromosomes.

Different mechanisms are involved in the repression of transcription by promoter methylation. In addition, methylation inhibits binding of transcription factors to the CpG containing recognition sites. The methyl–CpG-binding proteins, MeCP1, and MeCP2, bind specifically to methylated CpGs and inhibit the binding of transcription factors by limiting access to the promoter (Nan et al. 1998). Their inhibiting effect is mediated by the ability to recruit histone deacetylases (*HDACs*). MeCP1 recruits HDAC1, HDAC2, and the Rb-related proteins 46 and 48. MeCP2 binds to the Sin3-HDAC corepressor complex. HDACs deacetylate lysine residues in the N-terminal tails of the histones, thereby condensing and inactivating chromatin.

13.1.2
Methylation in Cancer: General Aspects

Pathologic activation and inactivation of genes controlling proliferation and cell death is a key feature of tumor cells. Activation of oncogenes may occur by gene amplification, translocation, and fusion of genes or by activating mutations. Inactivation of tumor suppressor genes may result from genomic deletions, mutations, and inappropriate promoter methylation. In fact, DNA methylation patterns necessary for maintaining gene expression and chromosomal stability are severely disrupted in cancer (Baylin and Bestor 2002; Herman and Baylin 2003; Feinberg and Tycko 2004; Jones 2005). Aberrant methylation of gene promoters is now recognized as a common mechanism for gene inactivation in human cancers. It is noteworthy that promoter hypermethylation leaves the physical structure of the gene untouched. Therefore, this process may be reversible and demethylation could reactivate both gene expression and gene function. Such reexpression of methylated genes has been demonstrated in experimental systems and renders methylated cancer-relevant genes potential targets for therapy.

Virtually all cancers, including gliomas, have both gains in methylation of CpG islands in gene promoters and loss of methylation in the CpG-depleted noncoding regions where most CpG dinucleotides are methylated in normal tissues (Feinberg and Vogelstein 1983; Goelz et al. 1985; Feinberg and Vogelstein 1987). Methylation of CpG islands in promoter regions results in aberrant silencing of transcription. Functionally, promoter hypermethylation can have the same effect as inactivating mutations in tumor suppressor genes. While in sporadic tumors, point mutations only rarely affect both copies of a tumor suppressor gene, hypermethylation of both copies of a gene is not infrequent in nonfamilial tumors (Esteller et al. 2001). *CDKN2A* (*p16*) in many types of cancer (including gliomas), *VHL* in renal cancer, and the mismatch repair gene *hMLH1* in colorectal cancer and other neoplasms are examples of cancer-related epigenetically silenced genes with classical tumor-suppressor gene function. Loss of methylation in noncoding regions of the genome also contributes to tumorigenesis. Such global reduction of methylation weakens the transcriptional repression of noncoding DNA regions. Thus, inserted and potentially harmful viral genes could be expressed (Walsh et al. 1998). Also, such hypomethylation could relax the tight control of imprinted genes and genes on the inactivated X chromosome, and either could be harmful because of increased transcription. Further, demethylation of pericentromeric regions disrupts the functional stability of chromosomes in cancer and leads to chromosomal instability and deficient DNA replication (Eden et al. 2003). Supporting evidence for this effect derives from a mouse model in which profound and long-standing loss of methylation from embryogenesis to adulthood is coupled with increasing genetic instability (Eden et al. 2003; Gaudet et al. 2003).

In addition, recent observations provide evidence that CpG methylation as a mechanism for silencing is not restricted to single genes but also occurs in stretches of DNA spanning larger chromosomal sections. Silencing of a 4-Mb band on chromosome *2q.14.2* has been observed, although not all genes in this region exhibited hypermethylation of CpGs in their respective promoter regions. In fact, hypermethylation was detected in only three distinct zones, resulting in heterochromatinization of adjacent genes (Frigola et al. 2006). It remains to be determined whether there are similarly repressed chromosomal bands elsewhere in the cancer epigenome and if so, if these are also common in gliomas.

13.2
Strategies of Epigenetic Studies in Gliomas

Methylation of promoter regions, with corresponding down-regulation of gene expression, has been implicated as an alternative mechanism to gene mutation for tumor-suppressor gene inactivation (Costello et al. 2000; Esteller 2003; Jain 2003; Ballestar and Esteller 2005; Esteller 2005). Most approaches to evaluate methylation as a means of tumor-suppressor gene inactivation in glioblastomas have focused on individual candidate genes (Li et al. 1998; 1999; Fan et al. 2002; Watanabe et al. 2002; Dallol et al. 2003; Gonzalez-Gomez et al. 2003a, b; Dickinson et al. 2004; Stone et al. 2004). Selection of the genes to be examined was mainly driven by evidence of a functional association with cell cycle regulation, tumor invasion, apoptosis, or tumor suppression. Further, the search for epigenetically regulated genes in gliomas focused on those genes shown to be hypermethylated in tumors outside the brain. An additional parameter for candidate selection was mapping to regions frequently deleted in glioma.

Comprehensive allelotyping of glioblastoma identified particular regions with common loss on chromosomal arms 6q, 9p, 10p, 10q, 13q, 14q, 15q, 17p, 18q, 19q, 22q, and Y (Kim et al. 1995; Mohapatra et al. 1998; Nishizaki et al. 1998; von Deimling et al. 2000; Collins 2004). However, only a few tumor-suppressor genes with inactivating mutations affecting both gene copies have been identified in these regions. Genes with such mutations include *TP53* on 17p (Chung et al. 1991; von Deimling et al. 1994; Ichimura et al. 2000), *PTEN* on 10q (Li et al. 1997; Steck et al. 1997; Wang et al. 1997), and, to a lesser extent, *RB1* on 13q (Henson et al. 1994; Ichimura et al. 1996); homozygous deletions have also been documented affecting *CDKN2A/p16/p14* on 9p (Ichimura et al. 1996, 2000; Ueki et al. 1996). The putative tumor-suppressor genes at all other loci remain elusive. Because promoter hypermethylation can functionally inactivate a gene copy as effective as a somatic mutation, much effort was put into the identification of epigenetic modifications in putative TSG mapping to these regions, with allelic losses particularly in candidates devoid of structural alterations (i.e., *CDKN2A/p16/p14* on chromosome 9p in human gliomas (Costello et al. 1996; Weber et al. 2007); *transcription factor 21 TCF21* on chromosome 6 in head, neck, and lung cancers (Smith et al. 2006); *oligodendrocyte transcription factor 1 (OLIG1)* on chromosome 21 in non-small cell lung cancer (Brena et al. 2007), and *DIRAS3* on chromosome 1p in oligodendrogliomas (Riemenschneider et al. 2008). Although such studies have implicated methylation as a tumorigenic event in human gliomas, these approaches do not provide a means to identify novel genes not considered *a priori* to be candidates. In this regard, it is important to note that gliomas are extensively methylated across the tumor genome (Costello et al. 2000) and that promoter hypermethylation is not necessarily tied to regions of allelic loss. In contrast, several studies on gliomas have shown that the distribution of promoter methylation is independent of regions with allelic deletions (Zardo et al. 2002; Hong et al. 2003). This calls for genome-wide screening tools able to provide an unbiased view on global promoter methylation patterns within defined tumor entities, including gliomas. Examples of some of these techniques are given in the following sections.

13.3
Methods of Epigenome Analysis

13.3.1
General Aspects of Methylation Analysis

Several techniques are available to detect and characterize DNA methylation. Which method to use depends on the specific question and aim of the study. Analyses of methylation in established markers for clinical evaluation require a different approach from that necessary to characterize novel target genes.

Protocols may be divided into two groups, with one including the techniques suitable for detection of qualitative and the other including techniques suitable for both qualitative and quantitative DNA methylation analysis. Techniques detecting qualitative change for distinction of methylated and unmethylated promoter sequences regardless of the methylation extent comprise MSP (Herman et al. 1996), and MSP-derived techniques such as melting curve analysis-based MSP (MCA-MSP) (Lorente et al. 2008b). Techniques to additionally determine the extent of DNA methylation can do so either in a quantitative or semiquantitative way. Techniques allowing a semiquantitative promoter methylation analysis include bisulfite-sequencing, melting curve analysis-based techniques implementing bisulfite sequencing primers (Worm et al. 2001; Guldberg et al. 2002; Lorente et al. 2008b), restriction landmark genomic scanning (RLGS), and methylation-specific multiplex ligation-dependent probe amplification (MS-MLPA). High-throughput methodologies have been developed, allowing quantitative methylation analyses targeting individual CpG-dinucleotide residues within an analyzed sequence. These techniques include pyrosequencing (Mikeska et al. 2007) and matrix-assisted laser desorption/ionization time-of-flight mass spectrometry (MALDI-TOF-MS) (Ehrich et al. 2005). However, both demand expensive hardware, which may not be easily accessible for many institutions, and they require time-consuming and sensitive sample preparation (MALDI-TOF) or are still limited to a rather short target sequence not suitable for screening purposes (pyrosequencing).

13.3.2
Bisulfite Sequencing

PCR and Sanger-sequencing do not distinguish between cytosines and methyl-cytosines. Therefore, most applications to identify methyl-cytosines require an initial step of conversion of cytosine to uracil by bisulfite treatment. Methyl-cytosine is not converted by this treatment. Consecutive PCR replaces uracil by thymidine in newly synthesized DNA strands. Sequencing bisulfite-modified DNA therefore allows establishing a comprehensive profile of cytosine methylation. The status of all CpG-dinucleotides within the promoter sequence, compared to normal tissue of the same type, allows for the distinction of cell-type from tumor-specific promoter methylation. Bisulfite conversion strongly depletes DNA sequence from cytosines and enriches for thymidines making primer design quite tedious and occasionally for some sequences impossible. Cloning of bisulfite modified DNA following PCR amplification successfully avoids mispriming and primer shifting during sequencing reactions. However, sequencing of one clone represents the methylation pattern of the promoter region in that particular clone only. Therefore, evaluation of promoter methylation profile requires sequencing of multiple clones with a typical analysis including ten clones. Sequencing of more clones will result in a better representation of the position and frequency of individually methylated cytosines in the region examined (Mueller et al. 2007). Once the methylation profile of a promoter sequence has been established by bisulfite sequencing, it is possible to identify CG-dinucleotides within the promoter sequence that readily and reliably enable the distinction between a methylated and an unmethylated promoter and correlate with transcriptional down-regulation or silencing of the respective gene. Once these CpGs are identified, a methylation-specific PCR (MSP) assay can be implemented.

13.3.3
Methylation-Specific PCR

This PCR-based technique takes advantage of the nucleotide differences between methylated and unmethylated DNA upon bisulfite treatment and was first described in 1996 (Herman et al. 1996). Primer sequences for unmethylated and methylated DNA reflect these differences. Nonmethylated cytosines within the primer sequences will be converted to thymidines and recognized by the so-called U-primers but not by the M-primers. On the contrary, methylated cytosines will not be affected and recognized by the M-primers but not by the U-primer pair.

In addition, both M- and U-primers are positioned in such a way that they contain cytosine residues other than CpG-dinucleotides. These will be converted regardless of CpG-site methylation. This will ensure amplification of converted DNA only and will avoid mispriming with genomic DNA.

Since this is a PCR-based technique, one has to be aware of its sensitivity to false-positive results. Because amplification of bisulfite-converted DNA requires longer annealing and extension times during amplification, higher cycle numbers as compared to conventional PCR protocols need to be programmed. This set-up requires stringent negative and positive controls for both methylated and unmethylated DNA. Another important factor influencing MSP is DNA quality and provenience. Reliable bisulfite conversion requires high-quality genomic DNA that preferably is isolated from snap-frozen tissue. Bisulfite modification degrades DNA. The amount of DNA entered into bisulfite modification should therefore reach or exceed 1 μg. Frequently, only formalin-fixed paraffin embedded (FFPE) tissue is available. DNA quantity and quality derived from these tissue samples often limit reliable interpretation of analyses downstream of bisulfite modification. In some studies, the drop-out rate of samples derived from FFPE tissues reached up to 50% (Hegi et al. 2005). In brief, MSP is a useful tool for analysis of larger samples for methylation in circumscribed regions for which clinical relevance has been established. DNA quality is a bottleneck for MSP analyses. MSP is not suitable for quantification.

13.3.4
Methods of Gene Identification

A number of screening methods have been developed for systematic analysis of differentially methylated genes that may be involved in tumorigenesis (Herman et al. 1996; Kohno et al. 1998; Liang et al. 1998; Curtis and Goggins 2005), including restriction landmark genome scanning (RLGS) (Smiraglia et al. 1999; Costello et al. 2000; Costello et al. 2000; Costello et al. 2002; Costello et al. 2002; Zardo et al. 2002; Hong et al. 2003), pharmaceutical unmasking of epigenetic alterations with 5-aza-dC coupled with cRNA microarray in tumor cell cultures (Yamashita et al. 2002; Lodygin et al. 2005; Morris et al. 2005), and array-based combination of BAC clones with methylation-sensitive restrictive enzymes NotI or BssHII (Ching et al. 2005).

Microarray chip technology (Affymetrix) allows genome-wide comparison of expression profiles of cell populations, including tumors. This, combined with the possibility to pharmacologically revoke the methylation pattern of tumor cell genomes by methylation inhibitors such as 5′aza-dC, permits an unbiased and functionally based approach to identify novel epigenetically silenced genes in cancer. Conceptually one argues that, as promoter methylation entails gene silencing, pharmacological inhibition of promoter methylation reconstitutes the expression of epigenetically silenced genes. Expression-profile comparison of native and pharmacologically demethylated tumor cell cultures should identify genes with reconstituted expression due to up-regulation following promoter activation. First described by Yamashita et al. (2002), multiple studies proved the feasibility of this technique in a variety of malignancies (Fukai et al. 2003; Chen et al. 2004; Lodygin et al. 2005; Dannenberg and Edenberg 2006; Ibanez de Caceres et al. 2006; Lind et al. 2006; Mori et al. 2006; Muthusamy et al. 2006; Okochi-Takada et al. 2006; Yamashita et al. 2006a, b; Yang et al. 2007).

Several studies applied this strategy to gliomas and successfully unveiled novel epigenetically regulated genes (Foltz et al. 2006; Kim et al. 2006; Mueller et al. 2007). Such approaches are powerful screening tools, albeit with some caveats. First, this method is sensitive to loss of gene function only and therefore designed and limited to the detection of tumor-associated epigenetically silenced genes with preferentially tumor suppressor capabilities. Another caveat is that gene expression results from interaction of multiple mechanisms. Proteins act as members of regulatory networks or pathways. Thus, promoter demethylation followed by increased expression of a distinct protein must indirectly affect expression changes in other members of the same network or pathway. It also means that these genes are likely to be detected in this type of microarray screen, even though their promoters are not epigenetically regulated. Thus, consecutive up-regulation of downstream targets of epigenetically silenced genes further complicates candidate gene prioritization.

Since the methylation inhibitor 5′aza-dC has effects beyond demethylation properties, it may up-regulate the expression of genes involved in counteracting or compensating for the toxicity of the drug itself. Cytidine deaminase (*CDA*) is a key enzyme in the catabolism of cytosine nucleoside analogs. It helps in the deamination of these analogs, including 5′aza-dC. The deamination of 5′aza-dC results in loss of its pharmacological activity. Thus *CDA* up-regulation in response to 5′aza-dC exposure inactivates 5′aza-dC and leads to 5′aza-dC resistance (Momparler 2005). Not surprisingly, *CDA* was found significantly up-regulated in two out of three studies on glioma using 5′aza-dC for demethylation of promoter sequences (Kim et al. 2006; Mueller et al. 2007).

Particular problems in interpreting the significance of such studies in malignant gliomas are lack of knowledge of cells of origin and inherent heterogeneity in these tumors (Louis 2006).

The comparison of expression profiles of short-term colon cancer cultures before and after demethylating treatment with colon mucosa culture before and after demethylating treatment has been shown to successfully identify genes specifically inactivated by methylation in colon cancer (Mori et al. 2006). Application of this approach to gliomas is more problematic because of the heterogeneous composition of normal brain and the limited knowledge on the cell of origin of gliomas. Therefore, additional validation of candidates for epigenetic regulation is required.

Database research on candidate gene expression in normal brain (gene expression omnibus, GEO, http://www.ncbi.nlm.nih.gov/geo/; SAGE, http://cgap.nci.nih.gov/SAGE) and comparative real-time PCR (RT-PCR) analyses of cDNA derived from normal brain and tumor tissues may help distinguish cell-type-specific from cancer-related gene silencing. Lack of expression in the normal brain, which integrates expression of all central nervous system cell types, suggests cell-type-specific rather than tumor-related gene silencing. Gene expression in nontumorous tissue, loss of expression in tumor-derived samples, and a significant up-regulation of expression after demethylation argues for tumor-specific promoter methylation.

Human glioma-derived cells have been studied following this conceptual approach in two studies (Foltz et al. 2006; Mueller et al. 2007), both taking into account that extensive passaging may have epigenetic effects (Matsumura et al. 1989). Immortalized glioma cell lines such as U87MG, LN-229, U-118MG, DBTRG-05MG, T98G, and LN-18 were used in another study (Kim et al. 2006). In order to distinguish between tumor-related and non-tumor-related gene silencing and in lieu of a cell or origin of glioma, cultured astrocytes were substituted as the originating cell type (Kim et al. 2006). In our experience, the analysis of randomly selected genes in U87MG indicates global hypermethylation rather than differential promoter hypermethylation, as found in short-term cultures of gliomas (Mueller et al. 2007). We therefore advocate the use of patient-derived glioma cell lines rather than established immortalized or extensively passaged glioma cell lines for candidate gene identification. Interestingly, even though the approach and the techniques used in these studies were comparable, and the tumors studied all were derived from high-grade gliomas, the identified epigenetically silenced genes showed minimal overlap. One possible reason for the lack of overlap is the limited number of short-term cultured primary gliomas that entered the analyses, as not all high-grade gliomas give rise to cell cultures suitable for multiple passages. Also, given the high sensitivity of chip expression analyses, interplatform comparison is very much dependent on a uniform experimental set-up. While the same chip technology was used in two of the three studies (Kim et al. 2006; Mueller et al. 2007), the third analysis was based on a 60-mer whole-genome oligonucleotide microarray (Applied Biosystems, Foster City, CA, USA). In addition, two of the three studies combined genome-wide demethylation with trichostatin induced histone deacetylation (Foltz et al. 2006; Kim et al. 2006). These were also the ones implementing different chip technologies for the gene expression analyses. These differences may explain the poor interplatform correlation in these studies.

13.3.5
Genome-Wide Methylation Profiling Implementing Methylation: Sensitive Restriction Enzymes

Restriction landmark genomic scanning (RLGS) is a technique that can be adapted for genome-wide qualitative and semiquantitative methylation profiling. Developed and first described in 1993 (Hayashizaki et al. 1993), it proved feasible for the detection of epigenetically regulated genes in gliomas and is still used in current studies (Costello et al. 2000; Costello et al. 2000). The technique is based on using restriction enzymes that cleave DNA dependent on the methylation status in the recognition site. Typical endonucleases with this property are *Not*I and *Asc*I. Following digestion with the enzyme, DNA fragments are end-labeled and separated by a two- dimensional electrophoresis. The advantages are (1) high-speed scanning ability, allowing simultaneous scanning of thousands of restriction landmarks; (2) extension of the scanning field using different kinds of landmarks in an additional series of electrophoresis; (3) application to any type of organism because of direct labeling of restriction enzyme sites and no hybridization procedure; and (4) reflection of the copy number of the restriction landmark by spot intensity, which enables distinction of haploid and diploid genomic DNAs. RLGS has various applications because it can be used to scan for physical genomic DNA alterations, such as amplification, deletion, and methylation. The copy number of the locus of a restriction landmark can be estimated by the spot intensity to find either an amplified or deleted region.

13.3.6
MS-MLPA: A Novel Technique for Methylation Analysis That Does Not Require Bisulfite Modification and Can Be Reliably Applied to FFPE Tissues

MS-MLPA is a robust and reliable method for methylation analysis that can be easily applied to differently processed tissues, including those fixed in formalin and embedded in paraffin (Nygren et al. 2005; Jeuken et al. 2007). In MS-MLPA, the ligation of MLPA probe oligonucleotides is combined with digestion of the genomic DNA–probe hybrid complexes with methylation-sensitive endonucleases. Both digestion of the genomic DNA–probe complex, rather than double-stranded genomic DNA, and the independence of MS-MLPA from bisulfite conversion, allow the use of DNA derived from the formalin fixed paraffin-embedded tissue (FFPE) samples. MS-MLPA can be used to evaluate the methylation status of multiple sequences (CpG dinucleotides) simultaneously, it provides semiquantitative data on the promoter methylation status, and in addition allows for a combined copy number detection and methylation-specific analysis. The semiquantitative aspect of MS-MLPA may prove to be of great value, especially in predicting response to treatment and its dependence on the extent of promoter methylation of specific genes. Glioblastomas with methylation of the *MGMT* promoter respond better to treatment with both alkylating drugs and irradiation than those tumors with unmethylated *MGMT* promoter.

13.3.7 Novel Platforms for Genome-Wide, High-Throughput Methylation Analyses in Cancer Samples

Illumina's GoldenGate Methylation Cancer Panel I is the first standard panel that allows high sample throughput and provides sufficiently high quality to perform methylation profiling (Bibikova et al. 2006). Bisulfite-treated DNA is amplified, labeled, and hybridized to a Sentrix Array Matrix (SAM) for simultaneous and quantitative analysis of the methylation status of up to 1,536 different CpG sites. Each sequence on this array is represented on average 30 times, which greatly increases sensitivity and reproducibility. The GoldenGate Methylation Cancer Panel I includes CpG loci from over 800 genes, including tumor suppressor genes, oncogenes, and genes involved in DNA repair, cell cycle control, cell differentiation, and apoptosis. The accuracy, speed, simplicity, and flexibility of this assay for methylation make it a valuable new tool for genome-wide profiling.

13.4 DNA: Methyltransferases and Methylation Pattern Maintenance

DNA methyltransferases (*DNMTs*) tightly control and regulate both cell-type-specific de novo DNA methylation during development and methylation pattern maintenance during DNA replication throughout the lifetime of the organism. In mammalian cells, three methyltransferases have been identified: *DNMT1*, *DNMT3A*, *DNMT3B*. Methylation is mostly maintained by *DNMT1*, while *DNMT3A* and *DNMT3B* regulate de novo methylation. Experimental germ line elimination of any one of these in mice is associated with a lethal phenotype. While homozygous *DNMT1* or *DNMT3B* deletion is lethal before birth, mice with homozygous loss of *DNMT3A* die after approximately 4 weeks after birth (Li et al. 1992; Okano et al. 1999). *DNMT* deregulation in tumors would in part explain genome-wide hypomethylation associated with promoter hypermethylation and epigenetic silencing of selected genes. Disruption of this tightly regulated process may also partly explain the epigenetic profile in tumors with multiple simultaneously methylated gene promoters in a single tumor.

Interestingly, *DNMT1* has been reported to be highly expressed in various cancer cells (el-Deiry et al. 1991; Issa et al. 1993; Belinsky et al. 1996) and notable increases in expression of de novo *DNMTs* have been found in diverse cancers and cancer cell lines (Robertson et al. 1999; Kanai et al. 2001; Saito et al. 2001; Girault et al. 2003). These findings indicate deregulation of both methylation maintenance and de novo methylation in these tumors.

To identify deregulated *DNMT* function in low- and high-grade gliomas and to elucidate possible associations between *DNMT* dysfunction and the promoter methylation status of selected genes, we have recently investigated the expression profile of three human *DNMTs* (*DNMT1*, *DNMT3A*, and *DNMT3B*) in relation to the promoter methylation status of selected TSG genes (Lorente et al. 2008a). Compared to normal brain samples, we observed higher expression levels of *DNMT1*, *DNMT3a*, and *DNMT3b* in tumor samples and glioma cell lines. Interestingly, the most overexpressed *DNMTs* were *DNMT3a* and *DNMT3b* responsible for de novo methylation. In our view, this might explain the methylation phenotype of tumor cells with simultaneous targeting promoters of many genes. Supporting evidence comes from lung and esophageal squamous cell carcinomas in which a significant correlation of *DNMT* overexpression and promoter methylation of selected TSG was observed (Simao Tde et al. 2006; Lin et al. 2007). To date, there is only a single report on *DNMT* expression in a small number of gliomas, including two established glioblastoma cell lines and two primary glioblastomas. This report described up-regulation of *DNMT1*, down-regulation of

DNMT3b and no significant changes of *DNMT3a* (Fanelli et al. 2008). It is difficult to interpret the significance of these data because only few samples were investigated. Our own analysis did not yield a correlation between methylation status of any tumor suppressor gene that we investigated and expression changes of the *DNMTs*. However, we still think that the observation of an association between *DNMT* deregulation and the epigenetic phenotype in other tumors, together with our results of overexpression of mainly the de novo *DNMTs3a* and *3b*, encourage further studies assessing the expression pattern of the *DNMTs* and its association with promoter methylation in gliomas.

Of note, *DNMT* inhibitors constitute the first line of clinically applicable therapeutic agents to overcome epigenetic silencing of TSGs in different cancers, including gliomas (see Chap. 8).

13.5 Epigenetically Regulated Genes of Interest in Gliomas

Numerous genes with frequent tumor-related promoter hypermethylation have been identified in gliomas. In glioblastomas, for instance, frequent promoter hypermethylation has been reported on for *p14arf* and *RB1* (Costello et al. 1996; Gonzalez-Gomez et al. 2003a, b). Novel candidate genes with potential TSG function, i.e., *RUNX3* and *TES* have been identified coupling 5′-aza-dC induced pharmacological reversal of promoter methylation in short-term cultured primary glioblastomas and array-based expression analysis (see above) (Mueller et al. 2007). As another example, in astrocytomas the *large tumor suppressor gene 1 (LATS1; 6q24-q25.1)* and *LATS2 (13q11-q12)* were found be methylated in 63.66% (56/88) and transcriptionally down-regulated in 71.5% in a total of 88 astrocytomas (Jiang et al. 2006). In glioma cell lines with silenced *LATS1* and *LATS2* expression, 5′-aza-dC was able to restore their expression and to induce apoptosis, supporting epigenetic silencing as the major means of inactivation of these genes. Frequent promoter hypermethylation coupled with gene silencing has been observed in gliomas affecting the *RASSF1A* gene *(3p21.3)*, its family members *(NORE1* and *RASSF3)*, as well as the genes *CACNA2D2, SEMA3B*, and *BLU* co-localizing with *RASSF1A* (Hesson et al. 2004; Ji et al. 2005). Demethylation treatment with 5′aza-dC restored *RASSF1A* expression and repressed tumor cell growth in glioma cell line H4 compatible with a TSG function. In oligodendrogliomas, promoter hypermethylation of genes located in commonly deleted chromosomal areas on *1p-19q* have been reported, including *CITED4* gene at *1p34.2* (Tews et al. 2007) and *ZNF342* (Hong et al. 2003) and *EMP3* on *19q13* (Alaminos et al. 2005; Kunitz et al. 2007). A microarray-based methylation analysis of astrocytomas identified a CpG island within the first exon of the *protocadherin-gamma subfamily A11 (PCDH-gamma-A11)* gene that showed hypermethylation compared to normal brain tissue (Waha et al. 2005). In a comprehensive analysis of gliomas and cell lines, hypermethylation was detected in 88% of astrocytomas (WHO grades II and III), 87% of glioblastomas (WHO grade IV), and in 100% of glioma cell lines (Waha et al. 2005). Therefore, *PCDH-gamma-A11* is a target epigenetically silenced in astrocytic gliomas. It was concluded that the inactivation of this cell–cell contact molecule might be involved in the invasive properties of astrocytoma cells. However, many of the other epigenetically regulated genes could not be associated with a function in tumor suppression.

Frequent promoter hypermethylation of *MGMT*, a gene coding for O(6)-methylguanine-DNA methyltransferase (MGMT), a DNA repair protein that confers tumor resistance to many anticancer alkylating agents, combined with its transcriptional down-regulation has been described for both oligodendrogliomas (Mollemann et al. 2005) and glioblastomas (Esteller et al. 2000; Hegi et al. 2005). It should be noted that the loss of function of *MGMT* by promoter hypermethylation in glioblastomas has been associated with a better response to chemotherapy with alkylating agents in general (Esteller et al. 2000) and temozolomide in particular (Hegi et al. 2005) in these patients. It is assumed that epigenetic down-regulation of *MGMT* prevents repair of guanine alkylated in the O(6) position, thus allowing efficient alkylation by the chemotherapeutic drug. *MGMT* promoter hypermethylation was also found prevalent in long-term survivors of glioblastomas (Krex et al. 2007; Martinez et al. 2007), possibly indicating that besides identifying tumors with a better chemotherapy response, *MGMT* promoter methylation may also indicate a genotypic subset of glioblastomas with a more favorable clinical course independent of therapeutic strategies. Even though there are abundant genes with promoter methylation in gliomas of which *p14arf* and *RB1* may be the most prominent examples, none of them has been shown to be of clinical relevance in patient care, tumor classification, identification, or therapeutic tumor surveillance. The clinical impact of *MGMT* analysis on treatment of GBM is limited because of a lack of data, indicating a better response to treatment alternative to combined radio- and chemotherapy. Interestingly, the investigation of secondary glioblastomas provided evidence that methylated *MGMT* may indeed be part of a genetic signature of glioblastomas with low-grade preceding lesions (secondary GBM) as promoter methylation coincided with loss of *17p* and or *19q* (Eoli et al. 2007). Data regarding *MGMT* methylation status and low-grade glioma prognosis and treatment response are conflicting. While *MGMT* promoter methylation was described as an independent predictor of shortened progression-free survival in patients with low-grade diffuse astrocytomas (Komine et al. 2003), it was found to be a favorable predictor of progression-free survival in low-grade astrocytomas treated with neoadjuvant temozolomide. The latter suggests that the assessment of *MGMT* status could help identify low-grade glioma patients who are more likely to respond to chemotherapy or to benefit from MGMT depletion strategies (Everhard et al. 2006).

MGMT promoter methylation silences *MGMT* expression. MGMT depletion in tumors prevents MGMT-dependent chemotherapy resistance to alkylating drugs. Ionizing radiation induces functional p53. Data suggest that overexpression of functional p53 depletes MGMT expression independent of the methylation status of *MGMT* (Grombacher et al. 1998; Blough et al. 2007). Radiation therapy is an integral part of glioma therapy. Thus, both *MGMT* promoter methylation and radiation-induced overexpression of functional p53 have a similar biological effect and augment chemosensitivity to alkylating drugs in gliomas. Tp53 is a negative regulator of *MGMT* gene expression and can create a MGMT-depleted state in human tumors similar to that achieved by O(6)-benzylguanine, a potent inhibitor of MGMT currently undergoing clinical trials (Srivenugopal et al. 2001). These data expose an additional benefit associated with p53 gene therapy and provide a strong biochemical rationale for combining the MGMT-directed alkylators with p53 gene transfer to achieve improved antitumor efficacy (Srivenugopal et al. 2001). Given these data, one could assume that patients harboring an unmethylated *MGMT* promoter in their glioma, but functional p53 should fare better than gliomas in which p53 function is disrupted. Although a significant increase in survival has been reported with combined radio- and chemotherapy with temozolomide, nearly all gliomas recur and in the course of the disease develop resistance to further treatment with this class of agents. There is recent evidence that a small subset of glioblastomas recurs during temozolomide therapy by expansion of tumor cell clones harboring inactivating somatic mutations in the mismatch repair gene *MSH6* (Cahill et al. 2007; Hunter et al. 2006). In this small subset of recurrent glioblastomas, continued exposure to alkylating agents in the presence of somatic

MSH6 mutations seemed to induce accelerated mutagenesis, resulting in early tumor progression and therapy resistance (Hunter et al. 2006).

13.6 Diagnostic and Prognostic Value of Epigenetic Analyses: *MGMT* Promoter Methylation in Glioblastomas, Current Concepts, and Possible Future Developments

Expression of MGMT results in resistance to alkylating agents and hypermethylation of the *MGMT* promoter is associated with higher chemosensitivity. Diagnostic testing for *MGMT* promoter methylation has to be fast, reliable, easy-to-handle, ubiquitously available, cost-effective, and easy to document. Furthermore, it should be possible to apply the test on routinely processed tissue. This usually involves FFPE tissue and therefore an immunohistochemistry to detect MGMT; estimating its amount would be ideal. However, immunohistochemistry for MGMT expression in tissue samples has proved to be difficult (Krex et al. 2007) and in our own experience, MGMT detection by Western blotting was not suitable to predict *MGMT* promoter methylation (Lorente et al. 2008a). Currently, MSP as specified by Hegi et al. is most widely applied test for *MGMT* promoter methylation analysis in glioma samples.

Future developments should be mentioned briefly. Quantitative analyses of promoter methylation may replace current protocols for analysis of *MGMT* promoter methylation. For example, pyrosequencing or melting curve analysis based methylation analyses (MCA-Meth) using bisulfite methylation primers to detect the extent of interpriming site methylation (Lorente et al. 2008a & b) may prove superior in the prediction by adding quantitative data. It may be possible to better predict likely responders based on quantitative rather than qualitative promoter methylation. Also, the near future will show whether bisulfite conversion-independent techniques, i.e., MS-MLPA, are sufficiently reliable and feasible for diagnostic routine.

13.7 Current Therapeutic Strategies to Overcome TSG Silencing

13.7.1 Chromatin Remodeling Agents

Promoter methylation functionally silences a TSG transcription but leaves the physical gene structure untouched. A great deal of excitement has therefore come from the possibility to chemically reactivate these dormant genes and thereby restore their tumor suppressor activity in cancer patients. Tumor suppressors silenced by methylation and transcriptional repression can be reactivated by a variety of chromatin remodeling drugs, such as methyltransferase inhibitors (including 5-aza-2′deoxicitidine, recently approved for therapeutic treatment) (Samlowski et al. 2005) and histone deacetylase inhibitors (such as suberoylanilide hydroxamic acid (SAHA). These drugs are able to relax the chromatin, enhancing the accessibility of the transcription machinery (Garber 2004). For example, a variety of epigenetically inactivated genes involved in cell growth, cell cycle control, differentiation, DNA repair, and cell death have been identified in patients with myelodysplastic syndrome. Therapeutic reversal of epigenetic silencing may become an effective treatment strategy in these patients (Beumer et al. 2007; Kantarjian et al. 2007; Oki and Issa 2007). Both inhibitors of DNA methyltransferases (5′aza-dC) and histone deacetylase (HDAC) inhibitors are the drugs of choice and studies demonstrated that low-dose treatment with 5′-aza-dC or HDAC inhibitors may be promising, particularly for elderly patients (Claus et al. 2005, 2006; Beumer et al. 2007; Kantarjian et al. 2007; Oki and Issa 2007). However, chemically induced demethylation or inhibition of histone deacetylation is not tumor suppressor gene-specific. Thus, it can be anticipated that global demethylation will be induced, including extensive regions that are normally methylated such as an entire X chromosome in female individuals. Therefore limitations for the use of these drugs in cancer patients include their toxicity, lack of target specificity, and, in addition, the development of acquired drug resistance (Juttermann et al. 1994).

13.7.1.1
Chromatin Remodeling Agents in Neuroectodermal Tumors

In glioblastomas, concomitant treatment with radiotherapy and adjuvant temozolomide has been shown to yield the best results. Patients with gliomas displaying hypermethylation of *MGMT* show the best response (Esteller et al. 2000; Paz et al. 2004; Hegi et al. 2005). The combination of MGMT-inhibiting agents with temozolomide in the treatment of glioblastomas may further enhance the efficacy of the chemotherapeutic treatment (Soffietti et al. 2007a, b). Thus O(6)-benzylguanine, a potent MGMT inhibitor, is currently in testing for therapy of recurrent glioblastomas (Hegi et al. 2004; Quinn et al. 2005; Koch et al. 2007; Weingart et al. 2007) and anaplastic gliomas (Schold et al. 2004). The tumor necrosis factor-related apoptosis-inducing ligand (TRAIL) has been proposed as a therapeutic agent for treatment of glioblastomas based on its ability to kill glioma cell lines *in vitro* and *in vivo*. However, glioblastomas show resistance to TRAIL stimulation due to down-regulation of caspase-8. It is known that exogenous caspase-8 expression is the main event able to restore TRAIL sensitivity in primary glioblastoma cells. Inhibition of methyltransferases by decitabine (5′-aza-dC) now resulted in considerable up-regulation of TRAIL receptor-1 and caspase-8. An inhibition of cell growth and sensitization of primary glioblastoma cells to TRAIL-induced apoptosis was observed following demethylation. Thus, the combination of TRAIL and demethylating agents may provide a key tool to overcome glioblastoma resistance to therapeutic treatments (Eramo et al. 2005). Similarly, 5′aza-dC and IFN-gamma cooperated at relatively low individual concentrations to restore caspase-8 expression and were able to sensitize resistant neuroblastoma and medulloblastoma cells again to TRAIL-induced apoptosis (Fulda and Debatin 2006). These findings have important implications for novel strategies targeting defective apoptosis pathways in neuroectodermal tumors.

In addition, cell sensitivity to TRAIL can be affected by several intracellular factors. Further downstream in the TRAIL apoptotic pathway, *Bax* mutations, or increased expression of IAP family members, in particularly XIAP and survivin, also cause TRAIL resistance. Therefore, researchers are currently seeking to identify effective sensitizers for TRAIL-induced apoptosis that may allow cancer cells to recover TRAIL sensitivity. Further successful attempts in sensitizing glioma cells to TRAIL-mediated apoptosis have been undertaken with Smac agonists, mammalian target of rapamycin inhibitors (mTOR), and celecoxib. The combination of TRAIL and Smac peptides proved to be successful in repressing glioma transplants in mice and both rapamycin and celecoxib enhanced TRAIL-mediated apoptosis in several glioma cell lines (Fulda et al. 2002; Panner et al. 2005; Gaiser et al. 2008).

13.7.1.2
Histone Deacetylase Inhibitors in Neuroectodermal and Embryonic Tumors

Data support the hypothesis that glioma therapy may benefit from the introduction of histone deacetylase (HDAC) inhibitors (Chinnaiyan et al. 2005). Loosening up the chromatin structure by histone acetylation may increase the efficiency of several anticancer drugs targeting

DNA. This may be advantageous for treating tumors intrinsically resistant to these DNA-targeting drugs (Kim et al. 2003).

For example, studies demonstrated that the treatment with the HDAC inhibitor SAHA enhances radiation-induced cytotoxicity in human glioma cells (Chinnaiyan et al. 2005), slows the growth of GBM *in vitro* and *in vivo* (Yin et al. 2007), and may be useful in the treatment of other neuroectodermal tumors such as medulloblastomas, particularly when applied in combination with radiation, appropriate cytostatic drugs, or with TRAIL (Sonnemann et al. 2006). Treatment of high-risk embryonal tumors with HDAC inhibitors induced the reactivation of growth regulatory genes and enhanced apoptosis (Furchert et al. 2007). These data warrant further studies and may help in the design of novel tumor tailored treatment protocols.

13.7.2
Gene Replacement Therapy as a Vision for Restoring Expression of Silenced Genes

Ectopic delivery of cDNA by viral vectors can reactivate silenced tumor suppressor genes (Duvshani-Eshet et al. 2007; Zarnitsyn et al. 2007). Modified herpes simplex virus type 1 (HSV-1) is one of these promising viral vectors for selective gene delivery in cancer therapy. Besides their ability to replicate *in situ*, spread, and exert oncolytic activity by a direct cytotoxic effect, these vectors can be used to transfer any foreign gene into host cells.

Interferon-beta (IFN-β) is a cytokine with antitumoral activity. Recently, a phase I trial employing an adenoviral vector expressing human IFN-β (hIFN-β) was conducted in gliomas (Chiocca et al. 2008). An increase in tumor cell apoptosis and development of tumor necrosis was observed (Chiocca et al. 2008).

Another phase I trial focused on cationic liposome-mediated hIFN-β gene delivery to high-grade gliomas (Wakabayashi et al. 2008). Gene therapy faces major obstacles in transgene delivery and suppression of the host immune response (Fulci et al. 2006, 2007; Chiocca 2008). In viral vectors, the type of vector is crucial and in nonviral vectors the transfection efficacy may limit suitability for clinical trials. Especially in highly infiltrative tumors, such as gliomas, transgene delivery remains a challenge. Viral vehicles tested in clinical trials often target tumor cells only adjacent to the injection site. Recently, the feasibility of human mesenchymal stem cells (hMSCs) to deliver a replication competent oncolytic adenovirus (CRAd) in a model of intracranial malignant glioma has been reported (Sonabend et al. 2008). Virus-loaded hMSCs effectively migrated *in vitro* and released CRAds that infected U87MG glioma cells. When injected away from the tumor site *in vivo*, hMSC migrated to the tumor and delivered 46-fold more viral copies than injection of CRAds alone (Sonabend et al. 2008). Taken together, these results indicate that hMSC migrate and deliver CRAd to distant glioma cells. The strategy using hMSC to deliver CRAds to distant tumor sites, in combination with gene delivery of selected target genes by these CRAds, should be further explored because it could improve the efficacy of oncolytic virotherapy in gliomas. Even though not explicitly reported to date, cDNA delivery of selected hypermethylated tumor suppressor genes to individual tumors with evidence of silencing of these genes may be able to restore their function and also contribute to the efficacy of chemo- and radiotherapy in gliomas.

13.7.3
Artificial Transcription Factors in Gliomas

One major disadvantage of demethylation therapy is the lack of specificity. The delivery of artificial transcription factors may be an interesting alternative. Recently, artificially designed transcription factors (ATFs) were successfully delivered to breast tumor cells. They targeted the epigenetically silenced TSG gene *MASPIN (SERPIN B5)* in these tumor cells. *MASPIN* was selectively reactivated by these ATFs *in vitro* (Beltran et al. 2007). Once successfully delivered to the breast tumor cells, they induced apoptosis and were able to reduce tumor cell invasion *in vitro*. Moreover, in a xenograft model in nude mice, the ATFs successfully suppressed tumor cell growth *in vivo* by selectively reactivating the tumor suppressor gene function of *MASPIN*. The ATFs themselves were made of six zinc finger domains (6ZF) targeting unique small sequences in the tumor suppressor gene promoter and were linked to an activator domain. The ATFs were found to interact with their cognate targets *in vitro* with high affinity and selectivity. In summary, these results encourage the hope that ATFs may be promising candidates for cancer therapeutics.

13.8 Conclusion and Perspective

Gene regulation in tumors by promoter methylation has been firmly established by now. Promoter methylation in distinct genes such as *MGMT* is of highly prognostic and predictive power in tumors. We can expect methylation analyses to become an important diagnostic tool for many types of cancer in the near future. Current research addresses the reactivation of genes that have been silenced by promoter methylation by different approaches including the development of demethylating drugs, direct gene transfer, and specific activation of promoters. These efforts will contribute to a more individualized tumor therapy.

References

Alaminos M, Davalos V, Ropero S, Setien F, Paz MF, Herranz M, Fraga MF, Mora J, Cheung NK, Gerald WL, Esteller M (2005) EMP3, a myelin-related gene located in the critical 19q13.3 region, is epigenetically silenced and exhibits features of a candidate tumor suppressor in glioma and neuroblastoma. Cancer Res 65(7):2565–2571

Antequera F, Bird A (1993) CpG islands. Exs 64:169–185

Antequera F, Bird A (1993) Number of CpG islands and genes in human and mouse. Proc Natl Acad Sci USA 90(24):11995–11999

Ballestar E, Esteller M (2005) The epigenetic breakdown of cancer cells: from DNA methylation to histone modifications. Prog Mol Subcell Biol 38:169–181

Baylin S, Bestor TH (2002) Altered methylation patterns in cancer cell genomes: cause or consequence? Cancer Cell 1(4):299–305

Belinsky SA, Nikula KJ, Baylin SB, Issa JP (1996) Increased cytosine DNA-methyltransferase activity is target-cell-specific and an early event in lung cancer. Proc Natl Acad Sci USA 93(9):4045–4050

Beltran A, Parikh S, Liu Y, Cuevas BD, Johnson GL, Futscher BW, Blancafort P (2007) Re-activation of a dormant tumor suppressor gene maspin by designed transcription factors. Oncogene 26(19):2791–2798

Beumer JH, Parise RA, Newman EM, Doroshow JH, Synold TW, Lenz HJ, Egorin MJ (2007) Concentrations of the DNA methyltransferase inhibitor 5-fluoro-2'-deoxycytidine (FdCyd) and its cytotoxic metabolites in plasma of patients treated with FdCyd and tetrahydrouridine (THU). Cancer Chemother Pharmacol J Clin Oncol (Meeting Abstracts) 2006; 24:2023

Bibikova M, Lin Z, Zhou L, Chudin E, Garcia EW, Wu B, Doucet D, Thomas NJ, Wang Y, Vollmer E, Goldmann T, Seifart C, Jiang W, Barker DL, Chee MS, Floros J, Fan JB (2006) High-throughput DNA methylation profiling using universal bead arrays. Genome Res 16(3):383–393

Bird A (2002) DNA methylation patterns and epigenetic memory. Genes Dev 16(1):6–21

Bird AP, Wolffe AP (1999) Methylation-induced repression – belts, braces, and chromatin. Cell 99(5):451–454

Blough MD, Zlatescu MC, Cairncross JG (2007) O6-methylguanine-DNA methyltransferase regulation by p53 in astrocytic cells. Cancer Res 67(2):580–584

Brena RM, Morrison C, Liyanarachchi S, Jarjoura D, Davuluri RV, Otterson GA, Reisman D, Glaros S, Rush LJ, Plass C (2007) Aberrant DNA methylation of OLIG1, a novel prognostic factor in non-small cell lung cancer. PLoS Med 4(3):e108

Cahill DP, Levine KK, Betensky RA, Codd PJ, Romany CA, Reavie LB, Batchelor TT, Futreal PA, Stratton MR, Curry WT, Iafrate AJ, Louis DN (2007) Loss of the mismatch repair protein MSH6 in human glioblastomas is associated with tumor progression during temozolomide treatment. Clin Cancer Res 13(7):2038–2045

Chen J, Rocken C, Klein-Hitpass L, Gotze T, Leodolter A, Malfertheiner P, Ebert MP (2004) Microarray analysis of gene expression in metastatic gastric cancer cells after incubation with the methylation inhibitor 5-aza-2'-deoxycytidine. Clin Exp Metastasis 21(5):389–397

Ching TT, Maunakea AK, Jun P, Hong C, Zardo G, Pinkel D, Albertson DG, Fridlyand J, Mao JH, Shchors K, Weiss WA, Costello JF (2005) Epigenome analyses using BAC microarrays identify evolutionary conservation of tissue-specific methylation of SHANK3. Nat Genet 37(6):645–651

Chinnaiyan P, Vallabhaneni G, Armstrong E, Huang SM, Harari PM (2005) Modulation of radiation response by histone deacetylase inhibition. Int J Radiat Oncol Biol Phys 62(1):223–229

Chiocca EA (2008) The host response to cancer virotherapy. Curr Opin Mol Ther 10(1):38–45

Chiocca EA, Smith KM, McKinney B, Palmer CA, Rosenfeld S, Lillehei K, Hamilton A, Demasters BK, Judy K, Kirn D (2008) A Phase I Trial of Ad.hIFN-beta Gene Therapy for Glioma. Mol Ther. 2008 Mar, 16(3):618–626

Chung R, Whaley J, Kley N, Anderson K, Louis D, Menon A, Hettlich C, Freiman R, Hedley-Whyte ET, Martuza R, et al. (1991) TP53 gene mutations and 17p deletions in human astrocytomas. Genes Chromosomes Cancer 3(5):323–331

Claus R, Almstedt M, Lubbert M (2005) Epigenetic treatment of hematopoietic malignancies: in vivo targets of demethylating agents. Semin Oncol 32(5):511–520

Claus R, Fliegauf M, Stock M, Duque JA, Kolanczyk M, Lubbert M (2006) Inhibitors of DNA methylation and histone deacetylation independently relieve AML1/ETO-mediated lysozyme repression. J Leukoc Biol 80(6):1462–1472

Collins VP (2004) Brain tumours: classification and genes. J Neurol Neurosurg Psychiatry 75(Suppl 2):ii2–11

Costello JF, Berger MS, Huang HS, Cavenee WK (1996) Silencing of p16/CDKN2 expression in human gliomas by methylation and chromatin condensation. Cancer Res 56(10):2405–2410

Costello JF, Fruhwald MC, Smiraglia DJ, Rush LJ, Robertson GP, Gao X, Wright FA, Feramisco JD, Peltomaki P, Lang JC, Schuller DE, Yu L, Bloomfield CD, Caligiuri MA, Yates A, Nishikawa R, Su Huang H, Petrelli NJ, Zhang X, O'Dorisio MS, Held WA, Cavenee WK, Plass C (2000) Aberrant CpG-island methylation has non-random and tumour-type-specific patterns. Nat Genet 24(2):132–138

Costello JF, Plass C, Cavenee WK (2000) Aberrant methylation of genes in low-grade astrocytomas. Brain Tumor Pathol 17(2):49–56

Costello JF, Plass C, Cavenee WK (2002) Restriction landmark genome scanning. Methods Mol Biol 200:53–70

Costello JF, Smiraglia DJ, Plass C (2002) Restriction landmark genome scanning. Methods 27(2):144–149

Costello JF, Vertino PM (2002) Methylation matters: a new spin on maspin. Nat Genet 31(2):123–124

Curtis CD, Goggins M (2005) DNA methylation analysis in human cancer. Methods Mol Med 103:123–36

Dallol A, Krex D, Hesson L, Eng C, Maher ER, Latif F (2003) Frequent epigenetic inactivation of the SLIT2 gene in gliomas. Oncogene 22(29):4611–4116

Dannenberg LO, Edenberg HJ (2006) Epigenetics of gene expression in human hepatoma cells: expression profiling the response to inhibition of DNA methylation and histone deacetylation. BMC Genomics 7:181

Dickinson RE, Dallol A, Bieche I, Krex D, Morton D, Maher ER, Latif F (2004) Epigenetic inactivation of SLIT3 and SLIT1 genes in human cancers. Br J Cancer 91(12):2071–2078

Duvshani-Eshet M, Benny O, Morgenstern A, Machluf M (2007) Therapeutic ultrasound facilitates antiangiogenic gene delivery and inhibits prostate tumor growth. Mol Cancer Ther 6(8):2371–2382

Eden A, Gaudet F, Waghmare A, Jaenisch R (2003) Chromosomal instability and tumors promoted by DNA hypomethylation. Science 300(5618):455

Ehrich M, Nelson MR, Stanssens P, Zabeau M, Liloglou T, Xinarianos G, Cantor CR, Field JK, van den Boom D (2005) Quantitative high-throughput analysis of DNA methylation patterns by base-specific cleavage and mass spectrometry. Proc Natl Acad Sci USA 102(44):15785–15790

el-Deiry WS, Nelkin BD, Celano P, Yen RW, Falco JP, Hamilton SR, Baylin SB (1991) High expression of the DNA methyltransferase gene characterizes human neoplastic cells and progression stages of colon cancer. Proc Natl Acad Sci USA 88(8):3470–3474

Eoli M, Menghi F, Bruzzone MG, De Simone T, Valletta L, Pollo B, Bissola L, Silvani A, Bianchessi D, D'Incerti L, Filippini G, Broggi G, Boiardi A, Finocchiaro G (2007) Methylation of O6-methylguanine DNA methyltransferase and loss of heterozygosity on 19q and/or 17p are overlapping features of secondary glioblastomas with prolonged survival. Clin Cancer Res 13(9):2606–2613

Eramo A, Pallini R, Lotti F, Sette G, Patti M, Bartucci M, Ricci-Vitiani L, Signore M, Stassi G, Larocca LM, Crino L, Peschle C, De Maria R (2005) Inhibition of DNA methylation sensitizes glioblastoma for tumor necrosis factor-related apoptosis-inducing ligand-mediated destruction. Cancer Res 65(24):11469–11477

Esteller M (2003) Cancer epigenetics: DNA methylation and chromatin alterations in human cancer. Adv Exp Med Biol 532:39–49

Esteller M (2005) Aberrant DNA methylation as a cancer-inducing mechanism. Annu Rev Pharmacol Toxicol 45:629–656

Esteller M, Fraga MF, Guo M, Garcia-Foncillas J, Hedenfalk I, Godwin AK, Trojan J, Vaurs-Barriere C, Bignon YJ, Ramus S, Benitez J, Caldes T, Akiyama Y, Yuasa Y, Launonen V, Canal MJ, Rodriguez R, Capella G, Peinado MA, Borg A, Aaltonen LA, Ponder BA, Baylin SB, Herman JG (2001) DNA methylation patterns in hereditary human cancers mimic sporadic tumorigenesis. Hum Mol Genet 10(26):3001–3007

Esteller M, Garcia-Foncillas J, Andion E, Goodman SN, Hidalgo OF, Vanaclocha V, Baylin SB, Herman JG (2000) Inactivation of the DNA-repair gene MGMT and the clinical response of gliomas to alkylating agents. N Engl J Med 343(19):1350–1354

Everhard S, Kaloshi G, Criniere E, Benouaich-Amiel A, Lejeune J, Marie Y, Sanson M, Kujas M, Mokhtari K, Hoang-Xuan K, Delattre JY, Thillet J (2006) MGMT methylation: a marker of response to temozolomide in low-grade gliomas. Ann Neurol 60(6):740–743

Fan X, Munoz J, Sanko SG, Castresana JS (2002) PTEN, DMBT1, and p16 alterations in diffusely infiltrating astrocytomas. Int J Oncol 21(3):667–674

Fanelli M, Caprodossi S, Ricci-Vitiani L, Porcellini A, Tomassoni-Ardori F, Amatori S, Andreoni F, Magnani M, De Maria R, Santoni A, Minucci S, Pelicci PG (2008) Loss of pericentromeric DNA methylation pattern in human glioblastoma is associated with altered DNA methyltransferases expression and involves the stem cell compartment. Oncogene 27(3):358–365

Feinberg AP, Tycko B (2004) The history of cancer epigenetics. Nat Rev Cancer 4(2):143–153

Feinberg AP, Vogelstein B (1983) Hypomethylation distinguishes genes of some human cancers from their normal counterparts. Nature 301(5895):89–92

Feinberg AP, Vogelstein B (1987) Alterations in DNA methylation in human colon neoplasia. Semin Surg Oncol 3(3):149–151

Foltz G, Ryu GY, Yoon JG, Nelson T, Fahey J, Frakes A, Lee H, Field L, Zander K, Sibenaller Z, Ryken TC, Vibhakar R, Hood L, Madan A (2006) Genome-wide analysis of epigenetic silencing identifies BEX1 and BEX2 as candidate tumor suppressor genes in malignant glioma. Cancer Res 66(13):6665–6674

Frigola J, Song J, Stirzaker C, Hinshelwood RA, Peinado MA, Clark SJ (2006) Epigenetic remodeling in colorectal cancer results in coordinate gene suppression across an entire chromosome band. Nat Genet 38(5):540–549

Fukai K, Yokosuka O, Chiba T, Hirasawa Y, Tada M, Imazeki F, Kataoka H, Saisho H (2003) Hepatocyte growth factor activator inhibitor 2/placental bikunin (HAI-2/PB) gene is frequently hypermethylated in human hepatocellular carcinoma. Cancer Res 63(24):8674–8679

Fulci G, Breymann L, Gianni D, Kurozomi K, Rhee SS, Yu J, Kaur B, Louis DN, Weissleder R, Caligiuri MA, Chiocca EA (2006) Cyclophosphamide enhances glioma virotherapy by inhibiting innate immune responses. Proc Natl Acad Sci USA 103(34):12873–12878

Fulci G, Dmitrieva N, Gianni D, Fontana EJ, Pan X, Lu Y, Kaufman CS, Kaur B, Lawler SE, Lee RJ, Marsh CB, Brat DJ, van Rooijen N, Stemmer-

Rachamimov AO, Hochberg FH, Weissleder R, Martuza RL, Chiocca EA (2007) Depletion of peripheral macrophages and brain microglia increases brain tumor titers of oncolytic viruses. Cancer Res 67(19):9398–9406

Fulda S, Debatin KM (2006) 5-Aza-2'-deoxycytidine and IFN-gamma cooperate to sensitize for TRAIL-induced apoptosis by upregulating caspase-8. Oncogene 25(37):5125–5133

Fulda S, Wick W, Weller M, Debatin KM (2002) Smac agonists sensitize for Apo2L/TRAIL- or anticancer drug-induced apoptosis and induce regression of malignant glioma in vivo. Nat Med 8(8):808–815

Furchert SE, Lanvers-Kaminsky C, Juurgens H, Jung M, Loidl A, Fruhwald MC (2007) Inhibitors of histone deacetylases as potential therapeutic tools for high-risk embryonal tumors of the nervous system of childhood. Int J Cancer 120(8):1787–1794

Gaiser T, Becker MR, Habel A, Reuss DE, Ehemann V, Rami A, Siegelin MD (2008) TRAIL-mediated apoptosis in malignant glioma cells is augmented by celecoxib through proteasomal degradation of survivin. Neurosci Lett 442(2):109–113

Garber K (2004) Purchase of Aton spotlights HDAC inhibitors. Nat Biotechnol 22(4):364–365

Gaudet F, Hodgson JG, Eden A, Jackson-Grusby L, Dausman J, Gray JW, Leonhardt H, Jaenisch R (2003) Induction of tumors in mice by genomic hypomethylation. Science 300(5618):489–492

Girault I, Tozlu S, Lidereau R, Bieche I (2003) Expression analysis of DNA methyltransferases 1, 3A, and 3B in sporadic breast carcinomas. Clin Cancer Res 9(12):4415–4422

Goelz SE, Vogelstein B, Hamilton SR, Feinberg AP (1985) Hypomethylation of DNA from benign and malignant human colon neoplasms. Science 228(4696):187–190

Gonzalez-Gomez P, Bello MJ, Arjona D, Lomas J, Alonso ME, De Campos JM, Vaquero J, Isla A, Gutierrez M, Rey JA (2003a) Promoter hypermethylation of multiple genes in astrocytic gliomas. Int J Oncol 22(3):601–608

Gonzalez-Gomez P, Bello MJ, Lomas J, Arjona D, Alonso ME, Aminoso C, De Campos JM, Vaquero J, Sarasa JL, Casartelli C, Rey JA (2003b) Epigenetic changes in pilocytic astrocytomas and medulloblastomas. Int J Mol Med 11(5):655–660

Goto Y, Gomez M, Brockdorff N, Feil R (2002) Differential patterns of histone methylation and acetylation distinguish active and repressed alleles at X-linked genes. Cytogenet Genome Res 99(1–4):66–74

Grombacher T, Eichhorn U, Kaina B (1998) p53 is involved in regulation of the DNA repair gene O6-methylguanine-DNA methyltransferase (MGMT) by DNA damaging agents. Oncogene 17(7):845–851

Guldberg P, Worm J, Gronbaek K (2002) Profiling DNA methylation by melting analysis. Methods 27(2):121–127

Hayashizaki Y, Hirotsune S, Okazaki Y, Hatada I, Shibata H, Kawai J, Hirose K, Watanabe S, Fushiki S, Wada S, et al. (1993) Restriction landmark genomic scanning method and its various applications. Electrophoresis 14(4):251–258

Hegi ME, Diserens AC, Godard S, Dietrich PY, Regli L, Ostermann S, Otten P, Van Melle G, de Tribolet N, Stupp R (2004) Clinical trial substantiates the predictive value of O-6-methylguanine-DNA methyltransferase promoter methylation in glioblastoma patients treated with temozolomide. Clin Cancer Res 10(6):1871–1874

Hegi ME, Diserens AC, Gorlia T, Hamou MF, de Tribolet N, Weller M, Kros JM, Hainfellner JA, Mason W, Mariani L, Bromberg JE, Hau P, Mirimanoff RO, Cairncross JG, Janzer RC, Stupp R (2005) MGMT gene silencing and benefit from temozolomide in glioblastoma. N Engl J Med 352(10):997–1003

Henson JW, Schnitker BL, Correa KM, von Deimling A, Fassbender F, Xu HJ, Benedict WF, Yandell DW, Louis DN (1994) The retinoblastoma gene is involved in malignant progression of astrocytomas. Ann Neurol 36(5):714–721

Herman JG, Baylin SB (2003) Gene silencing in cancer in association with promoter hypermethylation. N Engl J Med 349(21):2042–2054

Herman JG, Graff JR, Myohanen S, Nelkin BD, Baylin SB (1996) Methylation-specific PCR: a novel PCR assay for methylation status of CpG islands. Proc Natl Acad Sci USA 93(18):9821–9826

Hesson L, Bieche I, Krex D, Criniere E, Hoang-Xuan K, Maher ER, Latif F (2004) Frequent epigenetic inactivation of RASSF1A and BLU genes located within the critical 3p21.3 region in gliomas. Oncogene 23(13):2408–2419

Hong C, Bollen AW, Costello JF (2003) The contribution of genetic and epigenetic mechanisms to gene silencing in oligodendrogliomas. Cancer Res 63(22):7600–7605

Hunter C, Smith R, Cahill DP, Stephens P, Stevens C, Teague J, Greenman C, Edkins S, Bignell G, Davies H, O'Meara S, Parker A, Avis T, Barthorpe S, Brackenbury L, Buck G, Butler A, Clements J, Cole J, Dicks E, Forbes S, Gorton M, Gray K, Halliday K, Harrison R, Hills K, Hinton J, Jenkinson A, Jones D, Kosmidou V, Laman R, Lugg R, Menzies A, Perry J, Petty R, Raine K, Richardson D, Shepherd R, Small A, Solomon H, Tofts C, Varian J, West S, Widaa S, Yates A, Easton DF, Riggins G, Roy JE, Levine KK, Mueller W, Batchelor TT, Louis DN, Stratton MR, Futreal PA, Wooster R (2006) A hypermutation phenotype and somatic MSH6 mutations in recurrent human malignant gliomas after alkylator chemotherapy. Cancer Res 66(8):3987–3991

Ibanez de Caceres I, Dulaimi E, Hoffman AM, Al-Saleem T, Uzzo RG, Cairns P (2006) Identification of novel target genes by an epigenetic reactivation screen of renal cancer. Cancer Res 66(10): 5021–5028

Ichimura K, Schmidt EE, Goike HM, Collins VP (1996) Human glioblastomas with no alterations of the CDKN2A (p16INK4A, MTS1) and CDK4 genes have frequent mutations of the retinoblastoma gene. Oncogene 13(5):1065–1072

Ichimura K, Bolin MB, Goike HM, Schmidt EE, Moshref A, Collins VP (2000) Deregulation of the p14ARF/MDM2/p53 pathway is a prerequisite for human astrocytic gliomas with G1-S transition control gene abnormalities. Cancer Res 60(2):417–424

Issa JP, Vertino PM, Wu J, Sazawal S, Celano P, Nelkin BD, Hamilton SR, Baylin SB (1993) Increased cytosine DNA-methyltransferase activity during colon cancer progression. J Natl Cancer Inst 85(15):1235–1240

Jain PK (2003) Epigenetics: the role of methylation in the mechanism of action of tumor suppressor genes. Ann N Y Acad Sci 983:71–83

Jeuken JW, Cornelissen SJ, Vriezen M, Dekkers MM, Errami A, Sijben A, Boots-Sprenger SH, Wesseling P (2007) MS-MLPA: an attractive alternative laboratory assay for robust, reliable, and semiquantitative detection of MGMT promoter hypermethylation in gliomas. Lab Invest 87(10):1055–1065

Ji L, Minna JD, Roth JA (2005) 3p21.3 tumor suppressor cluster: prospects for translational applications. Future Oncol 1(1):79–92

Jiang Z, Li X, Hu J, Zhou W, Jiang Y, Li G, Lu D (2006) Promoter hypermethylation-mediated down-regulation of LATS1 and LATS2 in human astrocytoma. Neurosci Res 56(4):450–458

Jones PA (2005) Overview of cancer epigenetics. Semin Hematol 42(3 Suppl 2):S3–8

Juttermann R, Li E, Jaenisch R (1994) Toxicity of 5-aza-2'-deoxycytidine to mammalian cells is mediated primarily by covalent trapping of DNA methyltransferase rather than DNA demethylation. Proc Natl Acad Sci USA 91(25):11797–11801

Kanai Y, Ushijima S, Kondo Y, Nakanishi Y, Hirohashi S (2001) DNA methyltransferase expression and DNA methylation of CPG islands and peri-centromeric satellite regions in human colorectal and stomach cancers. Int J Cancer 91(2):205–212

Kantarjian H, Oki Y, Garcia-Manero G, Huang X, O'Brien S, Cortes J, Faderl S, Bueso-Ramos C, Ravandi F, Estrov Z, Ferrajoli A, Wierda W, Shan J, Davis J, Giles F, Saba HI, Issa JP (2007) Results of a randomized study of 3 schedules of low-dose decitabine in higher-risk myelodysplastic syndrome and chronic myelomonocytic leukemia. Blood 109(1):52–57

Kim DH, Mohapatra G, Bollen A, Waldman FM, Feuerstein BG (1995) Chromosomal abnormalities in glioblastoma multiforme tumors and glioma cell lines detected by comparative genomic hybridization. Int J Cancer 60(6):812–819

Kim MS, Blake M, Baek JH, Kohlhagen G, Pommier Y, Carrier F (2003) Inhibition of histone deacetylase increases cytotoxicity to anticancer drugs targeting DNA. Cancer Res 63(21):7291–7300

Kim TY, Zhong S, Fields CR, Kim JH, Robertson KD (2006) Epigenomic profiling reveals novel and frequent targets of aberrant DNA methylation-mediated silencing in malignant glioma. Cancer Res 66(15):7490–7501

Koch D, Hundsberger T, Boor S, Kaina B (2007) Local intracerebral administration of O(6)-benzylguanine combined with systemic chemotherapy with temozolomide of a patient suffering from a recurrent glioblastoma. J Neurooncol 82(1):85–89

Kohno T, Kawanishi M, Inazawa J, Yokota J (1998) Identification of CpG islands hypermethylated in human lung cancer by the arbitrarily primed-PCR method. Hum Genet 102(3):258–264

Komine C, Watanabe T, Katayama Y, Yoshino A, Yokoyama T, Fukushima T (2003) Promoter hypermethylation of the DNA repair gene O6-methylguanine-DNA methyltransferase is an independent predictor of shortened progression free survival in patients with low-grade diffuse astrocytomas. Brain Pathol 13(2):176–184

Krex D, Klink B, Hartmann C, von Deimling A, Pietsch T, Simon M, Sabel M, Steinbach JP, Heese O, Reifenberger G, Weller M, Schackert G (2007) Long-term survival with glioblastoma multiforme. Brain 130(Pt 10):2596–2606

Kunitz A, Wolter M, van den Boom J, Felsberg J, Tews B, Hahn M, Benner A, Sabel M, Lichter P, Reifenberger G, von Deimling A, Hartmann C (2007) DNA hypermethylation and aberrant expression of the EMP3 gene at 19q13.3 in Human Gliomas. Brain Pathol 17(4):363–370

Li E, Bestor TH, Jaenisch R (1992) Targeted mutation of the DNA methyltransferase gene results in embryonic lethality. Cell 69(6):915–926

Li J, Yen C, Liaw D, Podsypanina K, Bose S, Wang SI, Puc J, Miliaresis C, Rodgers L, McCombie R, Bigner SH, Giovanella BC, Ittmann M, Tycko B, Hibshoosh H, Wigler MH, Parsons R (1997) PTEN, a putative protein tyrosine phosphatase gene mutated in human brain, breast, and prostate cancer. Science 275(5308):1943–1947

Li Q, Ahuja N, Burger PC, Issa JP (1999) Methylation and silencing of the Thrombospondin-1 promoter in human cancer. Oncogene 18(21):3284–3289

Li Q, Jedlicka A, Ahuja N, Gibbons MC, Baylin SB, Burger PC, Issa JP (1998) Concordant methylation of the ER and N33 genes in glioblastoma multiforme. Oncogene 16(24):3197–3202

Liang G, Salem CE, Yu MC, Nguyen HD, Gonzales FA, Nguyen TT, Nichols PW, Jones PA (1998) DNA methylation differences associated with tumor tissues identified by genome scanning analysis. Genomics 53(3):260–268

Lin RK, Hsu HS, Chang JW, Chen CY, Chen JT, Wang YC (2007) Alteration of DNA methyltransferases contributes to 5'CpG methylation and poor prognosis in lung cancer. Lung Cancer 55(2):205–213

Lind GE, Skotheim RI, Fraga MF, Abeler VM, Esteller M, Lothe RA (2006) Novel epigenetically deregulated genes in testicular cancer include homeobox genes and SCGB3A1 (HIN-1). J Pathol 210(4):441–449

Lodygin D, Epanchintsev A, Menssen A, Diebold J, Hermeking H (2005) Functional epigenomics identifies genes frequently silenced in prostate cancer. Cancer Res 65(10):4218–4227

Lorente A, Mueller W, Urdangarin E, Lazcoz P, Lass U, von Deimling A, Castresana JS (2008a) RASSF1A-, BLU-, NORE1A-, PTEN- and MGMT expression and promoter methylation in gliomas and glioma cell lines and evidence of deregulated expression of de novo DNMTs. Brain Pathol (submitted)

Lorente A, Mueller W, Urdangarín E, Lázcoz P, von Deimling A, Castresana J (2008b) Detection of methylation in promoter sequences by melting curve analysis-based semiquantitative real time PCR. BMC Cancer 8:61

Louis DN (2006) Molecular pathology of malignant gliomas. Annu Rev Pathol 1:97–117

Martinez R, Schackert G, Yaya-Tur R, Rojas-Marcos I, Herman JG, Esteller M (2007) Frequent hypermethylation of the DNA repair gene MGMT in long-term survivors of glioblastoma multiforme. J Neurooncol 83(1):91–93

Matsumura T, Hunter JL, Farooq M, Holliday R (1989) Maintenance of DNA methylation level in SV40-infected human fibroblasts during their in vitro limited proliferative life span. Exp Cell Res 184(1):148–157

Mikeska T, Bock C, El-Maarri O, Hubner A, Ehrentraut D, Schramm J, Felsberg J, Kahl P, Buttner R, Pietsch T, Waha A (2007) Optimization of quantitative MGMT promoter methylation analysis using pyrosequencing and combined bisulfite restriction analysis. J Mol Diagn 9(3):368–381

Mohapatra G, Bollen AW, Kim DH, Lamborn K, Moore DH, Prados MD, Feuerstein BG (1998) Genetic analysis of glioblastoma multiforme provides evidence for subgroups within the grade. Genes Chromosomes Cancer 21(3):195–206

Mollemann M, Wolter M, Felsberg J, Collins VP, Reifenberger G (2005) Frequent promoter hypermethylation and low expression of the MGMT gene in oligodendroglial tumors. Int J Cancer 113(3):379–385

Momparler RL (2005) Pharmacology of 5-Aza-2'-deoxycytidine (decitabine). Semin Hematol 42(3 Suppl 2):S9–16

Mori Y, Cai K, Cheng Y, Wang S, Paun B, Hamilton JP, Jin Z, Sato F, Berki AT, Kan T, Ito T, Mantzur C, Abraham JM, Meltzer SJ (2006) A genome-wide search identifies epigenetic silencing of somatostatin, tachykinin-1, and 5 other genes in colon cancer. Gastroenterology 131(3):797–808

Morris MR, Gentle D, Abdulrahman M, Maina EN, Gupta K, Banks RE, Wiesener MS, Kishida T, Yao M, Teh B, Latif F, Maher ER (2005) Tumor suppressor activity and epigenetic inactivation of hepatocyte growth factor activator inhibitor type 2/SPINT2 in papillary and clear cell renal cell carcinoma. Cancer Res 65(11):4598–4606

Mueller W, Nutt CL, Ehrich M, Riemenschneider MJ, von Deimling A, van den Boom D, Louis DN (2007) Downregulation of RUNX3 and TES by hypermethylation in glioblastoma. Oncogene 26(4):583–593

Muthusamy V, Duraisamy S, Bradbury CM, Hobbs C, Curley DP, Nelson B, Bosenberg M (2006) Epigenetic silencing of novel tumor suppressors in malignant melanoma. Cancer Res 66(23): 11187–11193

Nan X, Cross S, Bird A (1998) Gene silencing by methyl-CpG-binding proteins. Novartis Found Symp 214:6–16; discussion 16–21, 46–50

Nishizaki T, Ozaki S, Harada K, Ito H, Arai H, Beppu T, Sasaki K (1998) Investigation of genetic alterations associated with the grade of astrocytic tumor by comparative genomic hybridization. Genes Chromosomes Cancer 21(4):340–346

Nygren AO, Ameziane N, Duarte HM, Vijzelaar RN, Waisfisz Q, Hess CJ, Schouten JP, Errami A (2005) Methylation-specific MLPA (MS-MLPA): simultaneous detection of CpG methylation and copy number changes of up to 40 sequences. Nucleic Acids Res 33(14):e128

Okano M, Bell DW, Haber DA, Li E (1999) DNA methyltransferases Dnmt3a and Dnmt3b are essential for de novo methylation and mammalian development. Cell 99(3):247–257

Oki Y, Issa JP (2007) Treatment options in advanced myelodysplastic syndrome, with emphasis on epigenetic therapy. Int J Hematol 86(4):306–314

Okochi-Takada E, Nakazawa K, Wakabayashi M, Mori A, Ichimura S, Yasugi T, Ushijima T (2006) Silencing of the UCHL1 gene in human colorectal and ovarian cancers. Int J Cancer 119(6): 1338–1344

Panner A, James CD, Berger MS, Pieper RO (2005) mTOR controls FLIPS translation and TRAIL sensitivity in glioblastoma multiforme cells. Mol Cell Biol 25(20):8809–8823

Paz MF, Yaya-Tur R, Rojas-Marcos I, Reynes G, Pollan M, Aguirre-Cruz L, Garcia-Lopez JL, Piquer J, Safont MJ, Balana C, Sanchez-Cespedes M, Garcia-Villanueva M, Arribas L, Esteller M (2004) CpG island hypermethylation of the DNA repair enzyme methyltransferase predicts response to temozolomide in primary gliomas. Clin Cancer Res 10(15):4933–4938

Quinn JA, Desjardins A, Weingart J, Brem H, Dolan ME, Delaney SM, Vredenburgh J, Rich J, Friedman AH, Reardon DA, Sampson JH, Pegg AE, Moschel RC, Birch R, McLendon RE, Provenzale JM, Gururangan S, Dancey JE, Maxwell J, Tourt-Uhlig S, Herndon JE, 2nd, Bigner DD, Friedman HS (2005) Phase I trial of temozolomide plus O6-benzylguanine for patients with recurrent or progressive malignant glioma. J Clin Oncol 23(28):7178–7187

Rideout WM, 3rd, Coetzee GA, Olumi AF, Jones PA (1990) 5-Methylcytosine as an endogenous mutagen in the human LDL receptor and p53 genes. Science 249(4974):1288–1290

Riemenschneider MJ, Reifenberger J, Reifenberger G (2008) Frequent biallelic inactivation and transcriptional silencing of the DIRAS3 gene at 1p31 in oligodendroglial tumors with 1p loss. Int J Cancer 122(11):2503–2510

Robertson KD, Uzvolgyi E, Liang G, Talmadge C, Sumegi J, Gonzales FA, Jones PA (1999) The human DNA methyltransferases (DNMTs) 1, 3a and 3b: coordinate mRNA expression in normal tissues and overexpression in tumors. Nucleic Acids Res 27(11):2291–2298

Saito Y, Kanai Y, Sakamoto M, Saito H, Ishii H, Hirohashi S (2001) Expression of mRNA for DNA methyltransferases and methyl-CpG-binding proteins and DNA methylation status on CpG islands and pericentromeric satellite regions during human hepatocarcinogenesis. Hepatology 33(3):561–568

Samlowski WE, Leachman SA, Wade M, Cassidy P, Porter-Gill P, Busby L, Wheeler R, Boucher K, Fitzpatrick F, Jones DA, Karpf AR (2005)

Evaluation of a 7-day continuous intravenous infusion of decitabine: inhibition of promoter-specific and global genomic DNA methylation. J Clin Oncol 23(17):3897–3905

Schold SC, Jr., Kokkinakis DM, Chang SM, Berger MS, Hess KR, Schiff D, Robins HI, Mehta MP, Fink KL, Davis RL, Prados MD (2004) O6-benzylguanine suppression of O6-alkylguanine-DNA alkyltransferase in anaplastic gliomas. Neuro Oncol 6(1): 28–32

Simao Tde A, Simoes GL, Ribeiro FS, Cidade DA, Andreollo NA, Lopes LR, Macedo JM, Acatauassu R, Teixeira AM, Felzenszwalb I, Pinto LF, Albano RM (2006) Lower expression of p14ARF and p16INK4a correlates with higher DNMT3B expression in human oesophageal squamous cell carcinomas. Hum Exp Toxicol 25(9):515–522

Smiraglia DJ, Fruhwald MC, Costello JF, McCormick SP, Dai Z, Peltomaki P, O'Dorisio MS, Cavenee WK, Plass C (1999) A new tool for the rapid cloning of amplified and hypermethylated human DNA sequences from restriction landmark genome scanning gels. Genomics 58(3):254–262

Smith LT, Lin M, Brena RM, Lang JC, Schuller DE, Otterson GA, Morrison CD, Smiraglia DJ, Plass C (2006) Epigenetic regulation of the tumor suppressor gene TCF21 on 6q23-q24 in lung and head and neck cancer. Proc Natl Acad Sci U S A 103(4):982–987

Soffietti R, Leoncini B, Ruda R (2007a) New developments in the treatment of malignant gliomas. Expert Rev Neurother 7(10):1313–1326

Soffietti R, Ruda R, Trevisan E (2007b) New chemotherapy options for the treatment of malignant gliomas. Anticancer Drugs 18(6):621–632

Sonabend AM, Ulasov IV, Tyler MA, Rivera AA, Mathis JM, Lesniak MS (2008) Mesenchymal Stem Cells Effectively Deliver an Oncolytic Adenovirus to Intracranial Glioma. Stem Cells 26(3):831–841

Sonnemann J, Kumar KS, Heesch S, Muller C, Hartwig C, Maass M, Bader P, Beck JF (2006) Histone deacetylase inhibitors induce cell death and enhance the susceptibility to ionizing radiation, etoposide, and TRAIL in medulloblastoma cells. Int J Oncol 28(3):755–766

Srivenugopal KS, Shou J, Mullapudi SR, Lang FF, Jr., Rao JS, Ali-Osman F (2001) Enforced expression of wild-type p53 curtails the transcription of the O(6)-methylguanine-DNA methyltransferase gene in human tumor cells and enhances their sensitivity to alkylating agents. Clin Cancer Res 7(5):1398–1409

Steck PA, Pershouse MA, Jasser SA, Yung WK, Lin H, Ligon AH, Langford LA, Baumgard ML, Hattier T, Davis T, Frye C, Hu R, Swedlund B, Teng DH, Tavtigian SV (1997) Identification of a candidate tumour suppressor gene, MMAC1, at chromosome 10q23.3 that is mutated in multiple advanced cancers. Nat Genet 15(4):356–362

Stone AR, Bobo W, Brat DJ, Devi NS, Van Meir EG, Vertino PM (2004) Aberrant methylation and down-regulation of TMS1/ASC in human glioblastoma. Am J Pathol 165(4):1151–1161

Tews B, Roerig P, Hartmann C, Hahn M, Felsberg J, Blaschke B, Sabel M, Kunitz A, Toedt G, Neben K, Benner A, Deimling A, Reifenberger G, Lichter P (2007) Hypermethylation and transcriptional downregulation of the CITED4 gene at 1p34.2 in oligodendroglial tumours with allelic losses on 1p and 19q. Oncogene 26(34):5010–5016

Ueki K, Ono Y, Henson JW, Efird JT, von Deimling A, Louis DN (1996) CDKN2/p16 or RB alterations occur in the majority of glioblastomas and are inversely correlated. Cancer Res 56(1):150–153

von Deimling A, Fimmers R, Schmidt MC, Bender B, Fassbender F, Nagel J, Jahnke R, Kaskel P, Duerr EM, Koopmann J, Maintz D, Steinbeck S, Wick W, Platten M, Muller DJ, Przkora R, Waha A, Blumcke B, Wellenreuther R, Meyer-Puttlitz B, Schmidt O, Mollenhauer J, Poustka A, Stangl AP, Lenartz D, von Ammon K (2000) Comprehensive allelotype and genetic analysis of 466 human nervous system tumors. J Neuropathol Exp Neurol 59(6):544–558

von Deimling A, Louis DN, Schramm J, Wiestler OD (1994) Astrocytic gliomas: characterization on a molecular genetic basis. Recent Results Cancer Res 135:33–42

Waha A, Guntner S, Huang TH, Yan PS, Arslan B, Pietsch T, Wiestler OD, Waha A (2005) Epigenetic silencing of the protocadherin family member PCDH-gamma-A11 in astrocytomas. Neoplasia 7(3):193–199

Wakabayashi T, Natsume A, Hashizume Y, Fujii M, Mizuno M, Yoshida J (2008) A phase I clinical trial of interferon-beta gene therapy for high-grade glioma: novel findings from gene expression profiling and autopsy. J Gene Med 10(4):329–339

Walsh CP, Chaillet JR, Bestor TH (1998) Transcription of IAP endogenous retroviruses is constrained by cytosine methylation. Nat Genet 20(2):116–117

Wang SI, Puc J, Li J, Bruce JN, Cairns P, Sidransky D, Parsons R (1997) Somatic mutations of PTEN in glioblastoma multiforme. Cancer Res 57(19): 4183–4186

Watanabe T, Huang H, Nakamura M, Wischhusen J, Weller M, Kleihues P, Ohgaki H (2002) Methylation of the p73 gene in gliomas. Acta Neuropathol 104(4):357–362

Weber RG, Hoischen A, Ehrler M, Zipper P, Kaulich K, Blaschke B, Becker AJ, Weber-Mangal S, Jauch A, Radlwimmer B, Schramm J, Wiestler OD, Lichter P, Reifenberger G (2007) Frequent loss of chromosome 9, homozygous CDKN2A/p14(ARF)/CDKN2B deletion and low TSC1 mRNA expression in pleomorphic xanthoastrocytomas. Oncogene 26(7):1088–1097

Weingart J, Grossman SA, Carson KA, Fisher JD, Delaney SM, Rosenblum ML, Olivi A, Judy K, Tatter SB, Dolan ME (2007) Phase I trial of polifeprosan 20 with carmustine implant plus continuous infusion of intravenous O6-benzylguanine in adults with recurrent malignant glioma: new approaches to brain tumor therapy CNS consortium trial. J Clin Oncol 25(4):399–404

Worm J, Aggerholm A, Guldberg P (2001) In-tube DNA methylation profiling by fluorescence melting curve analysis. Clin Chem 47(7): 1183–1189

Yamashita K, Upadhyay S, Osada M, Hoque MO, Xiao Y, Mori M, Sato F, Meltzer SJ, Sidransky D (2002) Pharmacologic unmasking of epigenetically silenced tumor suppressor genes in esophageal squamous cell carcinoma. Cancer Cell 2(6): 485–495

Yamashita K, Park HL, Kim MS, Osada M, Tokumaru Y, Inoue H, Mori M, Sidransky D (2006a) PGP9.5 methylation in diffuse-type gastric cancer. Cancer Res 66(7):3921–3927

Yamashita S, Tsujino Y, Moriguchi K, Tatematsu M, Ushijima T (2006b) Chemical genomic screening for methylation-silenced genes in gastric cancer cell lines using 5-aza-2'-deoxycytidine treatment and oligonucleotide microarray. Cancer Sci 97(1):64–71

Yang E, Kang HJ, Koh KH, Rhee H, Kim NK, Kim H (2007) Frequent inactivation of SPARC by promoter hypermethylation in colon cancers. Int J Cancer 121(3):567–575

Yin D, Ong JM, Hu J, Desmond JC, Kawamata N, Konda BM, Black KL, Koeffler HP (2007) Suberoylanilide hydroxamic acid, a histone deacetylase inhibitor: effects on gene expression and growth of glioma cells in vitro and in vivo. Clin Cancer Res 13(3):1045–1052

Zardo G, Tiirikainen MI, Hong C, Misra A, Feuerstein BG, Volik S, Collins CC, Lamborn KR, Bollen A, Pinkel D, Albertson DG, Costello JF (2002) Integrated genomic and epigenomic analyses pinpoint biallelic gene inactivation in tumors. Nat Genet 32(3):453–458

Zarnitsyn VG, Kamaev PP, Prausnitz MR (2007) Ultrasound-enhanced chemotherapy and gene delivery for glioma cells. Technol Cancer Res Treat 6(5):433–442

Brain Tumor Stem Cells

Christian Nern, Daniel Sommerlad, Till Acker and Karl H. Plate

Abstract The dogma that solid tumors are composed of tumor cells that all share the same ability to produce proliferating daughter cells has been challenged in recent years. There is growing evidence that many adult tissues contain a set of tissue stem cells, which might undergo malignant transformation while retaining their stem cell characteristics. These include the ability of indefinite self-renewal and the capability to differentiate into daughter cells of tissue-specific lineages. Brain tumors such as medulloblastomas or glioblastomas often contain areas of divergent differentiation, which raises the intriguing question of whether these tumors could derive from neural stem cells (NSCs).

This chapter reviews the current knowledge of NSCs and relates them to brain tumor pathology. Current therapy protocols for malignant brain tumors are targeted toward the reduction of bulk tumor mass. The concept of brain-tumor stem cells could provide new insights for future therapies, if the capacity for self-renewal of tumor cells and growth of the tumor mass would reside within a small subset of cancer cells.

14.1
The Concept of Cancer Stem Cells

The WHO classification of tumors of the central nervous system (CNS) defines a wide spectrum of different tumor entities including glial, neuronal, embryonal, and mixed glioneural tumors as well as tumors derived from meningeal and vascular structures. Most of these clinically malignant neoplasms show high infiltrative capacity, rendering curative therapies currently impossible. The histogenesis of brain tumors still remains poorly understood. The existence of tumor entities with mixed cellular differentiation points to a histogenetic origin from immature cell types. The most immature neoplastic cell type giving rise to tumor cell progeny would be a tumor cell with stem cell properties: a putative brain tumor stem cell (BTSC).

Already 150 years ago, the pathologists Rudolph Virchow and Julius Conheim observed histological similarities between fetal tissue and cancer cell types such as teratocarcinomas (Virchow 1855; Conheim 1867). This suggests an origin of certain tumor entities from embryonal undifferentiated cells, which is today discussed in terms of the cancer stem cell

D. Sommerlad (✉)
Neurological Institute (Edinger-Institute)
Neuroscience Center
Heinrich-Hoffmann-Str. 7
60528 Frankfurt am Main
E-mail: d.sommerlad@med.uni-frankfurt.de

hypothesis (Vescovi et al. 2006). However, solid tumors were interpreted as stochastically organized neoplasias, in which each tumor cell has the capacity to maintain tumor growth. In recent years, growing evidence for a hierarchical organization of different types of tumors was gathered. This hierarchical model suggests that only a certain subtype of tumor cells, a putative cancer stem cell, is able to preserve tumor expansion over a longer time period (Reya et al. 2001). These cells would show stem cell features including the two main functional criteria: unlimited self-renewal and multipotency. More committed progeny of such cancer stem cells would only be capable of proliferating for a very restricted period of time and would soon differentiate into cell types with a short lifespan (Fig. 14.1).

Preliminary evidence for the existence of cancer stem cells came from studies on acute myeloid leukemia (AML) (Bonnet and Dick 1997). In this study, the authors demonstrated that a small subpopulation of cells within the blood of AML patients was able to re-establish AML with hierarchical progeny in nude mice even after single-cell transplantation. These leukemia-initiating cells were exclusively found in the $CD34^+/CD38^-$ population and were independent of the phenotype of the leukemic blasts. Apart from their potential to proliferate and to differentiate, the authors also demonstrated the ability of leukemia-initiating cells to self-renew upon serial transplantation. Physiologically, the marker CD34 can be found on a subpopulation of hematopoietic stem cells that self-renew and are capable of giving rise to the complete spectrum of cell types found within the bone marrow and blood.

The early identification of cancer stem cells within the hematopoietic system was achieved

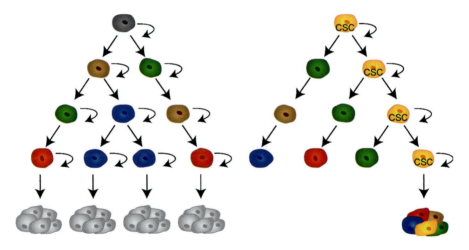

Fig. 14.1 Models of solid tumor organization. Two different models of solid tumor organization. *Left* Stochastic model. Within heterogenous tumors, each tumor cell exhibits the same capacity to proliferate and to sustain tumor growth. Tumor heterogeneity in this model is explained by the existence of multiple genetic tumor subclones, due to accumulative acquisition of genetic alterations. *Right* Hierarchical model. Unlimited self-renewal capacity exclusively resides in a subpopulation of tumor cells (*yellow*). Only these cancer stem cells (CSCs) can sustain or initiate tumor growth. The more differentiated progeny (*brown, blue, green, red*) have only limited proliferation potential and have lost the ability to initiate tumor growth. This hierarchy model adds a differentiation hierarchy as an additional factor to explain this heterogeneity (Adapted from Reya et al. 2001)

on the basis of a profound understanding of its physiological organization, because it had been discussed as an organ with the ability to renew itself in adulthood already decades ago (Till and McCulloch 1961). Further studies of the bone marrow revealed insights into its hierarchical structure during development and adulthood and definitions of its different cell types, including stem or progenitor cells that today can be tracked with the help of defined surface markers (Young and Hwang-Chen 1981; Bonnet 2002). More recently, the existence of cancer stem cells was also suggested for solid tumors including breast (Al-Hajj et al. 2003) and lung cancer (Kim et al. 2005) as well as tumors of the CNS (Singh et al. 2003). Mechanisms known to regulate stem cells in the corresponding tissue, from where the tumor is derived, seem to be preserved in cancer stem cells. In this review, the findings on brain-tumor stem cells are discussed in light of the current knowledge on neural stem cells (NSCs).

14.2
Neural Stem Cells in the Adult CNS

Tissue-specific stem cells have been described in different adult organs. However, the phenotype of organ-specific stem cells and their progeny in tissues other than the hematopoietic system is only poorly understood. Putative neural stem cells (NSCs) were first isolated from the adult CNS of rodents in the early 1990s (Reynolds and Weiss 1992) and some years later from humans (Johansson et al. 1999a).

In the adult rodent brain, two main neurogenic regions have been identified: the subventricular zone (SVZ) of the lateral wall of the lateral ventricles and the dentate gyrus (DG) of the hippocampus (Reynolds and Weiss 1992; Gage et al. 1995). Newborn cells have been shown to migrate from the SVZ via the rostral migratory stream to the olfactory bulb and become mature neurons (Lois and Alvarez-Buylla 1994). Within the hippocampus early progenitor cells reside in the granule cell layer of the DG and can give rise to neurons that integrate locally (Kuhn et al. 1996).

Different cell types have been controversially discussed to function as adult NSCs. These cell types include astrocytic (Doetsch et al. 1999), ependymal (Johansson et al. 1999b), and subependymal cells (Morshead et al. 1994). Interestingly, the development of brain tumors from putative cancer stem cells has been suggested for astrocytic, embryonal, and ependymal tumor entities (Hemmati et al. 2003; Singh et al. 2004; Taylor et al. 2005).

As the putative stem cells from neurogenic regions show structural and molecular characteristics of astrocytes, the most propagated hypothesis today is that astrocytes, which might derive from radial glia (Doetsch 2003), are stem cell candidates within the adult mammalian brain (Alvarez-Buylla and Lim 2004).

Within rodents' SVZ, three immature cell types have been characterized in more detail on the basis of morphological and functional studies: (1) putative slowly-dividing stem cells, the so-called type B astrocytes, that reside near the ependymal cell layer; (2) a population of rapidly dividing transit-amplifying progenitor cells (type C cells), which develop from type B cells and give rise to (3) migrating neuroblasts (type A cells) (Doetsch 2003) (Fig. 14.2). In a recent study a subtype of type B astrocytes, expressing the platelet-derived growth factor receptor alpha (PDGFR-α) was described (Jackson et al. 2006). Interestingly, stimulation with PDGF led to proliferation of these cells, arrest of neuroblast production, and induction of glioma-like atypical hyperplasias.

Within the granule cell layer of the hippocampus, neural progenitors have also been suggested to develop from regional astrocytes with stem cell properties (Seri et al. 2001). But more recently, it has been suggested that progenitors of the DG may derive from subependymal periventricular cells (Seaberg and van der Kooy 2002).

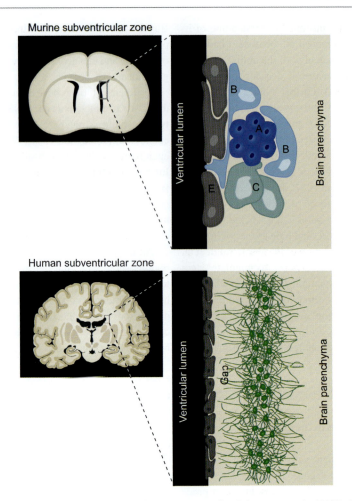

Fig. 14.2 Organization of the murine and human subventricular zone. Murine subventricular zone: Cellular organization of the subventricular zone (SVZ) in the adult mouse brain as suggested by Doetsch et al. (1999). Slowly dividing neural stem cells (**B**) give rise to rapidly dividing transit amplifying cells (**C**). These cells differentiate into committed neuroblasts (**A**). The ependymal cell layer (**E**) has also been discussed to harbor neural stem cells (Johansson et al. 1999b) (Adapted from Doetsch 2003). Human subventricular zone: In contrast to the rodent SVZ, the cellular organization of the human SVZ is poorly understood. As suggested by Sanai et al., local GFAP-expressing cells show stem cell properties in vitro (Sanai et al. 2004). These cells (*green*) are located within a ribbon, which is separated from the ependymal cell layer (*grey*) by a cell free area (*gap*)

The close contact of stem cells to the ventricular lumen can in principle be explained by the developmental origin from ventricular zone cells, but could also reflect a functional interaction of stem cells with the ventricular system. Factors such as vascular endothelial growth factor (VEGF), which are secreted by the choroid plexus, could influence stem cell maintenance and cell fate. Indeed, VEGF has been shown to increase neurogenesis and neuroprotection in mice after intraventricular injection (Jin et al. 2002; Schanzer et al. 2004).

The cerebrospinal fluid has also been shown to impair the rostral migratory abilities of neuroblasts by its flow direction (Sawamoto et al. 2006). Physiologically, neuroblasts are highly migratory and have been described to migrate in chains accompanied by astrocytes via long distances within the olfactory tracts. This process of chain migration has been demonstrated in adult rodents (Lois and Alvarez-Buylla 1994; Lois et al. 1996) and non-human primates (Pencea et al. 2001).

If brain tumors develop from neural stem or progenitor cells, the marked migratory capacities of stem cell progeny may explain why many brain tumors spread widely throughout the brain and are not only found within neurogenic regions.

The existence of stem or progenitor cells and neurogenesis in other regions of the adult brain is still controversially discussed (Emsley et al. 2005). Interestingly, the murine postnatal cerebellum has been shown to harbor neural progenitor cells (NPCs) (Lee et al. 2005). This observation may be relevant for the histogenesis of the classic medulloblastoma subtype (Kenney and Segal 2005), while desmoplastic medulloblastomas have been suggested to derive from residing NPCs within the external granule cell layer (Katsetos and Burger 1994; Pietsch et al. 2004).

While numerous studies identified newborn neurons in the adult rodent brain, evidence for in vivo neurogenesis in humans has only been observed in a single study (Eriksson et al. 1998). In this study, newborn neurons could be identified within the dentate gyrus in postmortem specimens from patients that had been treated with BrdU. However, neocortical neurogenesis in humans has been suggested to be restricted, at least under physiological conditions, to the developing brain (Bhardwaj et al. 2006).

The cellular architecture of neurogenic zones in humans differs markedly from that observed in rodents. In the adult human brain, SVZ astrocytes are located within a ribbon, which in contrast to the rodent system is separated from the ependymal cell layer (Sanai et al. 2004) (Fig. 14.2, bottom). Whether neuroblasts migrate from the SVZ to the olfactory bulbs in humans remains a controversial debate (Bedard and Parent 2004; Sanai et al. 2004).

Similar to the rodent brain, isolated astrocytes from the human SVZ show stem cell properties in vitro (Sanai et al. 2004). Interestingly, PDGFR-α-expressing SVZ astrocytes, which can give rise to atypical glial hyperplasias in rodents, can also be identified phenotypically within the adult human SVZ (Jackson et al. 2006). Additionally, isolation of multipotent progenitors from non-neurogenic regions has been described: glial progenitor cells isolated from the subcortical white matter of the adult human brain were shown to be multipotent in vitro (Nunes et al. 2003). Another study demonstrated the isolation of multipotent progenitors from the amygdala and frontal cortex (Arsenijevic et al. 2001). Such cells could also be relevant in the context of tumor initiation after neoplastic transformation.

14.3 Phenotypic and Functional Characterization of Neural Stem Cells

The identification and enrichment of putative brain tumor stem cells is based on methods also employed in neural stem cell research. In contrast to well characterized organs such as the hematopoietic system, unique NSC markers have not yet been identified within the adult mammalian nervous system. Most of the identified markers are not expressed solely by NSCs, but also by their downstream progeny and are insufficient to enrich a pure population with stem cell properties. Markers that have been used to identify or enrich stem cells from the adult mammalian brain include the intermediate filament protein nestin (Lendahl et al. 1990), CD133, which is also expressed by hematopoietic stem cells (Yin et al. 1997), sox-2 (Graham et al. 2003), the neural RNA-binding protein musashi-1 (Sakakibara et al. 1996), and LeX/ssea-1 (Capela and Temple 2002). Also, glial fibrillary acidic protein (GFAP) is expressed on neural stem cells (Doetsch et al. 1999). Other markers of more committed cell types have not been shown to be expressed by NSCs. These include markers of neuroblasts, like Dlx-2, calretinin (Brandt et al. 2003), doublecortin and polysialylated acidic neural cell adhesion molecule (PSA-NCAM) (Seki and Arai 1993). Dlx-2 is also found in type C cells (Doetsch 2003). Some of these proteins (e.g., nestin, sox-2, and CD133) are also expressed in brain tumors. Especially CD133 (Singh et al. 2004; Bao et al. 2006b) has been successfully used to enrich for putative cancer stem cells. During development, CD133 and its mouse homolog prominin are expressed in the apical cell membrane of mammalian neuroepithelial cells and are differentially distributed during asymmetric cell divisions. Neural stem cells retain CD133 while committed neural precursors do not (Weigmann et al. 1997). However, the precise function of CD133 is still unknown.

Because of the lack of a prospective marker profile, neural stem cells are typically defined by functional criteria, namely the ability to self-renew over an extended period of time and to generate a large number of progeny that can differentiate into the primary cell types of the tissue from which the cells are derived (multipotency). A common in vitro assay to analyze these properties is the neurosphere assay (Fig. 14.3). In principal, isolated cells are cultured in the presence of epidermal growth factor (EGF) and/or basic fibroblast growth factor (bFGF) and develop into floating heterogenous ball-like structures after a few days. These so-called neurospheres can be dissociated and recultured as single cells, which partially generate neurospheres again, suggesting that some of the cells self-renewed. Withdrawal of growth factors and

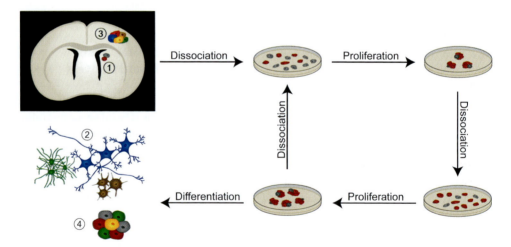

Fig. 14.3 Sphere-forming assay for neural stem cells and cancer stem cells. Isolated cells from neurogenic regions (**1**) can be grown as neurospheres in presence of growth factors (EGF, bFGF). Primary spheres may derive from neural stem cells (NSCs) and also from neural progenitor cells (NPCs). Only NSCs can be grown as spheres for an unlimited number of passages. Withdrawal of growth factors and addition of FCS induces differentiation of NSCs/NPCs into astrocytic, oligodendroglial, and neuronal cell types (**2**). Spheres can also be grown from different brain tumors (**3**). Similar to neurospheres, such tumorspheres might contain cells with stem cell properties. Such putative cancer stem cells (CSCs) possess the potential to self-renew and to differentiate into cells with the phenotypic characteristics of the tumor they are originally derived from (**4**)

addition of fetal cow serum (FCS) can induce cell adherence and differentiation. The detection of oligodendrocytes, astrocytes, and neurons after several days of differentiation is interpreted as the multipotent capacity of the neuroepithelial undifferentiated cells originally isolated. This assay is used in numerous studies investigating the characterization of neural stem cells, but one should be aware of several limitations.

For example, the assay is dependent on the culture conditions and only supports survival and expansion of cell populations that respond to the added growth factors. Not only stem cells, but also progenitor cells have been shown to form neurospheres after exposure to high concentrations of growth factors (Doetsch et al. 2002). Furthermore, oligodendrocyte precursor cells could be de-differentiated into multipotent progenitor cells (Kondo and Raff 2000). Cortical progenitor cells change their expression profile and lose their regional characteristics when cultured as neurospheres (Machon et al. 2005). The former view that one stem cell gives rise to one neurosphere and every secondary sphere derives from a stem cell again is obsolete, since the majority of spheres are in fact derived from non-stem cells (Reynolds and Rietze 2005). It has also been suggested that spheres are motile and able to fuse (Singec et al. 2006). This challenges the reliability of measuring the clonality, number, and fate of stem cells only through sphere-forming assays. Given these restrictions, results from these in vitro assays for the identification of BTSCs probably also have to be interpreted with caution.

14.4 Identification and Enrichment of Brain Tumor Stem Cells

During the isolation of tumor cells from solid tumors, several peculiarities have to be taken into account. Gathering the actual tumor cells from a tumor specimen requires biochemical or physical steps of tumor cell purification, which might alter the viability and the phenotype of the cells. Dense networks of glial fibrillary protein, collagen, reticulin, and other matrix proteins are present, which are usually removed through enzymatic digestion. This can damage epitopes of surface receptors. In addition, shearing forces during centrifugation may destroy subcellular components or the whole cell (Hill 2006). During the purification of tumor cells, it is therefore a major effort to eliminate nontumorous components without altering the tumor cells.

It has been proposed that all features of stem cells must be fulfilled in order to define a population of cancer stem cells (Vescovi et al. 2006). Apart from the stem cell properties of unlimited self-renewal and multipotency, cancer stem cells must additionally exhibit the capacity to initiate tumors while recapitulating the original phenotype upon orthotopic transplantation. Furthermore, the ability to differentiate into nontumorigenic progeny and the preservation of genetic alterations of the original tumor are required. Classic tumor cell lines might have met some of the above criteria before the concept of tumor stem cells was born. In a hierarchical model, the above criteria should only be fulfilled by a distinct subpopulation of cells: the cancer stem cells. Conversely, all other cells within the tumor should not have the ability to form tumors, self-renew, and differentiate into different lineages.

Methods commonly employed for the prospective isolation and characterization of tumor-initiating subpopulations in brain tumors comprise cell sorting for the CD133 antigen, the side population assay, and functional sphere-forming assays. By using one of these methods, brain cancer cell populations with stem cell properties were described in several tumor entities, including astrocytomas, glioblastomas, medulloblastomas, and ependymomas (Hemmati et al. 2003; Singh et al. 2003, 2004; Galli et al. 2004; Yuan et al. 2004; Patrawala et al. 2005; Taylor et al. 2005).

In most of these studies, the sphere-forming assay was used to identify cancer cells with stem cell properties within these tumors (Reynolds and Weiss 1992; Vescovi et al. 2006) (Fig. 14.3). Sphere formation occurred at variable rates of about 20% in glioblastomas and up to 80% in medulloblastomas, and was even shown to occur in pilocytic astrocytomas with rates of 0.3–1.5%.

Singh et al. showed a close correlation between the rate of sphere formation and CD133 expression in cancer cells freshly isolated from glioblastoma and medulloblastoma specimens, indicating that CD133 could act as a prospective marker for identifying sphere-forming tumor stem cells in human glioblastomas and medulloblastomas (Singh et al. 2004). Only CD133-positive (CD133$^+$) tumor cells were shown to act as tumor-initiating cells upon orthotopic xenotransplantation in nude mice, while marker negative cells did not. The tumor cell number needed to form xenografts was as few as 100 tumor cells in the CD133$^+$ fraction. Conversely, up to 10,000 tumor cells of the CD133-negative (CD133$^-$) fraction did not initiate tumors in this study. Similarly, an investigation conducted by Bao et al. showed no tumor-initiating capability of 10,000 freshly isolated, glioblastoma-derived CD133$^-$ tumor cells after FACS sorting (Bao et al. 2006b). However, the tumorigenicity of the CD133$^-$ fraction seemed to be culture-dependent in this study. When primary glioblastoma cells were expanded in vivo as murine xenografts prior to transplantation, the resulting CD133$^-$ tumor cell population was capable of forming small, barely vascularized tumors after transplantation in two out of six mice. Taken together, some residual tumorigenic potential could thus reside within a fraction of the CD133$^-$ tumor cell population, depending on the culture conditions of early passages.

These findings stress the importance of the microenvironment for stem cell features of putative cancer cells. Data from a study by Lee et al. suggest that the grade of "stemness" of the resulting cells of a tumor cell line is regulated by culturing conditions (Lee et al. 2006b). In this study, differences in proliferation kinetics, molecular expression patterns of stem cell markers and responsiveness to differentiation stimuli of primary tumor cells were dependent on propagation of the tumor cells in either serum-free or serum-containing media. It was shown that early passages of tumor cell lines cultured with serum did not form tumor xenografts upon orthotopic transplantation, while those cultured under serum-free conditions did so. During repeated passaging, tumor cells in serum-containing media rapidly regained genetic alterations, while concomitantly accumulating the ability to form tumor xenografts.

In the studies by Singh et al. and Bao et al. mentioned above, a proper calculation of cancer stem cell frequency is not possible, as unsorted tumor cells were not transplanted in cell dilution experiments. Determining stem cell frequency in solid tumors is possible from the data observed in a study of Al-Hajj et al. (2003). They prospectively isolated breast carcinoma cells in a CD44$^+$/ESA$^+$/CD24$^-$/lineage subpopulation, which led to tumor engraftment after transplantation of 100 cells. In the same study, 10,000 unsorted cells were necessary for tumor initiation. This calculates a tumor stem cell frequency of less than 0.01%. Bonnet and Dick estimated frequencies of 0.2–100 cancer stem cells per million mononuclear cells in the blood of AML patients (Bonnet and Dick 1997).

Considering the low tumor stem cell proportion in these cancers, the reported number of one in four tumor cells of a glioblastoma or medulloblastoma expressing CD133 exceeds the expected frequency of true cancer stem cells. Similarly, the high sphere-forming frequency of tumor cells derived from malignant brain tumors probably does not reflect the proportion of cancer stem cells.

Much lower frequencies of putative cancer stem cells are found using the side population assay. This assay was first described in 1997 when hematopoietic stem cells showed an active efflux of Hoechst dye 33342 in dual-wavelength FACS analysis (Goodell et al. 1996). This technique allows one to select for a subpopulation of cells that do not accumulate the dye and form a small low-signal population. The side population assay is used as a method to enrich putative stem cells in many different organs and cancers, including brain tumors. The formation of a side population depends on proteins of the ABC transporter family, which actively transport drugs and chemical substances such as the Hoechst dye against a gradient out of the cell. Although ABCG2 is a major player among ABC transporters, it is not generally accepted as a suitable marker to either describe the side population phenotype or to unequivocally define the phenotype of bona fide cancer-initiating stem cells. In fact, the side population isolated from tumors is heterogenous but is likely to contain a subset of cancer-initiating cells of a yet unknown phenotype (Patrawala et al. 2005).

Side populations are also found in long-term cultured glioma cell lines of rats and humans (Hirschmann-Jax et al. 2004; Kondo et al. 2004; Patrawala et al. 2005). These side populations are more tumorigenic and generate non-side-population progeny, reflecting important criteria of tumor stem cells, as mentioned above.

14.5
Brain Tumor Histogenesis

It has been suggested that the development of cancer requires the accumulation of numerous mutations within a cell, including mutations that affect self-renewal and proliferation (Hanahan and Weinberg 2000). Slowly dividing NSCs could therefore be interesting candidates for the origin of cancer stem cells. First, their ability to slowly and indefinitely divide over extended time periods makes the accumulation of different mutations necessary for tumorigenesis more likely. Second, the self-renewal program, which is essential for a cancer stem cell, is already a feature of stem cells and does not need to be acquired through mutations. Oncogenic mutations gathered during the long life of stem cells could also be passed on to their rapid amplifying progeny.

During development, progenitor cells derive from stem cells by asymmetric divisions. This mechanism ensures the generation of more committed progeny and the concomitant maintenance of the stem cell status. Mechanistically, intrinsic cues such as the asymmetric partitioning of cell components that determine cell fate can be distinguished from extrinsic cues resulting from, for example, asymmetric placement of daughter cells (Morrison and Kimble 2006). Two recent studies on nonvertebrates unraveled a mechanism by which loss of polarity in asymmetric divisions leads to tumorigenesis (Betschinger et al. 2006; Lee et al. 2006a). The generation of daughter cells via asymmetric divisions might therefore be another critical step in cancer development.

While certain tumor entities can be found predominantly in defined areas of the brain (Fig. 14.4, right), astrocytic tumors can occur at any location within the CNS. It has been shown that experimentally induced periventricular glioma microfoci lost their connection to the subventricular zone over time (Vick et al. 1977). If these neoplasias derived from an asymmetrically dividing cancer stem cell, the highly migratory potential of its progeny could explain this phenomenon. This implicates the possibility that the site of the lesion and the site of the cancer stem cell are not matched. In this type of model, the region where slowly dividing cancer stem cells reside could be clinically silent (Berger et al. 2004).

Early inactivation of p53 tumor suppressor gene in combination with NF1 loss has been shown to induce malignant gliomas in mice with a high penetrance (Zhu et al. 2005). In this study, early presymptomatic lesions were found predominantly within the SVZ. In animal models,

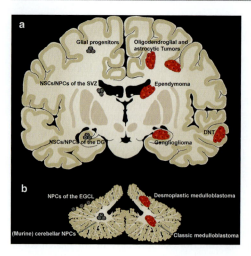

Fig. 14.4 Localization of neural stem/progenitor cells and tumors within the CNS. Astrocytic and oligodendroglial tumors are widely distributed throughout the brain. Malignant transformation of stem or progenitor cells of the adult brain may initiate the development of a wide spectrum of brain tumor entities. In addition to NSCs/NPCs from neurogenic regions (SVZ, DG), progenitor cells have been shown to reside also in non-neurogenic regions (**a**, *left*). It is yet unknown whether tumors that develop in the corresponding brain regions (**a**, *right*) originate from local NSCs/NPCs or from distant NSCs/NPCs, which after transformation migrate into these areas. **b** The possibility that different stem/progenitor cell populations give rise to different subtypes of brain tumors has been suggested in murine medulloblastoma models. While residual pluripotent cells of the external granule cell layer (EGCL) may give rise to desmoplastic medulloblastomas, postnatal progenitors of the cerebellar white matter might be involved in the development of the classic medulloblastoma subtype

brain regions with persistent neurogenesis were shown to be more susceptible to viral or chemical malignant transformation than regions with senescent cell populations (Sanai et al. 2005). Holland et al. showed that transfection of nestin-expressing cells with signal transduction molecules activated in gliomas such as K-Ras and Akt led to the formation of malignant gliomas in mice (Holland et al. 2000a). Transfection of mature GFAP-expressing cell types with the same vectors did not induce tumor formation. This points to a higher susceptibility to tumor initiation of nestin-expressing stem or progenitor cells in contrast to more committed cell types. Putative stem cells expressing GFAP within the SVZ (type B cells) were probably not targeted in this study, as the injections for transfection were placed in the frontal lobe parenchyma anterior to the striatum but not directly into the SVZ. As mentioned above, a PDGFR-α-expressing subtype of type B cells was recently shown to give rise to glioma-like hyperplasias (Jackson et al. 2006). These studies support the thesis that brain tumors derive predominantly in neurogenic regions of the brain and that stem cells residing in these regions might be involved in tumor initiation.

Restricted progenitor cells, which have been isolated from different locations of the adult brain, may also give rise to brain tumors (Figs. 14.4, left and 14.5). As these cells physiologically show only limited or no self-renewal capacity, the acquisition of this feature due to transformation might be crucial for tumorigenesis. Within rodent CNS, glial progenitors of the white matter gave rise to malignant gliomas after infection with PDGF-expressing retroviruses (Assanah et al. 2006). Acquisition of stem cell properties and concomitant malignant transformation of progenitor cells was also shown within the hematopoietic system: in a study by Huntly et al., transduction of certain leukemic oncogenes (MOZ-TIF2) conferred properties of leukemic stem cells to committed progenitors (Huntly et al. 2004).

However, a cancer stem cell does not obligatorily have to derive from a stem or progenitor cell. It has also been suggested that cancer stem cells could derive from more mature cell types. Mature GFAP-expressing astrocytes have been shown to give rise to astroglial but also to oligodendroglial and mixed tumors after infection with polyoma middle T virus antigen (MTA),

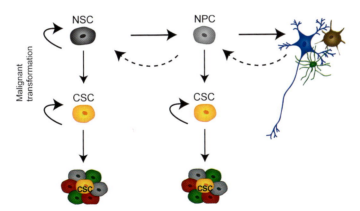

Fig. 14.5 Origin of cancer stem cells. Cancer stem cells (CSCs) have been proposed to develop from neural stem cells (NSCs) and also from progenitor cells (NPCs). As NSCs divide slowly and have a long life span, the accumulation of genetic alterations in these cells is facilitated. Due to their unlimited self-renewal capacity, fewer mutations are required to generate cancer cells with stem-like characteristics, as crucial stem cell programs are already in place. If CSCs derive from NPCs (or more committed cell types), re-acquisition of a self-renewal capacity concomitantly with inhibition of differentiation would be necessary for malignant transformation

which activates downstream effectors of PDGF signaling (Holland et al. 2000b). This suggests a de-differentiation of astrocytes into more immature cell types before giving rise to tumors of different lineages. It also has been observed that fate-restricted glial progenitors can acquire stem cell characteristics under certain conditions (Kondo and Raff 2000). Therefore more committed cell types might have the potential to de-differentiate into less restricted cell types, possibly into cells with (cancer) stem cell properties. Another interesting hypothesis is that cancer stem cells might be generated from horizontal gene transfer or cell fusion events (Bjerkvig et al. 2005).

14.6 Signaling Pathways of Neural Stem Cells and Brain Tumor Cells

The close relationship of neural stem cells and brain tumor (stem) cells is also reflected by their similar activation or depression of certain signaling pathways, including pathways that regulate self-renewal and proliferation. One of them is the sonic hedgehog (Shh) pathway. Shh signaling is a crucial morphogen during development and was shown to maintain proliferation of adult hippocampal neural progenitors in culture (Lai et al. 2003). Stimulation of the Shh pathway increased proliferation of adult NPCs also in vivo (Machold et al. 2003). Shh signaling regulates proliferation of progenitor cells within the external granule cell layer of the cerebellum by activation of certain transcription factors like N-myc and Gli family members (Kenney et al. 2003). Mutations that activate the Shh pathway were identified in human medulloblastomas (Wetmore 2003), while blockade of Shh signaling was shown to inhibit tumor growth in medulloblastomas (Berman et al. 2002). Furthermore, Gli expression can be found in neurogenic regions of the adult brain (Palma et al. 2005) and was suggested to regulate tumorigenesis of gliomas (Dahmane et al. 2001). Other pathways and regulatory molecules shared by neural stem cells and brain tumor cells include Wnt signaling (Yokota et al. 2002; Reya and Clevers 2005), the PTEN pathway, which is a regulator of neural stem cell proliferation and motility (Li et al. 2003), bmi-1 expression (Molofsky et al. 2003), and increased telomerase activity (Komata et al. 2002; Caporaso et al. 2003). Also, EGF receptors (EGFR) were shown to be expressed by neural stem cells and they are upregulated in primary gliomas. Under physiological conditions, EGF serves as a proliferative stimulus of transit-amplifying C cells (Doetsch et al. 2002). EGFR activation alone is insufficient to induce gliomas in mice (Holland 2001). However, EGFR activation leads to malignant transformation of astrocytes after disruption of cell cycle arrest pathways (Holland et al. 1998; Bachoo et al. 2002). Some intracellular pathways that are activated in brain tumors are hypoxia-regulated. This includes Notch-1 signaling as well as upregulation of the tyrosine kinase c-kit (Jogi et al. 2004; Purow et al. 2005).

14.7
The (Cancer) Stem Cell Niche

The characteristics of (cancer) stem cells and their progeny are not only given by unique molecular expression patterns of a defined cellular entity and their behavior in in vitro assays, but are influenced or even induced by the environment or niche in which these cells reside in vivo (Blau et al. 2001).

Such a stem cell niche is supported by different extrinsic stimuli provided by the ventricular system, interactions with basal laminae and endothelial cells, autocrine stimulation, cell–cell communication and influence through neurotransmitters via synaptic afferents (Watts et al. 2005).

An example for the relevance of a niche for stem cell function is the finding that astrocytes isolated from the adult hippocampus are able to increase neurogenesis from neural stem or progenitor cells in vitro, but astrocytes from the adult spinal cord are not (Song et al. 2002). This suggests fundamental differences in supportive cell function when cells of the same lineage are isolated either from a neurogenic or non-neurogenic niche. Even more importantly, it shows that the function of putative stem cells is dependent on subtle niche-associated distinctions concerning cellular interaction and extrinsic stimuli. In another study, transplantation of in vitro-generated multipotent cells from the rat spinal cord only generated neurons in vivo after transplantation into the hippocampus, but not after transplantation into the physiologically non-neurogenic spinal cord (Shihabuddin et al. 2000).

Such a complex environment may not only regulate physiological cell functions, but also prevent the development of cancer. It has been suggested that dysregulation of the stem cell niche may lead to uncontrolled proliferation of stem cells and consequently tumorigenesis (Li and Neaves 2006).

With regard to oxygenation, the microenvironment in tumors markedly differs from that in physiological stem cell niches. Because of their rapid growth, many solid tumors contain areas with insufficient vasculature, which leads to a decline in oxygen tension and a lack of nutrients. Tumor necrosis occurs as a result (Acker and Plate 2004). However, hypoxia was also shown to activate escape mechanisms that change the phenotype of the surviving tumor cells toward immaturity in some tumors (neuroblastoma, ductal breast carcinoma) (Jogi et al. 2002; Helczynska et al. 2003; Holmquist et al. 2005). Further signs of adaptation of tumor cells to this situation are the switch to anaerobic glycolysis and the induction of a neovasculature (Acker and Plate 2003).

Hypoxic tumors behave more aggressively and tend to metastasize (Brizel et al. 1996; Zhong et al. 1999; Rofstad 2000). They show increased therapeutic resistance due to impaired drug delivery and shorter persistence of free oxygen radicals after irradiation (Brown 2000, 2002).

14.8 Therapeutical Aspects

The prognosis of malignant brain tumors is still very poor today. The highly invasive capacity of brain tumor cells is one of the main limitations for the success of therapeutical strategies. Neither surgical treatment nor irradiation and chemotherapeutic approaches are sufficient to eradicate every single tumor cell that invades the brain parenchyma. In the case of glioblastomas, this can lead to a high rate of tumor recurrence and poor prognosis, with a mean total length of the disease of less than 1 year. As discussed in this review, it is possible that not all cells within a tumor and therefore not all invading tumor cells show similar tumorigenic capacities, but that a subpopulation of tumor-initiating cells exists. For future therapeutic strategies, it is essential to identify and characterize these putative tumor-initiating cells in more detail and analyze the environment from which they derive and in which they survive.

Current therapeutic approaches aim at reducing the heterogenous tumor mass, most likely missing this subpopulation of cells. Indeed, a recent study by Bao et al. indicates a preferential protection of CD133$^+$ cancer stem cells against radiotherapeutic strategies (Bao et al. 2006a). A profound knowledge of the processes regulating brain tumor stem cell growth could enable a direct therapeutic targeting of these cells that are responsible for tumor recurrence and growth (Fig. 14.6).

The observed similarities of neural stem or progenitor cells with tumor cells might also be useful for targeting invading tumor cells with the help of genetically modified NPCs. A study from Aboody et al. provided preliminary evidence that transplanted neural stem cells show tropism for neoplastic lesions of the adult rodent brain (Aboody et al. 2000). These cells (derived from a murine neural stem cell line) migrated over far distances to a glioblastoma cell line, surrounded the tumor, and furthermore were often found in direct juxtaposition to invading

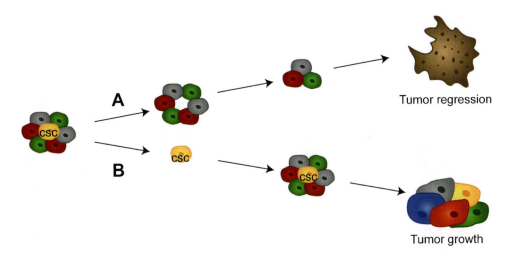

Fig. 14.6 Therapeutic perspectives. Targeting cancer stem cells might be crucial for the eradication of those cells, that initiate and sustain tumor growth and therefore could facilitate tumor regression in future therapies (**a**). In contrast, current less directed therapeutic approaches affect the bulk tumor mass, but not specifically CSCs, consequently leading to recurrent growth of the tumor (**b**)

glioma cells migrating away from the tumor center. NPCs therefore could provide a biological tool to follow invasive tumor cells widely into the brain parenchyma. Injections of genetically modified NPCs have been shown to increase the survival rate of glioma-bearing mice (Benedetti et al. 2000), supporting the thesis that NPCs might be used as vehicles for certain drugs or prodrugs in future therapies (Noble 2000; Yip et al. 2006). Not only transplanted, but also endogenous NPCs of adult rodents have been described to migrate to brain tumors, although this phenomenon was decreased in older animals. The survival time of old mice (age 6 months) after intracerebral injections of glioblastoma cells was significantly shorter than young animals (age 4 weeks). Interestingly, after co-injection of glioblastoma cells with nestin-expressing NPCs, the older animals reached the same survival time as young animals (Glass et al. 2005).

14.9 Outlook

Putative cancer stem cells have a great deal in common with neural stem cells. These include the capacity to self-renew, multipotency, and similarities in the molecular signature and comparable reactions to extracellular factors. These similarities and the approaches used to successfully enrich subpopulations of tumor cells with tumor-initiating capacities argue for the hypothesis that putative cancer stem cells could derive from physiological NSCs/NPCs. If distinct migratory capacities of neural stem or progenitor cells were inherited to neoplastic cells, this also could explain the invasive nature of certain brain tumor phenotypes. Furthermore, directly targeting cancer stem cells instead of a nontumorigenic cell population within the tumor mass could provide promising strategies for future selective therapies. However, the methods used for identification and enrichment of putative cancer stem cells still have restrictions. Further studies are needed to finally prove or disprove the cancer stem cell hypothesis and the existence of true brain tumor stem cells.

Acknowledgments

We thank S. Momma for lively discussions and critical proofreading of the manuscript. We also thank P. Janson for creating the figures.

Definitions as used in this review

Neural stem cell (NSC)	Multipotent, slowly dividing cell with capacity of unlimited self-renewal and ability to differentiate into committed progeny of all three neural lineages (astrocytic, oligondendroglial, neuronal)
Neural progenitor cell (NPC)	Derives from NSC and has limited self-renewal and differentiation capability
Brain tumor stem cell (BTSC)	Neoplastic neuroepithelial cell with all features of NSCs
Cancer stem cell (CSC)	Neoplastic cell with stem cell features
Tumor-initiating cell (TIC)	Tumor cell capable of initiating a tumor graft after transplantation

References

Aboody KS, Brown A, Rainov NG, Bower KA, Liu S, Yang W, Small JE, Herrlinger U, Ourednik V, Black PM, Breakefield XO, Snyder EY (2000) Neural stem cells display extensive tropism for pathology in adult brain: evidence from intracranial gliomas. Proc Natl Acad Sci USA 97:12846–12851

Acker T, Plate KH (2003) Role of hypoxia in tumor angiogenesis-molecular and cellular angiogenic crosstalk. Cell Tissue Res 314:145–155

Acker T, Plate KH (2004) Hypoxia and hypoxia inducible factors (HIF) as important regulators of tumor physiology. Cancer Treat Res 117:219–248

Al-Hajj M, Wicha MS, Benito-Hernandez A, Morrison SJ, Clarke MF (2003) Prospective identification of tumorigenic breast cancer cells. Proc Natl Acad Sci USA 100:3983–3988

Alvarez-Buylla A, Lim DA (2004) For the long run: maintaining germinal niches in the adult brain. Neuron 41:683–686

Arsenijevic Y, Villemure JG, Brunet JF, Bloch JJ, Deglon N, Kostic C, Zurn A, Aebischer P (2001) Isolation of multipotent neural precursors residing in the cortex of the adult human brain. Exp Neurol 170:48–62

Assanah M, Lochhead R, Ogden A, Bruce J, Goldman J, Canoll P (2006) Glial progenitors in adult white matter are driven to form malignant gliomas by platelet-derived growth factor-expressing retroviruses. J Neurosci 26:6781–6790

Bachoo RM, Maher EA, Ligon KL, Sharpless NE, Chan SS, You MJ, Tang Y, DeFrances J, Stover E, Weissleder R, Rowitch DH, Louis DN, DePinho RA (2002) Epidermal growth factor receptor and Ink4a/Arf: convergent mechanisms governing terminal differentiation and transformation along the neural stem cell to astrocyte axis. Cancer Cell 1:269–277

Bao S, Wu Q, McLendon RE, Hao Y, Shi Q, Hjelmeland AB, Dewhirst MW, Bigner DD, Rich JN (2006a) Glioma stem cells promote radioresistance by preferential activation of the DNA damage response. Nature

Bao S, Wu Q, Sathornsumetee S, Hao Y, Li Z, Hjelmeland AB, Shi Q, McLendon RE, Bigner DD, Rich JN (2006b) Stem cell-like glioma cells promote tumor angiogenesis through vascular endothelial growth factor. Cancer Res 66:7843–7848

Bedard A, Parent A (2004) Evidence of newly generated neurons in the human olfactory bulb. Brain Res Dev Brain Res 151:159–168

Benedetti S, Pirola B, Pollo B, Magrassi L, Bruzzone MG, Rigamonti D, Galli R, Selleri S, Di Meco F, De Fraja C, Vescovi A, Cattaneo E, Finocchiaro G (2000) Gene therapy of experimental brain tumors using neural progenitor cells. Nat Med 6:447–450

Berger F, Gay E, Pelletier L, Tropel P, Wion D (2004) Development of gliomas: potential role of asymmetrical cell division of neural stem cells. Lancet Oncol 5:511–514

Berman DM, Karhadkar SS, Hallahan AR, Pritchard JI, Eberhart CG, Watkins DN, Chen JK, Cooper MK, Taipale J, Olson JM, Beachy PA (2002) Medulloblastoma growth inhibition by hedgehog pathway blockade. Science 297:1559–1561

Betschinger J, Mechtler K, Knoblich JA (2006) Asymmetric segregation of the tumor suppressor brat regulates self-renewal in Drosophila neural stem cells. Cell 124:1241–1253

Bhardwaj RD, Curtis MA, Spalding KL, Buchholz BA, Fink D, Bjork-Eriksson T, Nordborg C, Gage FH, Druid H, Eriksson PS, Frisen J (2006) Neocortical neurogenesis in humans is restricted to development. Proc Natl Acad Sci USA 103:12564–12568

Bjerkvig R, Tysnes BB, Aboody KS, Najbauer J, Terzis AJ (2005) Opinion: the origin of the cancer stem cell: current controversies and new insights. Nat Rev Cancer 5:899–904

Blau HM, Brazelton TR, Weimann JM (2001) The evolving concept of a stem cell: entity or function? Cell 105:829–841

Bonnet D (2002) Haematopoietic stem cells. J Pathol 197:430–440

Bonnet D, Dick JE (1997) Human acute myeloid leukemia is organized as a hierarchy that originates from a primitive hematopoietic cell. Nat Med 3:730–737

Brandt MD, Jessberger S, Steiner B, Kronenberg G, Reuter K, Bick-Sander A, von der Behrens W, Kempermann G (2003) Transient calretinin expression defines early postmitotic step of neuronal differentiation in adult hippocampal neurogenesis of mice. Mol Cell Neurosci 24:603–613

Brizel DM, Scully SP, Harrelson JM, Layfield LJ, Bean JM, Prosnitz LR, Dewhirst MW (1996) Tumor oxygenation predicts for the likelihood of distant metastases in human soft tissue sarcoma. Cancer Res 56:941–943

Brown JM (2000) Exploiting the hypoxic cancer cell: mechanisms and therapeutic strategies. Mol Med Today 6:157–162

Brown JM (2002) Tumor microenvironment and the response to anticancer therapy. Cancer Biol Ther 1:453–458

Capela A, Temple S (2002) LeX/ssea-1 is expressed by adult mouse CNS stem cells, identifying them as nonependymal. Neuron 35:865–875

Caporaso GL, Lim DA, Alvarez-Buylla A, Chao MV (2003) Telomerase activity in the subventricular zone of adult mice. Mol Cell Neurosci 23:693–702

Conheim J (1867) Path Anat Physiol Klin Med 40:1–79

Dahmane N, Sanchez P, Gitton Y, Palma V, Sun T, Beyna M, Weiner H, Ruiz i Altaba A (2001) The Sonic Hedgehog-Gli pathway regulates dorsal brain growth and tumorigenesis. Development 128:5201–5212

Doetsch F (2003) The glial identity of neural stem cells. Nat Neurosci 6:1127–1134

Doetsch F, Caille I, Lim DA, Garcia-Verdugo JM, Alvarez-Buylla A (1999) Subventricular zone astrocytes are neural stem cells in the adult mammalian brain. Cell 97:703–716

Doetsch F, Petreanu L, Caille I, Garcia-Verdugo JM, Alvarez-Buylla A (2002) EGF converts transit-amplifying neurogenic precursors in the adult brain into multipotent stem cells. Neuron 36:1021–1034

Emsley JG, Mitchell BD, Kempermann G, Macklis JD (2005) Adult neurogenesis and repair of the adult CNS with neural progenitors, precursors, and stem cells. Prog Neurobiol 75:321–341

Eriksson PS, Perfilieva E, Bjork-Eriksson T, Alborn AM, Nordborg C, Peterson DA, Gage FH (1998) Neurogenesis in the adult human hippocampus. Nat Med 4:1313–1317

Gage FH, Coates PW, Palmer TD, Kuhn HG, Fisher LJ, Suhonen JO, Peterson DA, Suhr ST, Ray J (1995) Survival and differentiation of adult neuronal progenitor cells transplanted to the adult brain. Proc Natl Acad Sci USA 92:11879–11883

Galli R, Binda E, Orfanelli U, Cipelletti B, Gritti A, De Vitis S, Fiocco R, Foroni C, Dimeco F, Vescovi A (2004) Isolation and characterization of tumorigenic, stem-like neural precursors from human glioblastoma. Cancer Res 64:7011–7021

Glass R, Synowitz M, Kronenberg G, Walzlein JH, Markovic DS, Wang LP, Gast D, Kiwit J, Kempermann G, Kettenmann H (2005) Glioblastoma-induced attraction of endogenous neural precursor cells is associated with improved survival. J Neurosci 25:2637–2646

Goodell MA, Brose K, Paradis G, Conner AS, Mulligan RC (1996) Isolation and functional properties of murine hematopoietic stem cells that are replicating in vivo. J Exp Med 183:1797–1806

Graham V, Khudyakov J, Ellis P, Pevny L (2003) SOX2 functions to maintain neural progenitor identity. Neuron 39:749–765

Hanahan D, Weinberg RA (2000) The hallmarks of cancer. Cell 100:57–70

Helczynska K, Kronblad A, Jogi A, Nilsson E, Beckman S, Landberg G, Pahlman S (2003) Hypoxia promotes a dedifferentiated phenotype in ductal breast carcinoma in situ. Cancer Res 63:1441–1444

Hemmati HD, Nakano I, Lazareff JA, Masterman-Smith M, Geschwind DH, Bronner-Fraser M, Kornblum HI (2003) Cancerous stem cells can arise from pediatric brain tumors. Proc Natl Acad Sci USA 100:15178–15183

Hill RP (2006) Identifying cancer stem cells in solid tumors: case not proven. Cancer Res 66:1891–1895; discussion 1890

Hirschmann-Jax C, Foster AE, Wulf GG, Nuchtern JG, Jax TW, Gobel U, Goodell MA, Brenner MK (2004) A distinct "side population" of cells with high drug efflux capacity in human tumor cells. Proc Natl Acad Sci USA 101:14228–14233

Holland EC (2001) Gliomagenesis: genetic alterations and mouse models. Nat Rev Genet 2:120–129

Holland EC, Hively WP, DePinho RA, Varmus HE (1998) A constitutively active epidermal growth factor receptor cooperates with disruption of G1 cell-cycle arrest pathways to induce glioma-like lesions in mice. Genes Dev 12:3675–3685

Holland EC, Celestino J, Dai C, Schaefer L, Sawaya RE, Fuller GN (2000a) Combined activation of Ras and Akt in neural progenitors induces glioblastoma formation in mice. Nat Genet 25:55–57

Holland EC, Li Y, Celestino J, Dai C, Schaefer L, Sawaya RA, Fuller GN (2000b) Astrocytes give rise to oligodendrogliomas and astrocytomas after gene transfer of polyoma virus middle T antigen in vivo. Am J Pathol 157:1031–1037

Holmquist L, Jogi A, Pahlman S (2005) Phenotypic persistence after reoxygenation of hypoxic neuroblastoma cells. Int J Cancer 116:218–225

Huntly BJ, Shigematsu H, Deguchi K, Lee BH, Mizuno S, Duclos N, Rowan R, Amaral S, Curley D, Williams IR, Akashi K, Gilliland DG (2004) MOZ-TIF2, but not BCR-ABL, confers properties of leukemic stem cells to committed murine hematopoietic progenitors. Cancer Cell 6:587–596

Jackson EL, Garcia-Verdugo JM, Gil-Perotin S, Roy M, Quinones-Hinojosa A, VandenBerg S,

Alvarez-Buylla A (2006) PDGFR alpha-positive B cells are neural stem cells in the adult SVZ that form glioma-like growths in response to increased PDGF signaling. Neuron 51:187–199

Jin K, Zhu Y, Sun Y, Mao XO, Xie L, Greenberg DA (2002) Vascular endothelial growth factor (VEGF) stimulates neurogenesis in vitro and in vivo. Proc Natl Acad Sci USA 99:11946–11950

Jogi A, Vallon-Christersson J, Holmquist L, Axelson H, Borg A, Pahlman S (2004) Human neuroblastoma cells exposed to hypoxia: induction of genes associated with growth, survival, and aggressive behavior. Exp Cell Res 295:469–487

Jogi A, Ora I, Nilsson H, Lindeheim A, Makino Y, Poellinger L, Axelson H, Pahlman S (2002) Hypoxia alters gene expression in human neuroblastoma cells toward an immature and neural crest-like phenotype. Proc Natl Acad Sci USA 99:7021–7026

Johansson CB, Svensson M, Wallstedt L, Janson AM, Frisen J (1999a) Neural stem cells in the adult human brain. Exp Cell Res 253:733–736

Johansson CB, Momma S, Clarke DL, Risling M, Lendahl U, Frisen J (1999b) Identification of a neural stem cell in the adult mammalian central nervous system. Cell 96:25–34

Katsetos CD, Burger PC (1994) Medulloblastoma. Semin Diagn Pathol 11:85–97

Kenney AM, Segal RA (2005) Subtracting the Math: prominin-positive cerebellar stem cells in white matter. Nat Neurosci 8:699–701

Kenney AM, Cole MD, Rowitch DH (2003) Nmyc upregulation by sonic hedgehog signaling promotes proliferation in developing cerebellar granule neuron precursors. Development 130:15–28

Kim CF, Jackson EL, Woolfenden AE, Lawrence S, Barbar I, Vogel S, Crowley D, Bronson RT, Jacks T (2005) Identification of bronchioalveolar stem cells in normal lung and lung cancer. Proc Natl Acad Sci USA 102:14404–14409

Komata T, Kanzawa T, Kondo Y, Kondo S (2002) Telomerase as a therapeutic target for malignant gliomas. Oncogene 21:656–663

Kondo T, Raff M (2000) Oligodendrocyte precursor cells reprogrammed to become multipotential CNS stem cells. Science 289:1754–1757

Kondo T, Setoguchi T, Taga T (2004) Persistence of a small subpopulation of cancer stem-like cells in the C6 glioma cell line. Proc Natl Acad Sci USA 101:781–786

Kuhn HG, Dickinson-Anson H, Gage FH (1996) Neurogenesis in the dentate gyrus of the adult rat: age-related decrease of neuronal progenitor proliferation. J Neurosci 16:2027–2033

Lai K, Kaspar BK, Gage FH, Schaffer DV (2003) Sonic hedgehog regulates adult neural progenitor proliferation in vitro and in vivo. Nat Neurosci 6:21–27

Lee A, Kessler JD, Read TA, Kaiser C, Corbeil D, Huttner WB, Johnson JE, Wechsler-Reya RJ (2005) Isolation of neural stem cells from the postnatal cerebellum. Nat Neurosci 8:723–729

Lee CY, Wilkinson BD, Siegrist SE, Wharton RP, Doe CQ (2006a) Brat is a Miranda cargo protein that promotes neuronal differentiation and inhibits neuroblast self-renewal. Dev Cell 10:441–449

Lee J, Kotliarova S, Kotliarov Y, Li A, Su Q, Donin NM, Pastorino S, Purow BW, Christopher N, Zhang W, Park JK, Fine HA (2006b) Tumor stem cells derived from glioblastomas cultured in bFGF and EGF more closely mirror the phenotype and genotype of primary tumors than do serum-cultured cell lines. Cancer Cell 9:391–403

Lendahl U, Zimmerman LB, McKay RD (1990) CNS stem cells express a new class of intermediate filament protein. Cell 60:585–595

Li L, Neaves WB (2006) Normal stem cells and cancer stem cells: the niche matters. Cancer Res 66:4553–4557

Li L, Liu F, Ross AH (2003) PTEN regulation of neural development and CNS stem cells. J Cell Biochem 88:24–28

Lois C, Alvarez-Buylla A (1994) Long-distance neuronal migration in the adult mammalian brain. Science 264:1145–1148

Lois C, Garcia-Verdugo JM, Alvarez-Buylla A (1996) Chain migration of neuronal precursors. Science 271:978–981

Machold R, Hayashi S, Rutlin M, Muzumdar MD, Nery S, Corbin JG, Gritli-Linde A, Dellovade T, Porter JA, Rubin LL, Dudek H, McMahon AP, Fishell G (2003) Sonic hedgehog is required for progenitor cell maintenance in telencephalic stem cell niches. Neuron 39:937–950

Machon O, Backman M, Krauss S, Kozmik Z (2005) The cellular fate of cortical progenitors is not maintained in neurosphere cultures. Mol Cell Neurosci 30:388–397

Molofsky AV, Pardal R, Iwashita T, Park IK, Clarke MF, Morrison SJ (2003) Bmi-1 dependence distinguishes neural stem cell self-renewal from progenitor proliferation. Nature 425:962–967

Morrison SJ, Kimble J (2006) Asymmetric and symmetric stem-cell divisions in development and cancer. Nature 441:1068–1074

Morshead CM, Reynolds BA, Craig CG, McBurney MW, Staines WA, Morassutti D, Weiss S, van der Kooy D (1994) Neural stem cells in the adult mammalian forebrain: a relatively quiescent subpopulation of subependymal cells. Neuron 13:1071–1082

Noble M (2000) Can neural stem cells be used as therapeutic vehicles in the treatment of brain tumors? Nat Med 6:369–370

Nunes MC, Roy NS, Keyoung HM, Goodman RR, McKhann G, 2nd, Jiang L, Kang J, Nedergaard M, Goldman SA (2003) Identification and isolation of multipotential neural progenitor cells from the subcortical white matter of the adult human brain. Nat Med 9:439–447

Palma V, Lim DA, Dahmane N, Sanchez P, Brionne TC, Herzberg CD, Gitton Y, Carleton A, Alvarez-Buylla A, Ruiz i Altaba A (2005) Sonic hedgehog controls stem cell behavior in the postnatal and adult brain. Development 132:335–344

Patrawala L, Calhoun T, Schneider-Broussard R, Zhou J, Claypool K, Tang DG (2005) Side population is enriched in tumorigenic, stem-like cancer cells, whereas ABCG2 + and ABCG2- cancer cells are similarly tumorigenic. Cancer Res 65:6207–6219

Pencea V, Bingaman KD, Freedman LJ, Luskin MB (2001) Neurogenesis in the subventricular zone and rostral migratory stream of the neonatal and adult primate forebrain. Exp Neurol 172:1–16

Pietsch T, Taylor MD, Rutka JT (2004) Molecular pathogenesis of childhood brain tumors. J Neurooncol 70:203–215

Purow BW, Haque RM, Noel MW, Su Q, Burdick MJ, Lee J, Sundaresan T, Pastorino S, Park JK, Mikolaenko I, Maric D, Eberhart CG, Fine HA (2005) Expression of Notch-1 and its ligands, Delta-like-1 and Jagged-1, is critical for glioma cell survival and proliferation. Cancer Res 65:2353–2363

Reya T, Clevers H (2005) Wnt signalling in stem cells and cancer. Nature 434:843–850

Reya T, Morrison SJ, Clarke MF, Weissman IL (2001) Stem cells, cancer, and cancer stem cells. Nature 414:105–111

Reynolds BA, Weiss S (1992) Generation of neurons and astrocytes from isolated cells of the adult mammalian central nervous system. Science 255:1707–1710

Reynolds BA, Rietze RL (2005) Neural stem cells and neurospheres –re-evaluating the relationship. Nat Methods 2:333–336

Rofstad EK (2000) Microenvironment-induced cancer metastasis. Int J Radiat Biol 76:589–605

Sakakibara S, Imai T, Hamaguchi K, Okabe M, Aruga J, Nakajima K, Yasutomi D, Nagata T, Kurihara Y, Uesugi S, Miyata T, Ogawa M, Mikoshiba K, Okano H (1996) Mouse-Musashi-1, a neural RNA-binding protein highly enriched in the mammalian CNS stem cell. Dev Biol 176:230–242

Sanai N, Alvarez-Buylla A, Berger MS (2005) Neural stem cells and the origin of gliomas. N Engl J Med 353:811–822

Sanai N, Tramontin AD, Quinones-Hinojosa A, Barbaro NM, Gupta N, Kunwar S, Lawton MT, McDermott MW, Parsa AT, Manuel-Garcia Verdugo J, Berger MS, Alvarez-Buylla A (2004) Unique astrocyte ribbon in adult human brain contains neural stem cells but lacks chain migration. Nature 427:740–744

Sawamoto K, Wichterle H, Gonzalez-Perez O, Cholfin JA, Yamada M, Spassky N, Murcia NS, Garcia-Verdugo JM, Marin O, Rubenstein JL, Tessier-Lavigne M, Okano H, Alvarez-Buylla A (2006) New neurons follow the flow of cerebrospinal fluid in the adult brain. Science 311:629–632

Schanzer A, Wachs FP, Wilhelm D, Acker T, Cooper-Kuhn C, Beck H, Winkler J, Aigner L, Plate KH, Kuhn HG (2004) Direct stimulation of adult neural stem cells in vitro and neurogenesis in vivo by vascular endothelial growth factor. Brain Pathol 14:237–248

Seaberg RM, van der Kooy D (2002) Adult rodent neurogenic regions: the ventricular subependyma contains neural stem cells, but the dentate gyrus contains restricted progenitors. J Neurosci 22:1784–1793

Seki T, Arai Y (1993) Distribution and possible roles of the highly polysialylated neural cell adhesion molecule (NCAM-H) in the developing and adult central nervous system. Neurosci Res 17:265–290

Seri B, Garcia-Verdugo JM, McEwen BS, Alvarez-Buylla A (2001) Astrocytes give rise to new neurons in the adult mammalian hippocampus. J Neurosci 21:7153–7160

Shihabuddin LS, Horner PJ, Ray J, Gage FH (2000) Adult spinal cord stem cells generate neurons after transplantation in the adult dentate gyrus. J Neurosci 20:8727–8735

Singec I, Knoth R, Meyer RP, Maciaczyk J, Volk B, Nikkhah G, Frotscher M, Snyder EY (2006) Defining the actual sensitivity and specificity of the neurosphere assay in stem cell biology. Nat Methods 3:801–806

Singh SK, Clarke ID, Terasaki M, Bonn VE, Hawkins C, Squire J, Dirks PB (2003) Identification of a cancer stem cell in human brain tumors. Cancer Res 63:5821–5828

Singh SK, Hawkins C, Clarke ID, Squire JA, Bayani J, Hide T, Henkelman RM, Cusimano MD, Dirks PB (2004) Identification of human brain tumour initiating cells. Nature 432:396–401

Song H, Stevens CF, Gage FH (2002) Astroglia induce neurogenesis from adult neural stem cells. Nature 417:39–44

Taylor MD, Poppleton H, Fuller C, Su X, Liu Y, Jensen P, Magdaleno S, Dalton J, Calabrese C, Board J, Macdonald T, Rutka J, Guha A, Gajjar A, Curran T, Gilbertson RJ (2005) Radial glia cells are candidate stem cells of ependymoma. Cancer Cell 8:323–335

Till JE, McCulloch EA (1961) A direct measurement of the radiation sensitivity of normal mouse bone marrow cells. Radiat Res 14:213–222

Vescovi AL, Galli R, Reynolds BA (2006) Brain tumour stem cells. Nat Rev Cancer 6:425–436

Vick NA, Lin MJ, Bigner DD (1977) The role of the subependymal plate in glial tumorigenesis. Acta Neuropathol (Berl) 40:63–71

Virchow R (1855) Virchows Arch Pathol Anat Physiol Klin Med Editorial

Watts C, McConkey H, Anderson L, Caldwell M (2005) Anatomical perspectives on adult neural stem cells. J Anat 207:197–208

Weigmann A, Corbeil D, Hellwig A, Huttner WB (1997) Prominin, a novel microvilli-specific polytopic membrane protein of the apical surface of epithelial cells, is targeted to plasmalemmal protrusions of non-epithelial cells. Proc Natl Acad Sci USA 94:12425–12430

Wetmore C (2003) Sonic hedgehog in normal and neoplastic proliferation: insight gained from human tumors and animal models. Curr Opin Genet Dev 13:34–42

Yin AH, Miraglia S, Zanjani ED, Almeida-Porada G, Ogawa M, Leary AG, Olweus J, Kearney J, Buck DW (1997) AC133, a novel marker for human hematopoietic stem and progenitor cells. Blood 90:5002–5012

Yip S, Sabetrasekh R, Sidman RL, Snyder EY (2006) Neural stem cells as novel cancer therapeutic vehicles. Eur J Cancer 42:1298–1308

Yokota N, Nishizawa S, Ohta S, Date H, Sugimura H, Namba H, Maekawa M (2002) Role of Wnt pathway in medulloblastoma oncogenesis. Int J Cancer 101:198–201

Young NS, Hwang-Chen SP (1981) Anti-K562 cell monoclonal antibodies recognize hematopoietic progenitors. Proc Natl Acad Sci U S A 78:7073–7077

Yuan X, Curtin J, Xiong Y, Liu G, Waschsmann-Hogiu S, Farkas DL, Black KL, Yu JS (2004) Isolation of cancer stem cells from adult glioblastoma multiforme. Oncogene 23:9392–9400

Zhong H, De Marzo AM, Laughner E, Lim M, Hilton DA, Zagzag D, Buechler P, Isaacs WB, Semenza GL, Simons JW (1999) Overexpression of hypoxia-inducible factor 1alpha in common human cancers and their metastases. Cancer Res 59:5830–5835

Zhu Y, Guignard F, Zhao D, Liu L, Burns DK, Mason RP, Messing A, Parada LF (2005) Early inactivation of p53 tumor suppressor gene cooperating with NF1 loss induces malignant astrocytoma. Cancer Cell 8:119–130

Printing: Krips bv, Meppel, The Netherlands
Binding: Stürtz, Würzburg, Germany